AGING WELL WITH DIABETES

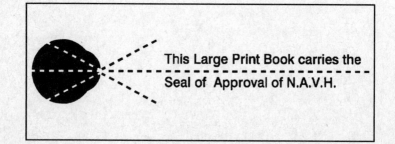

This Large Print Book carries the
Seal of Approval of N.A.V.H.

Aging Well with Diabetes

146 EYE-OPENING SECRETS THAT PREVENT AND CONTROL DIABETES

Bottom Line Inc.

THORNDIKE PRESS

A part of Gale, a Cengage Company

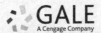

Farmington Hills, Mich • San Francisco • New York • Waterville, Maine
Meriden, Conn • Mason, Ohio • Chicago

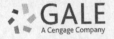

Copyright © 2017 by Bottom Line, Inc.
All brand names and product names used in this book are trademarks,
registered trademarks, or trade names of their respective holders. The
publisher is not associated with any product or vendor in this book.
Thorndike Press, a part of Gale, a Cengage Company.

Thorndike Press® Large Print Lifestyles.
The text of this Large Print edition is unabridged.
Other aspects of the book may vary from the original edition.
Set in 16 pt. Plantin.

LIBRARY OF CONGRESS CIP DATA ON FILE.
CATALOGUING IN PUBLICATION FOR THIS BOOK
IS AVAILABLE FROM THE LIBRARY OF CONGRESS

ISBN-13: 978-1-4328-4426-4 (hardcover)
ISBN-10: 1-4328-4426-1 (hardcover)

Published in 2017 by arrangement with Sourcebooks, Inc.

Printed in the United States of America
1 2 3 4 5 6 7 21 20 19 18 17

TABLE OF CONTENTS

13

PREFACE

More Americans than ever before are living with diabetes. In fact, 1.4 million people in the United States are diagnosed every year. Diabetes is a particular worry to people over the age of fifty, whose changing lifestyle and health concerns present different problems than those of younger men and women. Less activity, lower immunity, and the natural aging of the body increase risk enormously as adults mature. According to the American Diabetes Association, the percentage of American aged sixty-five and older with diabetes (or who remain undiagnosed) is estimated to be at over one-fourth of this population. This number is staggering! Yet, the resources for mature, health-conscious readers are scarce and scattered.*

The editors at Bottom Line are proud to

* American Diabetes Association, "Statistics about Diabetes," last modified December 12, 2016, http://www.diabetes.org/diabetes-basics/statistics/.

bring you *The Bottom Line Handbook for Aging Well with Diabetes,* the first book published to gather trustworthy and actionable life-saving information specifically for mature readers and their families and based on our bestselling book *Beat Diabetes Now!* In the pages of this collection, you'll find what you need to prevent type 2 diabetes from developing in the first place as well as easily actionable ways to keep your type 2 diabetes under control in your later years of life — whether it's natural foods and supplements or other nondrug approaches, breakthrough treatments for obesity, or solutions for the complications brought on by diabetes such as loss of eyesight, foot complications, or kidney disease.

How do we find all these top-notch medical professionals? Over the past four decades, we at Bottom Line have built a network of literally thousands of leading physicians in both alternative and conventional medicine. They are affiliated with the premier medical institutions and the best universities throughout the world. We read the important medical journals and follow the latest research that is reported at health conferences worldwide. And we regularly talk to our advisors in major teaching hospitals, private practices, and government health agencies for their insider perspectives.

The Bottom Line Handbook for Aging Well

with Diabetes is a result of our ongoing research and connection with these experts, and is a distillation of their latest findings and most important advice. We have worked with experts from the top diabetes clinics and research centers, such as Harvard's Joslin Diabetes Center and the Cleveland Clinic, to compile the information you need to know. We trust that you will glean new, helpful, and affordable information about living a healthy, diabetes-free life!

As a reader, please be assured that you are receiving well-researched information from a trusted source. But please use prudence in health matters. Always speak to your physician before taking vitamins, supplements, or over-the-counter medication; stopping a prescribed medication, changing your diet; or beginning an exercise program. If you experience side effects from any regimen, contact your doctor immediately.

Be well,

The Editors, Bottom Line Inc., Stamford, Connecticut

1
RISKS AND PREVENTION

Perhaps you've only just been diagnosed with diabetes, or you're a friend or family member who is hoping to better care for somebody else. There is so much information to contend with, even in simply understanding the concept of such a disease. The complications and details become even more varied when you're past the age of fifty.

In these articles, we'll provide a broad base of knowledge. This section explores the details of diagnosis — including risks like sugar, the APOE gene (which is also associated with Alzheimer's disease), and weight gain — along with ways to help prevent and improve control of diabetes through healthy daily habits and awareness.

The first step to wellness is through education and understanding, and it's never too late in your life to take the first step.

THE DANGERS OF DIABETES

More Americans than ever before have diabetes mellitus, a disorder characterized by elevated levels of blood sugar (glucose). About twenty-nine million Americans (approximately 9.3 percent of the U.S. population) are afflicted with the disease, according to the Centers for Disease Control and Prevention. More than eight million of these people don't even realize that they have it.

But that's not all. A staggering eighty-six million Americans show early signs of diabetes ("prediabetes") but don't know that they are at risk of developing the full-blown disease. This alarming trend is due, in part, to the ever-increasing number of Americans who are overweight, which sharply increases diabetes risk.

If you have been gaining weight, eating a lot of high-fat and high-sugar foods, and/or not getting much exercise, I'm afraid that you're already in danger of getting diabetes.

Even though this is a frightening scenario, there is some good news. If you identify the warning signs early enough, you can prevent diabetes from developing. If you already have diabetes, proper monitoring and healthful eating can help you control your glucose levels and avoid many of the disease's serious complications, such as heart failure, stroke, kidney failure, eye disease, nerve damage, and/or amputation.

What is Diabetes?

Whenever we eat or drink, the food or liquid we ingest is broken down into nutrients that our bodies need to function. Glucose (a simple sugar that acts as the main energy source for our bodies) is one of the key nutrients. When glucose is absorbed into the bloodstream, it stimulates the pancreas to produce insulin. This hormone transports glucose into our body's cells, where it is then converted to energy for immediate or later use.

There are two main types of diabetes.

Type 1 (formerly known as juvenile-onset) diabetes affects only about 10 percent of people with diabetes. Although the disorder usually develops in childhood or early adulthood (before age thirty), an increasing number of adults are now being affected.

Researchers theorize that the increasing incidence of obesity in adults may accelerate the autoimmune destruction that characterizes type 1 diabetes — specifically, the body's immune system attacks and destroys the insulin-producing cells of the pancreas.

People with type 1 diabetes need frequent doses of insulin, which is typically delivered by injection with thin needles, a pen that contains an insulin-filled cartridge, or a small special "pump" that delivers a continuous dose of insulin.

Type 2 (once known as adult-onset) diabetes affects 90 percent of people who suffer from the disease. Most cases occur during adulthood, and risk increases with age. In recent years, many overweight children and teenagers have been diagnosed with type 2 diabetes.

In type 2 diabetes, the pancreas produces insulin (sometimes more than the usual amounts), but fat and tissue cells are resistant, preventing the hormone from doing what it's supposed to do — which is to unlock cells so that blood glucose can enter.

Your risk of type 2 diabetes increases significantly if you eat a lot of foods that are high in simple carbohydrates (which are rapidly transformed into sugar) and foods that are low in dietary fiber (needed to slow the absorption of sugars from the food we eat and digest). Also, people who don't get much exercise are more likely to develop type 2 diabetes because of the insulin resistance that results from weight gain and an imbalance of stress hormones.

In addition to obesity, risk factors for type 2 diabetes include a family history of the disease (especially in parents or siblings), apple-shaped body type, high blood pressure, high cholesterol, or, among women, a history of diabetes during pregnancy (gestational diabetes, which usually disappears after delivery). People with type 2 diabetes who have difficulty controlling their glucose levels may require oral medication, such as metformin and/ or insulin injections.

Heading Off Diabetes

Prediabetes affects 35 percent of Americans between the ages of forty and seventy-four — well into your older years. In these people, blood glucose levels are elevated but not enough to be considered type 2 diabetes. Detecting the telltale signs of prediabetes — which show up in blood tests — helps you prevent the full-blown disease. Without these measures, there's a good chance that a person diagnosed with prediabetes will develop type 2 diabetes within ten years.

I advise my patients (and readers) to get yearly blood tests to help identify many early-stage diseases, including diabetes. Diabetes-related tests should include fasting blood glucose to determine whether you are showing signs of prediabetes. Before you go to your doctor's office for the test, you will need to fast for at least eight hours. Then blood is drawn and sent to a lab for a measurement of the glucose concentration, which is expressed in milligrams of glucose per deciliter (mg/ dL). A fasting level of 100 to 125 mg/dL is considered prediabetes. (For more on the diagnostic criteria for diabetes, see "Test for Diabetes" on page 6.)

Too often, patients who have glucose levels

of 100 to 115 mg/dL are told by their doctors that they don't have a problem. In my view, a fasting blood glucose level in this range indicates prediabetes. I consider my patients to be free of any immediate risk only if their glucose levels are in the range of 70 to 86 mg/dL. If a patient's glucose level is 87 to 100 mg/dL, I recommend some of the same strategies that I prescribe for people with prediabetes.

An oral glucose tolerance test can be used to check for prediabetes. After fasting for eight to twelve hours, a blood sample is taken to determine your fasting blood glucose level. Then your doctor will ask you to drink a solution with a high sugar content. After one, two, and three hours, your doctor draws a blood sample and checks your glucose reading. A level of 140 to 199 mg/dL for any of the readings indicates prediabetes. A reading of 200 mg/dL or above indicates diabetes.

I recommend that doctors also check insulin levels with the blood sample used for the glucose tolerance test. If insulin levels are abnormally high (15 to 20 microunits per milliliter or higher), it's a sign that you are developing insulin resistance — which is often a step on the road to diabetes.

Better Diabetes Monitoring
If you have diabetes, proper monitoring of your condition can literally save your life.

Blood sugar levels can change dramatically within a matter of minutes, causing confusion, dizziness, fatigue, and, in serious cases, a life-threatening coma. People with diabetes can easily measure their blood sugar levels with a small portable device that analyzes a drop of blood obtained by pricking a fingertip with a lancet. I recommend self-monitoring at least twice daily (upon awakening and thirty to sixty minutes after dinner). In addition, people with diabetes should make regular visits to their primary care doctors, have annual physicals, and get yearly eye exams from their ophthalmologists.

Other tests for people with diabetes include:

- **Hemoglobin A1C.** This test measures the amount of glucose sticking to the hemoglobin in red blood cells. It can be used as a marker of average blood glucose level over the past two to three months. Studies show that for every percentage point drop in A1C blood levels, risks for circulatory disorders as well as eye, kidney, and nerve diseases drop by 40 percent. Most doctors say that a hemoglobin A1C reading below 7 percent is acceptable. However, I believe that a reading below 6 percent is more desirable, because it shows better blood glucose control. People with an A1C reading of 7 percent or less should have this test twice a year. If your reading is above 8 percent, you should have it every three months.

- **Oxidative stress analysis.** This test measures the amount of tissue damage, or oxidative stress, caused by free radicals (harmful, negatively charged molecules). Few medical doctors know about oxidative stress testing, but I recommend it for patients with diabetes because they have high levels of oxidative stress, which accelerates the disease's progression. The markers of free radical activity can be measured by blood or urine tests. Elevated levels mean that the antioxidants that are normally produced in the body and ingested via foods and supplements are not effectively neutralizing the overabundance of free radicals.

  Your doctor can use Genova Diagnostics (800-522-4762, www.gdx.net) for the test. It costs about one hundred dollars, but most health insurers will cover it. People with diabetes should receive this test every six months until their values are normal.

- **Cardiovascular markers.** People with diabetes are more susceptible to heart disease. That's because elevated glucose levels accelerate the buildup of plaque in the arteries. For this reason, I recommend blood tests for homocysteine, C-reactive protein, fibrinogen, lipoprotein A, apolipoprotein A and B, and iron. Abnormal levels of these markers are linked to the development of heart disease. I recommend a baseline test and yearly follow-up testing for people who have abnormal readings for any of these markers. Most health insurers will cover the costs of these tests.

The Sugar Connection

Everyone knows that people who have diabetes or who are at risk for it should pay close attention to their diet. However, I'm convinced that few people realize just how damaging certain foods can be.

For example, about 20 percent of the average American's energy intake comes from foods such as burgers, pizza, chips, pastries, and soft drinks. A study published in the *American Journal of Clinical Nutrition* found that between 1980 and 1997, the average American's daily calorie consumption increased by five hundred calories. Eighty percent of this increase was due to increases in carbohydrates, which include almost all sweet and starchy foods. During the same period, the prevalence of type 2 diabetes increased by 47 percent, and the prevalence of obesity increased by 80 percent.

One of the worst culprits in the war on diabetes is the simple sugar fructose, which is naturally found in fruit and honey. Table sugar is half fructose (the other half is glucose, which is chemically the same as blood glucose). A type of fructose known as high-fructose corn syrup (HFCS) is especially harmful because it worsens insulin resistance. It has become the sweetener of choice for many soft drinks, ice creams, baked goods, candies/sweets, jams, yogurts, and other sweetened products. My recommendation is to put a strict limit on your consumption of foods that contain HFCS. This can be done by reducing your intake of packaged, processed foods, avoiding drinks that are high in fructose, and eating as many fresh foods as possible. (Natural sources of fructose, such as fruit and honey, can be safely consumed in moderation.)

There is one exception — some liquid nutritional supplements, such as liquid vitamin formulas, contain crystalline fructose, a natural sweetener that is far less processed than HFCS and is not believed to cause dramatic increases in insulin levels.

Symptoms of Diabetes
• Increased thirst
• Frequent urination (especially at night)
• Unexplained increase in appetite
• Fatigue
• Erection problems
• Blurred vision
• Tingling or numbness in the hands and/or feet

Test for Diabetes

You have diabetes if any one of the following test results occurs on at least two different days:*

- A fasting blood glucose level of 126 mg/dL or higher.
- A two-hour oral glucose tolerance test result of 200 mg/dL or higher.
- Symptoms of diabetes (see previous list) combined with a random (nonfasting) blood glucose test of 200 mg/dL or higher.

Mark A. Stengler, NMD, a naturopathic medical doctor and leading authority on the practice of alternative and integrated medicine. Dr. Stengler is author of the *Health Revelations* newsletter, *The Natural Physician's Healing Therapies,* and *Bottom Line's Prescription for Natural Cures.* He is also the founder and medical director of the Stengler Center for Integrative Medicine in Encinitas, California, and former adjunct associate clinical professor at the National College of Natural Medicine in Portland, Oregon. MarkStengler.com.

* American Diabetes Association, "Diagnosing Diabetes and Learning about Prediabetes," last modified November 21, 2016, http://www.diabetes.org/diabetes-basics/diagnosis/.

HOW AMERICA'S TOP DIABETES DOCTOR AVOIDS DIABETES

You might think that a diabetes researcher would never develop the disease that he's dedicated his life to studying. But I can't count on it.

My family's story: My father was diagnosed with diabetes at age seventy-two and was promptly placed on three medications to control his insulin levels.

What my father did next made all the difference: Even though he began taking diabetes medication, he simultaneously went into action — walking an hour a day and going on the diet described below. A year and a half later, he no longer needed the prescriptions. He still had diabetes, but diet and exercise kept it under control.

As a diabetes researcher and physician whose own diabetes risk is increased by his family history, I've got a lot at stake in finding the absolute best ways to avoid and fight this disease.

Here are the steps I take to prevent diabetes — all of which can benefit you whether you want to avoid this disease or have already been diagnosed with it and are trying to control or even reverse it:

Step 1: **Follow a rural Asian diet.** This diet includes the most healthful foods of a traditional Asian diet — it consists of 70 percent complex carbohydrates, 15 percent fat, 15 percent protein, and fifteen grams of fiber for every thousand calories. Don't worry too much about all these numbers — the diet is actually pretty simple to follow once you get the hang of it.

You might be surprised by 70 percent complex carbohydrates, since most doctors recommend lower daily intakes of carbohydrates. The difference is, I'm recommending high amounts of complex, unrefined (not processed) carbohydrates. This type of carb is highly desirable because it's found in foods — such as whole grains, legumes, vegetables, and fruits — that are chock-full of fiber. If your goal is to reduce diabetes risk, fiber is the holy grail.

Why I do it: The rural Asian diet has been proven in research to promote weight loss, improve insulin sensitivity (a key factor in the development and treatment of diabetes) and glucose control, and decrease total cholesterol and LDL "bad" cholesterol levels.

To keep it simple, I advise patients to follow a 2-1-1 formula when creating meals — two portions of nonstarchy veggies (such as spinach, carrots, or asparagus); one portion of whole grains (such as brown rice or quinoa), legumes (such as lentils or chickpeas), or starchy veggies (such as sweet potatoes or winter squash); and one portion of protein (such as salmon, lean beef, tofu, or eggs). Have a piece of fruit (such as an apple or a pear) on the side. Portion size is also important. Portions fill a nine-inch-diameter plate, which is smaller than a typical twelve-inch American dinner plate.

Helpful: I take my time when eating — I chew each bite at least ten times before swallowing. Eating too quickly can cause glucose levels to peak higher than usual after a meal.

Step 2: **Fill up on dark green vegetables.** I include dark, leafy greens in my diet every day. These leafy greens are one of the two portions of nonstarchy veggies in the 2-1-1 formula.

Why I do it: Dark green vegetables contain antioxidants and compounds that help your body fight insulin resistance (a main driver of diabetes).

My secret "power veggie": a Chinese vegetable called bitter melon. It is a good source of fiber and has been shown to lower blood sugar. True to its name, bitter melon tastes a little bitter but is delicious when used in soups and stir-fries. It is available at Asian groceries. Eat bitter melon as one of the two portions of nonstarchy veggies in the 2-1-1 formula.

Step 3: **Adopt an every-other-day workout routine.** I try to not be sedentary and to walk as much as I can (by using a pedometer, I can tell whether I've reached my daily goal of ten thousand steps).

While this daily practice helps, it's not enough to significantly affect my diabetes risk. For that, I have an every-other-day workout routine that consists of thirty minutes of jogging on the treadmill (fast enough so that I'm breathing hard but can still carry on a conversation), followed by thirty minutes of strength training (using handheld weights, resistance bands, or weight machines).

Why I do it: Working out temporarily reduces your insulin resistance and activates enzymes and proteins that help your muscles use glucose instead of allowing the body to accumulate fat — a beneficial effect that lasts for forty-eight hours (the reason for my every-other-day routine).Strength training is crucial — your muscles are what really kick your body's glucose burning into high gear. A weekly game of tennis helps shake up my routine.

Step 4: **Keep the temperature chilly.** At the courts where I play tennis, the temperature is naturally cool, but I wear a very thin T-shirt that leaves my neck exposed. This helps activate the "brown fat" in my body. Most people have this special type of body fat — mainly around the neck, collarbone, and shoulders.

Why I do it: Brown fat burns calories at high rates when triggered by the cold. To help burn brown fat, exercise in temperatures of 64°F or lower, set your home's thermostat in the mid-60s, and dress as lightly as possible in cool weather. Walking for fifty to sixty minutes a day in cool weather also helps.

Step 5: **Get the "sleep cure."** I make a point to sleep at least six hours a night during the week and seven hours nightly on weekends.

Why I do it: Lack of sleep has been proven to dramatically harm the body's ability to properly metabolize glucose — a problem that sets the stage for diabetes. Research shows that seven to eight hours a night are ideal. However, because of my work schedule, I'm not always able to get that much sleep on weekdays. That's why I sleep a bit longer on weekends.

Research now shows that the body has some capacity to catch up on lost sleep and reverse some — but not all — of the damage that occurs to one's insulin sensitivity when one is sleep deprived.

George L. King, MD, research director and chief scientific officer of Harvard's Joslin Diabetes Center, where he heads the vascular cell biology research section, and professor of medicine at Harvard Medical School in Boston. Dr. King is coauthor, with Royce Flippin, of *The Diabetes Reset: Avoid It, Control It, Even Reverse It — A Doctor's Scientific Program.*

THE BEST WAY TO PREVENT DIABETES — NO DRUGS NEEDED

Approximately 9.3 percent of Americans have diabetes; the percentage of Americans age sixty-five and older remains high, at 25.9 percent, or 11.8 million people (diagnosed and undiagnosed). So if your doctor ever tells you (or has already told you) that you have prediabetes, you'd be wise to consider it a serious red flag. It means that your blood sugar level is higher than normal — though not yet quite high enough to be classified as diabetes — because your pancreas isn't making enough insulin and/or your cells have become resistant to the action of insulin.

A whopping 35 percent of American adults now have prediabetes. Nearly one-third of them will go on to develop full-blown diabetes, with all its attendant risks for cardiovascular problems, kidney failure, nerve damage, blindness, amputation, and death.

That's why researchers have been working hard to figure out the best way to keep prediabetes from progressing to diabetes. And according to an encouraging new study, one particular approach involving some fairly quick action has emerged as the winner — slashing prediabetic patients' risk for diabetes by an impressive 85 percent, without relying on drugs.

New Look at the Numbers

The new study draws on data from the National Diabetes Prevention Program, the largest diabetes prevention study in the United States, which began back in 1996. The program included 3,041 adults who had prediabetes and were at least somewhat overweight.

Participants were randomly divided into three groups. One group was given a twice-daily oral placebo and general lifestyle modification recommendations about the importance of healthful eating, losing weight, and exercising. A second group was given twice-daily oral metformin (a drug that prevents the liver from producing too much glucose) and those same lifestyle recommendations. The third group was enrolled in an intensive lifestyle modification program, with the goal of losing at least 7 percent of their body weight and exercising at moderate intensity for at least 150 minutes each week.

The original analysis of the data, done after 3.2 years, showed that intensive lifestyle modification reduced diabetes risk by 58 percent, and metformin use reduced diabetes risk by 31 percent, as compared with the placebo group.

Updated analysis: Researchers wanted to know whether those odds could be improved even further, so they did a new analysis, this time looking specifically at what happened in the first six months after prediabetes patients began treatment and then following up for ten years. What they found:

- **At the six-month mark,** almost everyone (92 percent) in the intensive lifestyle-modification group had lost weight, while more than 25 percent in the metformin group (and nearly 50 percent in the placebo group) had gained weight. The average percentage of body weight lost in each group was 7.2 percent in the lifestyle group, 2.4 percent in the metformin group, and 0.4 percent in the placebo group. Ten years later, most of those in the lifestyle group had maintained their substantial weight loss — quite an accomplishment, given how common it is for lost pounds to be regained.
- **In the intensive lifestyle-modification group,** those who lost 10 percent or more of their body weight in the first six months reduced their diabetes risk by an impressive 85 percent. But even those who fell short of the 7 percent weight loss goal benefited. For instance, those who lost 5 percent to 6.9 percent of their body weight reduced their risk by 54 percent, and those who lost just 3 percent to 4.9 percent reduced their risk by 38 percent.

If you have prediabetes: Don't assume that diabetes is an inevitable part of your future, and don't assume that you necessarily have to take drugs. By taking action now, you can greatly reduce your risk of developing this deadly disease. So talk with your doctor about joining a program designed to help people with prediabetes adopt healthful dietary and exercise habits that will promote safe, speedy, and permanent weight loss. Ask your doctor or health insurer for a referral, or to find a YMCA Diabetes Prevention Program near you, go to www.ymca.net/diabetes-prevention.

Nisa M. Maruthur, MD, assistant professor of medicine, The Johns Hopkins School of Medicine and the Welch Center for Prevention, Epidemiology, and Clinical Research, both in Baltimore. Her study was published in the *Journal of General Internal Medicine*.

THE SHOCKING DIABETES TRIGGER THAT CAN STRIKE ANYONE

Everyone knows about high blood sugar and the devastating effects it can have on one's health and longevity. But low blood sugar (hypoglycemia) can be just as dangerous — and it does not get nearly the attention that it should.

Simply put, hypoglycemia occurs when the body does not have enough glucose to use as fuel. It most commonly affects people with type 2 diabetes who take medication that sometimes works too well, resulting in low blood sugar.

Who gets overlooked: In other people, hypoglycemia can be a precursor to diabetes that is often downplayed by doctors and/or missed by tests. Having low blood sugar might even make you think that you are far from having diabetes when, in fact, the opposite is true.

Hypoglycemia can also be an underlying cause of anxiety that gets mistakenly treated with psychiatric drugs rather than the simple steps (see page 13) that can stabilize blood sugar levels. That's why anyone who seems to be suffering from an anxiety disorder needs to be seen by a doctor who takes a complete medical history and orders blood tests. When a patient comes to me complaining of anxiety, hypoglycemia is one of the first things I test for.

What's the link between hypoglycemia and anxiety? A sudden drop in blood sugar deprives the brain of oxygen. This, in turn, causes the adrenal glands to release adrenaline, the "emergency" hormone, which may lead to agitation, or anxiety, as the body's fight-or-flight mechanism kicks in.

The Dangers of Hypoglycemia

Hypoglycemia has sometimes been called carbohydrate intolerance, because the body's insulin-releasing mechanism is impaired in a manner similar to what occurs in diabetics. In people without diabetes, hypoglycemia is usually the result of eating too many simple carbohydrates (such as sugar and white flour). The pancreas then overreacts and releases too much insulin, thereby excessively lowering blood sugar.

The good news is that hypoglycemia — if it's identified — is not that difficult to control through diet and the use of specific supplements. Hypoglycemia should be considered a warning sign that you must adjust your carbohydrate intake or risk developing type 2 diabetes.

Caution: An episode of hypoglycemia in a person who already has diabetes can be life-threatening and requires prompt care, including the immediate intake of sugar — a glass of orange juice or even a sugar cube can be used.

***Common symptoms of hypoglycemia in-
clude:*** Fatigue, dizziness, shakiness and faint-
ness; irritability and depression; weakness or
cramps in the feet and legs; numbness or
tingling in the hands, feet, or face; ringing in
the ears; swollen feet or legs; tightness in the
chest; heart palpitations; nightmares and
panic attacks; "drenching" night sweats (not
menopausal or perimenopausal hot flashes);
constant hunger; headaches and migraines;
impaired memory and concentration; blurred
vision; nasal congestion; abdominal cramps;
loose stools; and diarrhea.

A Tricky Diagnosis

Under-the-radar hypoglycemia (known as
subclinical hypoglycemia) is difficult to
diagnose because symptoms may be subtle
and irregular, and test results can be within
normal ranges. Technically, if your blood
sugar drops below 70 milligrams per deciliter
(mg/dL), you are considered hypoglycemic.
But people without diabetes do not check
their blood sugar levels on their own, so it is
important to be aware of hypoglycemia symptoms.

If you suspect that you may have hypoglycemia, talk to your physician. Ideally, you
should arrange to have your blood glucose
levels tested when you are experiencing
symptoms. You will then be asked to eat food
so that your blood glucose can be tested

43

again. If this approach is impractical for you, however, talk to your doctor about other testing methods.

The Right Treatment

If you have been diagnosed with diabetes, hypoglycemia may indicate that your diabetes medication dose needs to be adjusted. The sugar treatment described earlier can work in an emergency but is not recommended as a long-term treatment for hypoglycemia. Left untreated, hypoglycemia in a person with diabetes can lead to loss of consciousness and even death.

In addition to getting their medication adjusted, people with diabetes — and those who are at risk for it due to hypoglycemia — can benefit from the following:

- **A high-protein diet and healthful fats.** To keep your blood sugar levels stabilized, consume slowly absorbed, unrefined carbohydrates, such as brown rice, quinoa, oatmeal, and sweet potatoes. Also, get moderate amounts of healthful fats, such as those found in avocado, olive oil, and fatty fish, including salmon, and protein, such as fish, meat, chicken, soy, and eggs.
  Recommended protein intake: 10 to 35 percent of daily calories. If you have kidney disease, get your doctor's advice on protein intake.

44

- **Eat several small meals daily.** Start with breakfast to give your body fuel for the day (if you don't, stored blood sugar will be released into your bloodstream) and then have a small meal every three to four waking hours.
- **Avoid tobacco, and limit your use of alcohol and caffeine.** They cause an excessive release of neurotransmitters that, in turn, trigger the pancreas to deliver insulin inappropriately.
- **Add supplements.** The supplements below also help stabilize blood sugar levels (and can be used in addition to a daily multivitamin).*

  ▶ **Chromium and vitamin B-6.** Chromium helps release accumulated sugars in the liver, which can lead to a dangerous condition called fatty liver. Vitamin B-6 supports chromium's function and helps stabilize glucose levels.
  Typical daily dose: 200 micrograms (mcg) of chromium with 100 milligrams (mg) of vitamin B-6.

  ▶ **Glutamine.** As the most common amino acid found in muscle tissue, glutamine plays a vital role in controlling blood

* Consult your doctor before trying any supplements, especially if you take prescription medication and/or have a chronic medical condition, including diabetes.

sugar. Glutamine is easily converted to glucose when blood sugar is low.

Typical daily dose: Up to four 500-mg capsules daily, or add glutamine powder to a protein drink or a smoothie that does not contain added sugar — these drinks are good options for your morning routine. Glutamine is best taken thirty minutes before a meal to cut your appetite by balancing your blood sugar.

Hyla Cass, MD, a board-certified psychiatrist and nationally recognized expert on integrative medicine based in Los Angeles. She is author of numerous books, including *8 Weeks to Vibrant Health* and *The Addicted Brain and How to Break Free*. CassMD.com.

The Secret Invasion
That Causes Diabetes

It's easy to get the impression that diabetes is all about blood sugar. Most people with diabetes check their glucose levels at least once a day. Even people without diabetes are advised to have glucose tests every few years — just to make sure that the disease isn't creeping up on them.

But glucose is only part of the picture. Scientists now know that chronic inflammation increases the risk that you'll develop diabetes. If you already have insulin resistance (a precursor to diabetes) or full-blown diabetes, inflammation will make your glucose levels harder to manage.

A common mistake: Unfortunately, many doctors still don't test for inflammation even though it accompanies all of the main diabetes risk factors, including smoking, obesity, and high-fat/sugar diets.

Silent Damage

You hear a lot about inflammation, but what exactly is it — and when is it a problem? Normal inflammation is protective. It comes on suddenly and lasts for just a few days or weeks — usually in response to an injury or infection. Inflammation kills or encapsulates microbes, assists in the formation of protective scar tissue, and helps regenerate damaged tissues.

But chronic inflammation — caused, for example, by infection or injuries that lead to continuously elevated levels of toxins — does not turn itself off. It persists for years or even decades, particularly in those who are obese, eat poor diets, don't get enough sleep, or have chronic diseases, including seemingly minor conditions such as gum disease.

The diabetes link: Persistently high levels of inflammatory molecules interfere with the ability of insulin to regulate glucose — one cause of high blood sugar. Inflammation also appears to damage beta cells, the insulin-producing cells in the pancreas.

Studies have shown that when inflammation is aggressively lowered — with salsalate (an anti-inflammatory drug), for example — glucose levels can drop significantly. Inflammation is typically identified with a blood test that measures a marker known as CRP, or C-reactive protein (see page 17).

How to Fight Inflammation

Even though salsalate reduces inflammation, when taken in high doses, it causes too many side effects, such as stomach bleeding and ringing in the ears, to be used long term. Here are some *safer ways to reduce inflammation and keep it down:*

- **Breathe clean air.** Smoke and smog threaten more than just your lungs. Recent research has shown that areas with the highest levels of airborne particulates that are small enough to penetrate deeply into the lungs have more than 20 percent higher rates of type 2 diabetes than areas with the lowest levels of these particulates.

Air pollution (including cigarette smoke) increases inflammation in fatty tissues and in the vascular system. In animal studies, exposure to air pollution increases both insulin resistance and the risk for full-fledged diabetes.

My advice: Most people — and especially those who live in polluted areas — could benefit from using an indoor HEPA filter or an electrostatic air filter. They will trap nearly 100 percent of harmful airborne particulates from indoor air.

If you live in a large metropolitan area, avoid outdoor exercise during high-traffic times of day.

- **Take care of your gums.** Even people who take good care of their teeth often neglect their gums. It's estimated that almost half of American adults have some degree of periodontal (gum) disease.

Why it matters: The immune system can't always eliminate infections that occur in gum pockets, the areas between the teeth and gums. A persistent gum infection causes equally persistent inflammation that contributes to other illnesses. For example, research shows that people with gum disease were twice as likely to develop diabetes as those without it.

My advice: After every meal (or at least twice a day), floss and brush, in that order. And clean your gums — gently use a soft brush. Twice a day, also use an antiseptic mouthwash (such as Listerine).

It's particularly important to follow these steps before you go to bed to remove bacteria that otherwise will remain undisturbed until morning.

- **Get more exercise.** It's among the best ways to control chronic inflammation because it burns fat. When you have less fat, you'll also produce fewer inflammation-promoting cytokines.

  Data from the Nurses' Health Study and the Health Professionals Follow-Up Study found that walking briskly for a half hour daily reduced the risk of developing diabetes by nearly one-third.

  My advice: Take ten thousand steps per day. To do this, walk whenever possible for daily activities, such as shopping, and even walk inside your home if you don't want to go out. Wear a pedometer to make sure you reach your daily goal.

- **Enjoy cocoa.** Cocoa contains a type of antioxidant known as flavanols, which have anti-inflammatory properties. Known primarily for their cardiovascular benefits, flavanols are now being found to help regulate insulin levels.

My advice: For inflammation-fighting effects, have one square of dark chocolate (with at least 70 percent cocoa) daily.

• **Try rose hip tea.** Rose hips are among the richest sources of vitamin C, with five times as much per cup as what is found in one orange. A type of rose hip known as *Rosa canina* is particularly potent, because it may contain an additional anti-inflammatory compound known as glycoside of mono and diglycerol (GOPO). It inhibits the production of a number of inflammatory molecules, including chemokines and interleukins.

My advice: Drink several cups of tangy rose hip tea a day. It's available both in bags and as a loose-leaf tea. If you're not a tea drinker, you can take rose hip supplements. Follow the directions on the label.

• **Season with turmeric.** This spice contains curcumin, one of the most potent anti-inflammatory agents. It inhibits the action of eicosanoids, signaling molecules that are involved in the inflammatory response.

My advice: Eat more turmeric — it's a standard spice in curries and yellow (not Dijon) mustard. You will want something more potent if you already have diabetes and/or elevated CRP. I often recommend Curamin, a potent form of curcumin that's combined with boswellia, another anti-inflammatory herb.

Important: Be sure to talk to your doctor before trying rose hip or turmeric supplements if you take medication or have a chronic health condition.

Check Your CRP Level

An inexpensive and accurate blood test that is often used to estimate heart attack risk is also recommended for people who have diabetes or are at increased risk for it. The blood test measures C-reactive protein (CRP), a marker for inflammation, which can lead to heart disease and impair the body's ability to regulate glucose.

A high-sensitivity CRP (hs-CRP) test typically costs about twenty dollars and is usually covered by insurance. A reading of less than 1 mg/L is ideal. Levels above 3 mg/L indicate a high risk for insulin resistance and diabetes as well as for heart attack.

If the first test shows that your CRP level is elevated, you'll want to do everything you can to lower it — for example, through exercise, a healthful diet, and weight loss. Repeat the test every four to six months to see how well your lifestyle improvements are working.

George L. King, MD, research director and chief scientific officer of Harvard's Joslin Diabetes Center, where he heads the vascular cell biology research section, and professor of medicine at Harvard Medical School in Boston. Dr. King is coauthor, with Royce Flippin, of *The Diabetes Reset: Avoid It, Control It, Even Reverse It — A Doctor's Scientific Program.*

How Your APOE Genes Lead to Diabetes or Heart Disease

If you have a family history of diabetes or heart disease, you no doubt have been told to watch your diet — to consume whole grains, olive oil, lean protein, tons of produce, and maybe some red wine. But could some of those supposedly heart-healthy foods actually be increasing your risk? Yes, depending on a particular gene that you may have, a gene that even many doctors don't know about.

Your family's ailments may be linked to a gene known as apolipoprotein E (APOE), which determines how your body metabolizes certain foods. According to cardiologist Suzanne Steinbaum, DO, author of *Dr. Suzanne Steinbaum's Heart Book,* if your diet suits your APOE type, you should be able to avoid following in your family's unfortunate medical footsteps. "The APOE genotype is like a light switch — it is going to activate only if you turn it on by eating foods that are wrong for your type," she says.

There are three genotypes (gene subtypes) associated with the gene — APOE-2, APOE-3, and APOE-4. A person inherits one of these from each parent.

About two-thirds of people have a "3/3" pairing, meaning they inherited APOE-3 from their mother and APOE-3 from their father. These lucky folks don't need to adhere too closely to any particular type of diet in order to avoid heart disease and diabetes, provided they follow a reasonably healthful diet, control their weight, exercise regularly, and don't smoke.

However, people who inherited the APOE-2 gene from one or both parents (a bit more than 10 percent of the population) have trouble metabolizing carbohydrates. **This makes them prone to diabetes.**

People who inherited the APOE-4 gene from one or both parents (just over 20 percent of the population) can't handle fat. **This increases their risk for coronary artery disease.**

An unlucky minority (less than 2 percent of the population) have a "2/4" pairing — meaning they inherited APOE-2 from one parent and APOE-4 from the other parent — **and thus are prone to both diabetes and coronary artery disease.**

Telling Your Type

A blood test can determine which genotype you have inherited. Dr. Steinbaum often recommends the test because she has found that patients generally comply better with dietary advice when there's a scientific indication that a particular diet will be especially protective for them. Some insurance policies cover the test (which costs about $150 or more, depending on the lab), so ask your insurance company.

If you choose not to get the blood test, you can get some idea — though not with certainty — of whether you carry the APOE-2 and/or APOE-4 genes.

People who inherited the APOE-2 gene from one or both parents tend to have:

• High triglycerides and blood sugar
• A family history of diabetes and obesity

Diet recommendations: People with APOE-2 often crave foods like cookies, jelly beans, bread, and soda — but their bodies cannot metabolize sugars and simple carbohydrates, and they often wind up overweight or obese, Dr. Steinbaum says. Lean proteins and moderate amounts of complex carbohydrates (such as whole grains and legumes) are the keys to good health for these people.

Note: Even though a glass of red wine with dinner is often said to be heart-healthy, Dr. Steinbaum advises APOE-2 carriers against drinking wine because it is loaded with sugars.

People who inherited the APOE-4 gene from one or both parents tend to have:

• High LDL "bad" cholesterol
• A family history of coronary artery disease

Recommended: If this is your profile, you're likely to gravitate toward Buffalo wings, cheeseburgers, rich ice cream, and other fatty foods — yet your body has a hard time breaking down and absorbing fats, and the receptors that are supposed to sweep up LDL "bad" cholesterol are suppressed. Dr. Steinbaum says, "For these people, I usually advise following an extremely low-fat diet, preferably a vegetarian or vegan diet, with less than 7 percent of calories coming from saturated fats." Even plant-based fats such as olive oil and nuts, which are considered heart-healthy for other people, should be consumed only in moderate amounts by people with the APOE-4 gene. You should also be aware that cholesterol-lowering statin drugs are less effective in APOE-4 individuals than in other people, so even if you take a statin, a low-fat diet is still very important for you.

People who inherited the APOE-2 gene from one parent and the APOE-4 gene from the other parent tend to have:

- High triglycerides, high blood sugar, and high LDL cholesterol
- A family history of both diabetes and coronary artery disease

Recommended: If you have a "2/4" pairing, you're in the unfortunate minority of people who have trouble metabolizing not only sugars and simple carbohydrates but also fats. Your best choice is to be a vegetarian, Dr. Steinbaum says. Focus primarily on vegetables, legumes, whole grains, and other complex carbohydrates, and avoid sweets, wine, white bread, white pasta, and other simple carbs. You also need to keep your fat intake quite low, consuming only modest amounts of plant-based fats and little or no animal fat. Your healthiest food options are vegetables, legumes, whole grains, and other complex carbohydrates.

Knowing your APOE gene can be very empowering. "When you think of heart disease as being genetic, you might assume, 'Well, my dad got it, my aunts got it, and my grandfather got it, so I'm going to get it too.' But if your dad's whole family had eggs for breakfast, chicken for lunch, and beef for dinner most days, the real problem lies in the fact that everyone was eating the wrong way for their gene type," Dr. Steinbaum says. The same goes for a family legacy of diabetes when the family diet tended toward high-carb foods.

So remember — whether your genetic legacy leaves you vulnerable to heart disease, diabetes, or both, committing to the right type of diet for you might well be enough to break that chain.

Suzanne Steinbaum, DO, attending cardiologist and director of Women's Heart Health, Lenox Hill Hospital, New York City. SRSHeart.com.

COULD ANTIBIOTICS
GIVE YOU DIABETES?

Antibiotics can cure. They kill infectious bacteria and save lives. Type 2 diabetes is a chronic disease. It shortens lives. But older men and women generally have to be extra careful when it comes to antibiotics, and now there is disturbing evidence that the cure may be contributing to the disease — in other words, certain antibiotics may increase the risk of developing diabetes.

The connection is the ecosystem of bacteria in our gut that scientists call the microbiome. It affects digestion and immunity, and an unhealthy microbiome has been linked to diseases as diverse as obesity, certain cancers, inflammatory bowel disease, rheumatoid arthritis, and diabetes. Several studies have shown that type 2 diabetes, the kind that affects most people, is more common in people who have microbiomes with altered or low bacteria diversity. What we eat and drink changes the composition of the bacteria, and so can the medication we take, especially antibiotics.

Penicillin, the original wonder drug, saved soldiers from battlefield infections in World War II and later revolutionized medicine by curing once-fatal infections. But antibiotics by their very nature disturb the microbiome by killing bacteria, including beneficial bacteria in the gut.

Now, the newest research finds an association between the repeated use of certain antibiotics and the diabetes epidemic that affects thirty million Americans . . . and counting.

A Strong Association in a Million People

In the latest study, researchers had access to nearly complete medical records of almost ten million people living in the United Kingdom. The records included medical diagnoses, tests and procedures, prescription medications, and lifestyle factors, including smoking and drinking history.

The research team identified 208,002 people who were diagnosed with diabetes (either type 1 or 2). Each case was matched with four controls, people of the same age and sex who did not have diabetes. In all, the study included more than one million men and women, with an average age of sixty.

Looking deeper into the medical records of the participants, the researchers searched for prescriptions for several different antibiotics, including, yes, penicillin, still the most popular choice. They excluded antibiotics prescribed in the year before a diabetes diagnosis, since many of these patients may have had undiagnosed diabetes already. They adjusted statistically for many variables, including smoking, high cholesterol, obesity, heart disease, skin and respiratory infections, and previous blood sugar measurement. The results:

- **In most cases,** a single course of antibiotics was not associated with any increased risk for diabetes, compared with taking no antibiotics at all.
- **The exception was a class of antibiotics called cephalosporins,** broad-spectrum antibiotics often prescribed for strep throat and urinary tract infections (UTIs). Even taking a single course of these antibiotics was associated with a 9 percent increase in type 2 diabetes risk.
- **For the antibiotics linked with type 2 diabetes,** the more courses people took in any one year, the greater the risk. Taking two to five courses of penicillin in a single year was linked to an 8 percent increase in diabetes risk, for example, while taking more than five courses was linked to a raised risk of 23 percent. Similarly, taking two to five courses of quinolones, prescribed for skin and respiratory infections as well as UTIs, was linked to a 15 percent increase in diabetes risk, while taking more than five courses raised risk 37 percent.
- **Tetracyclines** were associated with a raised type 2 diabetes risk only in people who took them for five or more courses in a year.
- **Nitroimidazoles,** prescribed for vaginal infections as well as skin infections such as rosacea, were not associated with increased diabetes risk when taken at any frequency.

- **Neither antiviral nor antifungal medications were linked with diabetes risk.**
- **While there appeared to be an association between some antibiotics and type 1 diabetes,** an autoimmune condition, for some antibiotics, the results were inconclusive.

With Antibiotics, Do the Right Thing

This study, while big and statistically powerful, doesn't tell us whether using antibiotics actually cause diabetes. That's because it's observational. It looks back and draws connections. A prospective study would assign one group of people to take antibiotics whether they need them or not, deny them to another group, and follow them for years to see who gets diabetes. For practical and ethical reasons, of course, that's impossible.

So it's possible that people who would go on to develop diabetes even years later are more prone to infections and so would need more antibiotics. On the other side, prospective animal studies have shown that antibiotics promote the growth of bacteria that promote diabetes. Because diabetes is so common and such a damaging disease, researchers are looking for other ways to tease out whether and how antibiotics contribute to diabetes.

You don't have to wait to do the right thing though. These wonder drugs have been overused, both for human medicine and animal livestock, and many are losing their effectiveness due to rising antibiotic resistance, a scary prospect. Using antibiotics only when they are really needed not only protects your own health but helps keep these drugs effective when they are really needed.

By all means, take an antibiotic if it's the right treatment. But there are already many good reasons to avoid antibiotics if possible, and the truth is, they are often prescribed for health conditions for which they can't possibly work. Antibiotics kill bacteria, so they won't help with, say, the common cold, which is caused by a virus. Most sinus infections, even those caused by bacterial infections, don't require antibiotics either.

In many cases, doctors prescribe antibiotics when they're not needed because a patient insists on it for almost any sort of infection or even suspected infection.

Don't be that patient!

Yu-Xiao Yang, MD, associate professor of medicine, division of gastroenterology, department of medicine, department of epidemiology and biostatistics, Perelman School of Medicine at University of Pennsylvania, Philadelphia. His study was published in the *European Journal of Endocrinology*.

THESE DRUGS CAN RAISE
DIABETES RISK

When your doctor pulls out his/her prescription pad, you probably assume that your health problem will soon be improving. Sure, there may be a side effect or two — perhaps an occasional upset stomach or a mild headache. But overall, you will be better off, right?

Not necessarily. While it's true that many drugs can help relieve symptoms and sometimes even cure certain medical conditions, a number of popular medications actually cause disease — not simply side effects — while treating the original problem.

Here's what happens: Your kidney and liver are the main organs that break down drugs and eliminate them from your body. But these organs weaken as you age. Starting as early as your twenties and thirties, you lose 1 percent of liver and kidney function every year. As a result, drugs can build up in your body (particularly if you take more than one), become toxic, damage crucial organs, such as the heart and brain — and trigger disease, such as diabetes.

Older adults are at greatest risk for this problem because the body becomes increasingly less efficient at metabolizing drugs with age. But no one is exempt from the risk.

Many commonly prescribed drugs increase risk for type 2 diabetes. These medications include statins, beta blockers, anti-depressants, antipsychotics, steroids, and alpha blockers prescribed for prostate problems and high blood pressure.

There are a number of safer alternatives to discuss with your doctor, consultant pharmacist, or other health-care professional.

If you're prescribed a beta blocker: Ask about using a calcium-channel blocker instead. Diltiazem has the fewest side effects. The twenty-four-hour sustained-release dose provides the best control.

If you're prescribed an antidepressant: Ask about venlafaxine, a selective serotonin and norepinephrine reuptake inhibitor (SSNRI) antidepressant that treats depression and anxiety and has been shown to cause fewer problems for diabetic patients than any of the older selective serotonin reuptake inhibitor (SSRI) drugs.

If you're prescribed an alpha blocker: For prostate problems, rather than taking the alpha blocker tamsulosin, ask about using dutasteride or finasteride. For high blood pressure, ask about a calcium-channel blocker drug.

The Very Best Drug Self-Defense

If you're over age sixty — especially if you take more than one medication or suffer drug side effects — it's a good idea to ask your physician to work with a consulting pharmacist who is skilled in medication management. A consulting pharmacist has been trained in drug therapy management and will work with your physician to develop a drug management plan that will avoid harmful drugs. These services are relatively new and may not be covered by insurance, so be sure to check with your provider.

To find a consulting pharmacist in your area, go to the website of the American Society of Consultant Pharmacists, www.ascp.com, and click on "Find a Senior Care Pharmacist."

Also helpful: Make sure that a drug you've been prescribed does not appear on the Beers Criteria for Potentially Inappropriate Medication Use in Older Adults. Originally developed by the late Mark Beers, editor of the *Merck Manual of Medical Information,* the list has been recently updated by the American Geriatrics Society. To download the list for free, go to www.geriatricscareonline.org and click on Clinical Guidelines & Recommendations.

Armon B. Neel Jr., PharmD, a certified geriatric pharmacist, adjunct instructor in clinical pharmacy at Mercer University College of Pharmacy and Health Sciences in Atlanta. Dr. Neel is also coauthor of *Are Your Prescriptions Killing You? How to Prevent Dangerous Interactions, Avoid Deadly Side Effects, and Be Healthier with Fewer Drugs.* MedicationXpert.com.

GET MORE OF THIS MINERAL TO SHIELD AGAINST DIABETES

Diabetes — the disease of chronically high levels of blood sugar — is an epidemic.

Ten percent of American adults have it, including 40 percent of people sixty-five and older. In fact, the rate of diabetes is rising so fast, the Centers for Disease Control predict the number of Americans with the disease will triple by 2050.

Key fact not widely reported: One reason so many of us get diabetes may be that so few of us get enough of the mineral magnesium in our diets.

In a recently completed twenty-year study of nearly forty-five hundred Americans, researchers from the University of North Carolina at Chapel Hill found that those with the biggest intake of magnesium (200 mg per every one thousand calories consumed) had a 47 percent lower risk of diabetes than those with the smallest intake (100 mg per every one thousand calories consumed). The study also linked lower magnesium intake to higher levels of a biomarker of insulin resistance and three biomarkers of chronic inflammation (C-reactive protein, interleukin-6, fibrinogen).

What happens: Insulin is the hormone that ushers blood sugar (glucose) out of the bloodstream and into cells. In insulin resistance, cells don't respond to the hormone, and blood glucose levels stay high — often leading to diabetes. And inflammatory bio-chemicals trigger the manufacture of proteins that increase insulin resistance.

"Magnesium has an anti-inflammatory effect, and inflammation is one of the risk factors for diabetes," says Ka He, MD, the study leader. "Magnesium is also a cofactor in the production of many enzymes that are a must for balanced blood sugar levels."

Compelling Scientific Evidence

Other recent studies also link magnesium intake and diabetes:

- **Ten times more magnesium deficiency in people with diabetes.** Compared with healthy people, people with newly diagnosed diabetes were ten times more likely to have low blood levels of magnesium, and people with "known diabetes" were eight times more likely to have low levels, reported researchers from Cambridge University in the journal *Diabetes Research and Clinical Practice.*

- **Low magnesium, high blood sugar.** People with diabetes and low intake of magnesium had poorer blood sugar control than people with a higher intake of magnesium, reported Brazilian scientists. "Magnesium plays an important role in blood glucose control," they concluded in the journal *Clinical Nutrition.*

- **More nerve damage.** Nerve damage —

70

diabetic neuropathy, with pain and burning in the feet and hands — is a common complication of diabetes. Indian researchers found that people with diabetic neuropathy had magnesium levels 23 percent lower than people without the problem.

- **Magnesium protects diabetic hearts.** High blood sugar damages the circulatory system, with diabetes doubling the risk of heart attack or stroke. In a study from Italian researchers, taking a magnesium supplement strengthened the arteries and veins of older people with diabetes. The results were in the journal *Magnesium Research.*

A magnesium supplement balances blood sugar — even if you're not diabetic. In a study of fifty-two overweight people with insulin resistance (but not diabetes), those who took a daily magnesium supplement of 365 mg had a greater drop in blood sugar levels and insulin resistance than those who took a placebo, reported German researchers in *Diabetes, Obesity and Metabolism.*

Bottom line: "Based on evidence from the study I led and other studies, increasing the intake of magnesium may be beneficial in diabetes," says Dr. He.

More Magnesium

The recommended dietary allowance (RDA) for magnesium is 420 mg a day for men and

320 mg a day for women.

However: In a study conducted by the Centers for Disease Control, no group of U.S. citizens tested — including Caucasian, African American, Hispanic American, men, or women — consumed the RDA for magnesium. "Substantial numbers of U.S. adults fail to consume adequate magnesium in their diets," concluded researchers in the journal *Nutrition.*

They also found that magnesium intake decreased as age increased — a troublesome finding, since diabetes is usually diagnosed in middle-aged and older people.

Healthful strategy: "I recommend increasing the intake of foods rich in magnesium, such as whole grains, nuts, legumes, vegetables, and fruits," says Dr. He.

Best food sources of magnesium include:

- **Nuts and seeds** (almonds, cashews, pumpkin seeds, sunflower seeds, sesame seeds)
- **Leafy green and other vegetables** (spinach, Swiss chard, kale, collard greens, mustard greens, turnip greens, cabbage, broccoli, cauliflower, Brussels sprouts, green beans, asparagus, cucumber, celery, avocado, beets)
- **Whole grains** (whole-grain breakfast cereals, wheat bran, wheat germ, oats, brown rice, buckwheat)
- **Beans and legumes** (soybeans and soy

products, lentils, black-eyed peas, kidney
beans, black beans, navy beans)
- **Fruit** (bananas, kiwi fruit, watermelon,
raspberries)
- **Fish** (salmon, halibut)

Consider a Magnesium Supplement

But magnesium-rich food may not be sufficient to protect you from diabetes, says Michael Wald, MD, director of nutritional services at the Integrated Medicine and Nutrition clinic in Mt. Kisco, New York. That's because many factors can deplete the body of magnesium or block its absorption. They include:

- Overcooking greens and other magnesium-rich foods
- Eating too much sugar
- Emotional and mental stress
- Taking magnesium-draining medications, such as diuretics for high blood pressure
- Exposure to environmental toxins such as pesticides
- Bowel diseases and bowel surgery

"Low blood levels of magnesium are very common," says Dr. Wald. And conventional doctors rarely test magnesium levels.

Recommended: To help guarantee an adequate blood level of magnesium, Dr. Wald recommends taking PERQUE Magnesium

Plus Guard. For maximum absorption and effectiveness, this doctor-developed supplement contains four different forms of the mineral (magnesium glycinate, magnesium ascorbate, magnesium citrate, magnesium stearate). It also contains nutritional cofactors that help the mineral work in the body.

The supplement is available at www.perque .com and through many other retail outlets, both online and in stores where supplements are sold. Follow the dosage recommendations on the label.

Ka He, MD, chair and professor, epidemiology and biostatistics, Indiana University, Bloomington. Environmental Nutrition. EnvironmentalNutrition.com.

Michael Wald, MD, physician and director of nutritional services at the Integrated Medicine and Nutrition clinic in Mt. Kisco, New York. IntMedNy.com.

SUPPLEMENT SAFELY WITH MAGNESIUM

If you feel that you are one of the majority of Americans who don't get enough magnesium from their diets, it may make sense to take a daily supplement, but always check with your doctor before taking any supplements.

If you decide to get your magnesium level checked, ask your doctor for a magnesium red blood cell (RBC-Mg) test. It measures the magnesium that is inside cells. It's a more accurate measure of magnesium than the standard serum magnesium test. An optimal RBC-Mg level is more than 5.5 mg/dL.

The test isn't essential. If you are generally healthy, you can't go wrong with extra magnesium. The Institute of Medicine advises women thirty-one years old and older to get 320 mg of magnesium daily. For men, the recommended amount is 420 mg. These are conservative estimates based on your minimal needs. I recommend that you multiply your weight in pounds by 3 mg to determine the optimal dose.

Example: A 140-pound woman would take 420 mg of magnesium. During times of stress, when your need for magnesium is higher, multiply your weight by five instead of three. Keep taking the higher dose until things calm down again. You will start to feel the benefits within a few days.

When you're shopping for supplements,

look for products that end with "ate" — magnesium glycinate, taurate, malate, etc. These forms are readily absorbed into the bloodstream and less likely to cause diarrhea.

Dennis Goodman, MD, board-certified cardiologist, clinical associate professor of medicine at New York University School of Medicine. He is author of *Magnificent Magnesium: Your Essential Key to a Healthy Heart and More.* DennisGoodman MD.com.

Don't Let Artificial Sweeteners Sabotage Your Health

In recent news, it was reported that sucralose — the artificial sweetener marketed as Splenda — interferes with insulin secretion and glucose metabolism. That report knocked sucralose out of the water as a sweet alternative for people who need to keep their blood sugar in check. Now, a more recent study has found that the problem is much broader — it goes well beyond Splenda — and the study also got to the bottom of what exactly you're doing to your body when you opt for artificial sweeteners.

The Sugar-Free Truth

After decades of thinking that artificial sweeteners were the answer to weight and sugar control, nutritionists and scientists are now realizing that it's not so. Sucralose isn't the only culprit — and glucose intolerance (a reduced ability to remove sugar from the blood) is not the only damage caused by artificial sweeteners. No-calorie artificial sweeteners in general have been linked to weight gain, as illogical as that sounds. And if you are thinking that folks who drink diet soda gain weight because they otherwise load up on other sugary foods, that's not so, says the research.

So how do you get fat on sugar-free edibles?

That part of the research equation wasn't clear until Israeli scientists discovered what artificial sweeteners do to the gut microbiome — the galaxy of bacteria that live in the gut, aid digestion, and play a big role in whether someone is healthy.

The researchers conducted a series of experiments that began with mice. Some mice were fed water spiked with one of three different artificial sweeteners — saccharin, sucralose, or aspartame. Then these mice were compared with mice fed either plain water or sugar water.

Result: Glucose intolerance developed within eleven weeks in the mice given each of the artificial sweeteners. Meanwhile, the mice given plain water — and even those given sugar water — were just fine.

Why that's bad: Glucose intolerance can lead to prediabetes.

When the researchers delved into whether the gut microbiome had something to do with these findings, they discovered that it sure did. Mice treated with antibiotics to wipe out their gut microbiomes didn't become glucose intolerant when fed artificial sweeteners, because the artificial sweetener had nothing to react with once it hit the gut. But water-fed mice that lost their microbiomes became glucose intolerant when gut bacteria from mice fed artificial sweeteners was transplanted into them to repopulate their microbiomes.

Translation: The artificial sweeteners transformed the gut microbiomes to include a very unhealthful mixture of organisms.

Mice are mice, but what about people? Experiments in humans delivered the same results. The researchers already knew, from an earlier study they had done, that nondiabetic people who consumed artificial sweeteners were more likely than people who didn't use artificial sweeteners to gain weight and show signs of impaired glucose tolerance. They reconnected with a portion of those study participants to examine their microbiomes. Sure enough, just as in the mice, the microbiomes of people who consumed artificial sweeteners were altered compared with the microbiomes of people who didn't touch fake sugar.

Sugar-Free Challenge

Going sugar-free but then consuming edibles that mimic or try to taste exactly like the food and drink you give up is the kind of trickery where the joke is on you. Not only are you *not* losing weight from substituting sugar with artificial sweeteners, you're training your body to be diabetic! There is a much better way. You can retrain your taste buds to simply stop craving or expecting sugary flavors.

Jotham Suez et al., "Artificial Sweeteners Induce Glucose Intolerance by Altering the Gut Microbiota," *Nature* 514, no. 7521 (October 9, 2014): 181–186.

THIN PEOPLE GET DIABETES TOO

It's widely known that type 2 diabetes tends to strike people who are overweight. In fact, about 85 percent of people with diabetes are carrying extra pounds, and one out of four Americans who are sixty-five or older have type 2 diabetes. But what about those who aren't overweight?

A popular misconception: It's commonly believed — even by many doctors — that lean and normal-weight people don't have to worry about diabetes. The truth is, you can develop diabetes regardless of your weight.

An unexpected risk: For those who have this "hidden" form of diabetes, recent research is now showing that they are at even greater risk of dying than those who are overweight and have the disease.

The Extra Danger No One Expected

No one knows exactly why some people who are not overweight develop diabetes. There's some speculation that certain people are genetically primed for their insulin to not function properly, leading to diabetes despite their weight.

Still, because diabetes is so closely linked to being overweight, even researchers were surprised by the results of a recent analysis of twenty-six hundred people with type 2 diabetes who were tracked for up to fifteen years.

Startling new finding: Among these people with diabetes, those who were of normal weight at the time of diagnosis were twice as likely to die of non-heart-related causes, primarily cancer, during the study period as those who were overweight or obese.* The normal-weight people were also more likely to die of cardiovascular disease, but there weren't enough heart-related events to make that finding statistically significant.

Possible reasons for the higher death rates among normal-weight people with diabetes include:

- **The so-called obesity paradox.** Even though overweight and obese people have a higher risk of developing diabetes, kidney disease, and heart disease, they tend to weather these illnesses somewhat better, for unknown reasons, than lean or normal-weight people.
- **Visceral fat,** a type of fat that accumulates around the internal organs, isn't always apparent. Unlike the fat you can grab, which is largely inert, visceral fat causes metabolic disturbances that increase the risk for

* Normal weight is defined as a body mass index (BMI) of 18.5 to 24.9, overweight is 25 to 29.9, and obese is 30 or above. To calculate your BMI, go to http://www.nhlbi.nih.gov/health/educational/lose_wt/BMI/bmicalc.htm.

diabetes, heart disease, and other conditions. You can have high levels of visceral fat even if you're otherwise lean. Visceral fat can truly be measured only by imaging techniques such as a CT scan (but the test is not commonly done for this reason). However, a simple waist measurement can help indicate whether you have visceral fat (see below).

- **Lack of good medical advice.** In normal-weight people who are screened and diagnosed with diabetes, their doctors might be less aggressive about pursuing treatments or giving lifestyle advice than they would be if treating someone who is visibly overweight.

How to Protect Yourself

It's estimated that about 25 percent of the roughly twenty-nine million Americans with diabetes haven't been diagnosed. Whether you're heavy or lean:

- **Get tested at least once every three years** — regardless of your weight. That's the advice of the American Diabetes Association (ADA).

Remember: If your weight is normal, your doctor may have a lower clinical suspicion of diabetes — a fancy way of saying he/she wouldn't even wonder if you have the condition. As a result, the doctor might think it's OK to skip the test or simply forget to recommend it. Ask for diabetes testing — even if your doctor doesn't mention it.

A fasting glucose test, which measures blood sugar after you have gone without food for at least eight hours, is typically offered. *Alternative:* The HbA1C blood test. It's recommended by the ADA because it shows your average blood glucose levels over the previous two to three months. Many people prefer the A1C test because it doesn't require fasting. Both types of tests are usually covered by insurance.

- **Pull out the tape measure.** Even if you aren't particularly heavy, a large waist circumference could indicate high levels of visceral fat. Abdominal obesity is defined as a waist circumference of more than thirty-five inches in women and more than forty inches in men. Even if you are under these limits, any increase in your waist size could be a warning sign. Take steps such as diet and exercise to keep it from increasing.

  To get an accurate measurement: Wrap a tape measure around your waist at the level of your navel. Make sure that the tape is straight and you're not pulling it too tight. And don't hold in your stomach!
- **Watch the sugar and calories.** The Harvard Nurses' Health Study found that

women who drank just one daily soft drink (or fruit punch) had more than an 80 percent increased risk of developing diabetes.

Research has consistently linked sweetened beverages with diabetes. But it's not clear whether the culprits are the sweeteners (such as high-fructose corn syrup) or just the extra calories, which lead to weight gain. Either way, it's smart no matter what you weigh to eliminate soda and other supersweet beverages from your diet — or if you don't want to give them up, have no more than one soft drink a week, the amount that wasn't associated with weight gain in the study.

Remember: A single soft drink often contains hundreds of calories.

• **Get the right type of exercise.** People who want to lose weight often take up aerobic workouts, such as swimming or biking, which burn a lot of calories. But if you don't need to lose weight, strength training might be a better choice. When you add muscle, you significantly improve insulin sensitivity and enhance the body's ability to remove glucose from the blood.

Walking may not sound very sexy, but it's one of the best exercises going because it has both aerobic and muscle-building effects. In fact, walking briskly (at a pace that causes sweating and mild shortness of breath) for half an hour daily reduces the risk for diabetes by nearly one-third. That's pretty impressive!

Mercedes Carnethon, PhD, associate professor of preventive medicine and epidemiology at Northwestern University Feinberg School of Medicine in Chicago, where she specializes in population studies of diabetes, obesity, cardiovascular disease, and fitness.

SKIPPING BREAKFAST RAISES RISK FOR TYPE 2 DIABETES BY 21 PERCENT

Skipping breakfast is associated with a 21 percent increase in type 2 diabetes risk. And the best breakfast is a combination of low-saturated-fat protein and low-glycemic-index carbohydrates.

Example: A western omelet with peppers, low-fat cheese, and ham. Eating fruit is common at breakfast but not ideal — it contains too much sugar and may leave you hungry again within as little as an hour.

Other ways to avoid type 2 diabetes: Increase physical activity and intake of omega-3s and vitamin D.

The late Frederic J. Vagnini, MD, a cardiovascular surgeon at the Heart, Diabetes and Weight Loss Centers of New York, New Hyde Park.

HIGH TRIGLYCERIDES: THIS HEART DISEASE THREAT CAN INCREASE YOUR DIABETES RISK

The medical mantra for people age fifty or over is to "know your numbers," which is to say, your cholesterol, blood pressure, and blood sugar levels as they relate to cardiac risk, so that you can take action to address potential problems. While many people pay attention to this advice, and because there is enduring truth to this medical sound bite, it is important to mention that there is one number that eludes even the savviest health consumers. It is tested right along with cholesterol and blood sugar and is becoming increasingly respected as a marker for cardiac risk — triglycerides.

Like cholesterol, triglycerides are a type of fat in the blood, but they are quite different from their more famous cousin. Triglycerides are produced by the body and ingested from food, as is cholesterol, but they serve a different purpose. If the body's energy needs are exceeded by food intake, the body converts the excess calories into triglycerides and stores them to provide extra energy when called for.

However, for a variety of reasons, triglyceride levels can rise to unhealthy levels in the blood, sometimes along with a rise in cholesterol, sometimes independently of that.

Normal fasting levels of triglycerides are less than 150 mg/dL, and when triglycerides rise to a fasting level of 200 mg/dL or over, the level is considered high. Occasionally, levels go to even 500 mg/dL or higher, though this is usually because of genetic disorders or an underlying disease.

A good deal of controversy exists about the exact role of high triglycerides and atherosclerosis, but there is definitely an association between high levels of them and heart disease. People who have triglycerides over 150 mg/dL and HDL "good" cholesterol under 40 mg/dL have a higher risk for heart disease. And high triglycerides are associated with a number of other diseases as well, all of which make it important to pay attention.

According to cardiologist Helene Glassberg, MD, physician at the University of Pennsylvania Health System, high triglycerides are especially associated with insulin resistance — a prediabetic state — and diabetes, in particular when it is poorly controlled. In fact, high levels of triglycerides signal the need to check for the presence of diabetes. Other problems that are sometimes associated with high levels are hypothyroidism or kidney disease. Pancreatitis is also associated with high triglycerides, which Dr. Glassberg says can exacerbate or even cause this disease.

Lowering Your Triglycerides

The good news is that this is one problem that lifestyle can often turn around. Dr. Glassberg recommends the following:

- **Normalize your weight.** Obesity is a risk factor for elevated levels, especially if you carry excess pounds in your abdomen.
- **Reduce or eliminate alcohol.** Excessive drinking has been directly associated with elevated triglycerides. In some people, even modest amounts of alcohol can affect the level.
- **Eat a nutritious diet.** Pay special attention to getting plenty of omega-3s and eliminate excess carbohydrates, saturated fat, and all trans fat.
- **Exercise at least thirty minutes each day.** Push away from the table before dessert and go for a walk instead.
- **Avoid smoking.**

When lifestyle changes are not enough to lower levels sufficiently, Dr. Glassberg says that there are excellent medications patients can take that address the problem in addition to lifestyle changes. Of course, pharmaceutical treatments often come with associated risks as well.

The Natural Approach

For more natural ways to manage triglycerides, Mark Stengler, NMD, advises all individuals with high triglycerides to talk with a trained professional before trying any supplements. His favorites include aged garlic extract (AGE) — the most commonly available brand is Kyolic — with the caveat that people on blood-thinning medications clear it with their doctor first. And those on the muscle-relaxant drug chlorzoxazone or the antiplatelet drug ticlopidine must not take garlic supplements. Pantethine has also been shown to lower triglycerides.

Dr. Stengler adds his advice to Dr. Glassberg's in emphasizing how important it is to treat insulin resistance and diabetes, since triglycerides tend to be high in these people. In addition to a careful diet and regular exercise, Dr. Stengler suggests taking chromium picolinate, which research has shown may lower levels significantly. And to end on a tasty note, a recent study in Norway showed that eating two or three kiwi fruits each day lowered triglyceride levels by as much as 15 percent.

Helene Glassberg, MD, physician, University of Pennsylvania Health System.

Mark A. Stengler, NMD, a naturopathic medical doctor and author of the *Health Revelations* newsletter, *The Natural Physician's Healing Therapies,* and *Bottom Line's Prescription for Natural Cures.* He is also the founder and medical director of the Stengler Center for Integrative Medicine in Encinitas, California, and former adjunct associate clinical professor at the National College of Natural Medicine in Portland, Oregon. MarkStengler.com.

CERTAIN STATINS ARE LINKED TO DIABETES . . . IS YOURS?

Has your doctor put you on cholesterol-lowering statin medication or suggested that it's time to start? If so, you probably know that statins can have some very serious side effects, such as muscle aches, liver problems, and perhaps impaired memory. But you may not have heard that the medication can increase your risk for developing a very common and potentially deadly disease — diabetes.

Now, thanks to a major recent study, we've learned that all statins are not created equal when it comes to diabetes risk. As it turns out, some are significantly riskier than others.

Which type are you taking?

Studying Statins Up North

Statin drugs reduce blood cholesterol levels by interfering with an enzyme that helps the liver make cholesterol. However, different types of statins work in slightly different ways, and their effects on the body vary somewhat. Earlier studies suggested that statins in general made people more likely to get diabetes, but that one type, pravastatin, made people less likely to get diabetes.

So for the recent study, researchers set out to determine more specifically how the most commonly used types of statins affected the risk for diabetes relative to each other. With access to health and pharmacy records of 1.5 million older Canadians, researchers identified 471,250 people age sixty-six and up who did not have diabetes when they first started taking statins. Then they followed each statin user for up to five years to see which ones got diabetes. (Though this study took place in Canada, the same statin drugs are prescribed in the United States.)

An earlier study suggested that patients taking pravastatin had a lower risk for diabetes compared with people taking a placebo. For that reason, in the new study, the researchers used pravastatin as the basis of comparison in gauging the diabetes risk associated with five other types of statins. After adjustments were made for various other diabetes risk factors (age, sex, health status, other medication use), here's how each drug fared relative to pravastatin:

- **Atorvastatin**, which accounted for more than half of all new statin prescriptions, was associated with a 22 percent increase in diabetes risk.
- **Rosuvastatin** was associated with an 18 percent increase in diabetes risk. However, the researchers noted that this risk may be dose-dependent, meaning present at higher dosages but not at lower dosages.
- **Simvastatin** was associated with a 10

percent increase in diabetes risk.

- Both **lovastatin** and **fluvastatin** were comparable to pravastatin.

The Statin/Insulin Connection

There are several possible explanations for why patients taking certain statins are more prone to develop diabetes. Some statins may cause damage to beta cells, which are responsible for storing and secreting insulin, and/or these statins may interfere with the process that transports glucose from the blood through the cell membrane and into the body's cells.

As for why pravastatin might reduce diabetes risk, animal studies have suggested that it improves cells' sensitivity to insulin. Lovastatin and fluvastatin may have similar beneficial effects on insulin sensitivity.

Bottom line: If you are taking or have been advised to take one of the statins associated with increased risk for diabetes (atorvastatin, rosuvastatin, simvastatin), talk with your doctor about the diet and lifestyle changes that could lower your cholesterol and perhaps reduce your need for the medication. Also, discuss whether it's appropriate to consider switching to pravastatin (or perhaps lovastatin or fluvastatin), particularly if you have other risk factors for type 2 diabetes, such as excess weight, high blood pressure, high triglycerides, a history of gestational diabetes or polycystic ovary syndrome, or a family history of diabetes.

Muhammad M. Mamdani, PharmD, MPH, professor, University of Toronto, director, Applied Heath Research Centre, St. Michael's Hospital, and adjunct scientist, Institute for Clinical Evaluative Sciences, all in Toronto, Canada. His study was published in *BMJ*.

DON'T LET STRESS RAISE YOUR BLOOD SUGAR . . . AND MORE

It's widely known that acute stress can damage the heart. For example, the risk for sudden cardiac death is, on average, twice as high on Mondays as on other days of the week, presumably because of the stress many people feel about going back to work after the weekend. People also experience more heart attacks in the morning because of increased levels of cortisol and other stress hormones.

Important recent research: In a study of almost one thousand adult men, those who had three or more major stressful life events in a single year, such as the death of a spouse, had a 50 percent higher risk of dying over a thirty-year period.

But even low-level, ongoing stress, such as that from a demanding job, marriage or other family conflicts, financial worries, or chronic health problems, can increase inflammation in the arteries. This damages the inner lining of the blood vessels, promotes the accumulation of cholesterol, and increases risk for clots, the cause of most heart attacks.

Among the recently discovered physical effects of stress:

• **Increased blood sugar.** The body releases blood sugar (glucose) during physical and emotional stress. It's a survival mechanism that, in the past, gave people a jolt of energy when they faced a life-threatening emergency.

However, the same response is dangerous when stress occurs daily. It subjects the body to constantly elevated glucose, which damages blood vessels and increases the risk for insulin resistance (a condition that precedes diabetes) as well as heart disease.

What helps: Get regular exercise, which decreases levels of stress hormones.

• **More pain.** Studies have shown that people who are stressed tend to be more sensitive to pain, regardless of its cause. In fact, imaging studies show what's known as stress-induced hyperalgesia, an increase in activity in areas of the brain associated with pain. Similarly, patients with depression seem to experience more pain — and pain that's more intense — than those who are mentally healthy.

What helps: To help curb physical pain, find a distraction. One study found that postsurgical patients who had rooms with views of trees needed less pain medication than those who had no views. On a practical level, you can listen to music. Read a light-hearted book. Paint. Knit. These steps will also help relieve any stress that may be exacerbating your pain.

Also helpful: If you have a lot of pain that isn't well-controlled with medication, ask your doctor if you might be suffering from anxiety or depression. If so, you may benefit from taking an antidepressant, such as duloxetine or venlafaxine, which can help reduce pain along with depression.

- **Impaired memory.** After just a few weeks of stress, nerves in the part of the brain associated with memory shrink and lose connections with other nerve cells, according to laboratory studies.

Result: You might find that you're forgetting names or where you put things. These lapses are often due to distraction — people who are stressed and always busy find it difficult to store new information in the brain. This type of memory loss is rarely a sign of dementia unless it's getting progressively worse.

What helps: Use memory tools to make your life easier. When you meet someone, say that person's name out loud to embed it in your memory. Put your keys in the same place every day.

Also helpful: Make a conscious effort to pay attention. It's the only way to ensure that new information is stored. Sometimes, the guidance of a counselor is necessary to help you learn how to manage stress. Self-help materials, such as tapes and books, may also be good tools.

- **Weight gain.** The fast-paced American life-style may be part of the reason why two-thirds of adults in this country are over-weight or obese. People who are stressed tend to eat more — and the "comfort" foods they choose often promote weight gain. Some people eat less during stressful times, but they're in the minority.

  What helps: If you tend to snack or eat larger servings when you're anxious, stressed, or depressed, talk to a therapist. People who binge on "stress calories" usu-ally have done so for decades — it's dif-ficult to stop without professional help.

  Also helpful: Pay attention when you find yourself reaching for a high-calorie snack even though you're not really hungry.

  Healthy zero-calorie snack: Ice chips.

  Low-calorie options: Grapes, carrots, and celery sticks. Once you start noticing the pattern, you can make a conscious effort to replace eating with nonfood activities — working on a hobby, taking a quick walk, etc.

Stress-Fighting Plan

There are a number of ways to determine whether you are chronically stressed — you may feel short-tempered, anxious most of the time, have heart palpitations, or suffer from insomnia.

However, I've found that many of my patients don't even realize how much stress they have in their lives until a friend, family member, coworker, or doctor points it out to them. Once they understand the degree to which stress is affecting their health, they can explore ways to unwind and relax.

In general, it helps to:

• **Get organized.** Much of the stress that we experience comes from feeling overwhelmed. You can overcome this by organizing your life.

Examples: Use a day calendar to keep your activities and responsibilities on track, and put reminder notes on the refrigerator.

• **Ask for help.** You don't have to become overwhelmed. If you're struggling at work, ask a mentor for advice. Tell your partner/ spouse that you need help with the shopping or housework. Taking charge of your life is among the best ways to reduce stress — and asking for help is one of the smartest ways to do this.

• **Write about your worries.** The anxieties

and stresses floating around in our heads often dissipate, or at least seem more manageable, once we write them down.

- **Sleep for eight hours.** No one who is sleep-deprived can cope with stress effectively.

Irene Louise Dejak, MD, an internal medicine specialist who focuses on preventive health, including counseling patients on the dangers of chronic stress. She is a clinical assistant professor at the Cleveland Clinic Lerner College of Medicine of Case Western Reserve University in Cleveland and an associate staff member at the Cleveland Clinic Family Health Center in Strongsville, Ohio.

ANOTHER REASON TO QUIT

Smoking increases risk for type 2 diabetes. Smoking can lead to insulin resistance, a precursor to type 2 diabetes.

Recent finding: Smokers have a 44 percent higher risk for developing diabetes than non-smokers.

Self-defense: If you smoke, get help quitting from a health professional. Also, maintain a healthy diet and exercise regularly.

Carole Willi, MD, chief resident, department of community medicine and public health, University of Lausanne, Switzerland, and leader of a meta-analysis of twenty-five studies, published in the *Journal of the American Medical Association.*

CAN YOUR TOILETRIES AND COSMETICS GIVE YOU DIABETES?

We've known for years that chemicals called phthalates — types of plasticizers contained in many products, including furniture, toys, plastic bags, and detergents, as well as in some cosmetics, including lotions, hair sprays, and perfumes — can knock our endocrine systems out of whack, potentially raising our risk for obesity and hardening of the arteries.

What's worse, a recent study suggests that we can now add type 2 diabetes to the list of phthalate dangers.

The cosmetics part is especially creepy, since we do more than simply touch that stuff — we often massage lotions or makeup into our skin and spray perfume onto our necks, where we breathe it right in. And if you should kiss someone wearing phthalate-containing cosmetics or perfume, what's getting into your mouth?

The chemical and cosmetics industries dispute the latest research and tell us that we should be perfectly happy to smear and spray their phthalates onto our bodies. It might be that they turn out to be right and the products are safe. But that's a long-term result that's not worth the risk to find out. We spoke with the researchers who found the diabetes link and then learned how to find phthalate-free cosmetics and perfumes.

What Lurks In Our Cosmetics?

The phthalates are put into many types of cosmetics because they do have some benefits. In perfume, for example, they help the scent linger longer; in nail polish, the chemicals reduce cracking by making polishes less brittle; and in hair spray, phthalates allow the spray to form a flexible film on hair, avoiding stiffness. But phthalates in these products can be either absorbed through the skin or inhaled, which causes them to enter the bloodstream . . . and then, watch out!

In the study, the researchers from Uppsala University in Sweden drew fasting blood samples from more than one thousand adults, looking for several toxins, including four substances specifically formed when the body breaks down phthalates. Even after adjusting for typical type 2 diabetes risk factors such as obesity, cholesterol levels, smoking, and exercise habits, researchers found that participants whose phthalate levels were among the highest 20 percent of the group were twice as likely to have type 2 diabetes when compared with those whose phthalate levels fell into the lowest 20 percent of the group.

Study author Monica Lind, PhD, an associate professor of occupational and environmental medicine at the university, says that since she and her colleagues are among the first scientists to measure phthalate levels in blood, "high" and "low" are relative to this study — in other words, it's difficult to discern whether the levels of phthalates in this study were high on any kind of absolute scale. And researchers didn't track the amount of phthalate-containing products that participants used. But the study does suggest that the higher the levels of phthalates in the blood, the higher the risk of getting type 2 diabetes, and that might reflect a greater use of products that contain them.

Check the Labels

Phthalates may increase the risk for type 2 diabetes by disrupting insulin production and/or inducing insulin resistance, Dr. Lind says. But those ideas are disputed by the FDA, which states that "it's not clear what effect, if any, phthalates have on health."

In the United States, the FDA does not require cosmetics or perfumes to be phthalate-free. It does require nonfragrance ingredients to be listed on cosmetic products, but the loophole is that any ingredients that are parts of a fragrance don't have to be listed — a manufacturer can simply put "fragrance" on the label. As a result, according to the nonprofit Campaign for Safe Cosmetics, most cosmetics and perfumes that contain phthalates don't list them on the label. In other words, if the word "fragrance" is listed, then you won't know for sure what's in the product, unfortunately.

If this is a concern for you, go through your makeup, perfumes, and lotions. Search online for cosmetics that are fragrance-free using the nonprofit Environmental Working Group's Skin Deep cosmetics database at www.ewg.org/skindeep, and then choose among the products that are also phthalate-free. For perfumes, specifically, search online using the phrase "phthalate-free perfumes," which should lead to many brands, such as Zorica of Malibu, Kai, Pacifica, Agape & Zoe Naturals, Rich Hippie, Honoré des Prés, Blissoma Blends, Red Flower Organic Perfumes, Tsi-La Organic Perfume, and Ayala Moriel Parfums.

Monica Lind, PhD, associate professor of occupational and environmental medicine, Uppsala University, Uppsala, Sweden. Her research was published in *Diabetes Care*.

How to Keep the Toxic Chemical BPA Out of Your Food

BPA (bisphenol A) is used in many plastic food and beverage containers, particularly those made of hard, clear polycarbonate plastic. BPA is also an additive in polyvinyl chloride (PVC) plastic, which is used in some plastic food wraps.

Surprising news: BPA is in the epoxy resins found in the lining of almost all cans used by the food industry (including baby formula cans!). In fact, canned food is the primary food source of BPA for adults.

The problem: BPA molecules that escape their chemical bonds can migrate into the foods and beverages they contact, especially if the container is heated or the food inside is acidic. We then ingest the BPA, thereby increasing our risk for numerous health problems. There's even BPA on the coated paper from cash registers — the toxin gets into our bodies when we touch the paper and then handle the food we're about to eat. BPA can also be absorbed through the skin.

Frederick S. vom Saal, PhD, curators' professor of biological sciences at the University of Missouri and a leading BPA researcher, explains that this chemical has estrogen-like effects on the body. It acts as an endocrine disruptor, interrupting our hormonal patterns and actually reprogramming our genes. Roughly one thousand published, peer-reviewed studies have linked BPA to negative health consequences. These include:

- Breast cancer, ovarian cysts, and uterine fibroids in females (and prostate cancer, sexual dysfunction, and altered sperm in males)
- Type 2 diabetes and its precursor, insulin resistance
- Heart disease and heart rhythm abnormalities
- Liver disease
- Thyroid dysfunction
- Obesity and greater accumulation of fat in cells

Unborn babies, infants, and children are especially susceptible to BPA's harmful effects because they are still growing. Exposure before birth and/or during childhood has been linked to:

- Birth defects
- Cognitive problems, including learning deficits
- Behavioral problems (e.g., hyperactivity)
- Early puberty in females
- Increased risk for cancer in adulthood

How much is too much? The EPA estimates that exposure of up to 50 micrograms (mcg) of BPA per kilogram (kg) of body weight per day is safe. However, recent studies suggest that even a tiny fraction of this amount — as little as 0.025 mcg/kg per day — may be dangerous.

Dr. vom Saal says, "No matter what you might hear from the plastics industry, which is trying to convince consumers that BPA is safe, hundreds of published papers show that BPA is a toxin with no safe levels."

Scary: When the CDC studied urine samples of more than twenty-five hundred Americans age six and older, 93 percent of those tested had BPA in their urine.

BPA Self-Defense

Here are Dr. vom Saal's suggestions for minimizing your exposure to BPA:

- **Avoid canned foods as much as possible.**

    Note: It does not help to store cans in the refrigerator or to use canned goods soon after you buy them. The harm is already done even before the cans reach the market, because high heat must be used to sterilize the food during canning.

    Exceptions: Several manufacturers — including Eco Fish, Eden Organic, Edward & Sons, Muir Glen, Oregon's Choice, and Wild Planet — have begun using BPA-free cans for some of their products. (See a manufacturer's website for information on its BPA-free canned products, or contact the company directly.)

- **Choose cardboard over metal.** Cardboard cartons (such as those used for juice or milk) and cardboard cylindrical "cans" (such as those used for raisins) generally are better options than metal cans — but they are not ideal, because they may contain some recycled paper (which is loaded with BPA), or they may be lined with a resin that contains BPA.

Best: Opt for foods that are fresh or frozen or that come in glass bottles or jars or in foil pouches.

- **Never give canned liquid formula to an infant.** Powdered is much safer.

- **When microwaving, never let plastic wrap come in contact with your food.** If a product has a plastic film covering that is supposed to be left in place during microwave cooking, remove the film and replace it with a glass or ceramic cover instead.

- **Transfer prepackaged food to a glass or ceramic container before cooking,** even if the instructions say to microwave the product in the plastic pouch it comes in.

- **Check the triangle-enclosed recycling numeral** on plastic items that come in contact with foods or beverages — storage containers, water pitchers, baby bottles, sippy cups, utensils, and tableware. The numeral 7 indicates a plastic that may or may not contain BPA. To be safe, Dr. vom Saal says, "If you see a numeral 7 and it doesn't say BPA-free, assume there is BPA." The letters "PC" stamped near the recycling number are another indication that the plastic contains BPA.

- **Recheck what's in your cupboards.** Those new travel mugs? They might be made from number-seven plastic. Plastics labeled number two or five, which are also often used for food containers, do not have BPA. But they may contain other potentially harmful chemicals that can leach out, especially when heat breaks down the molecular bonds of plastic. To be safe, wash all plastic kitchenware in cold to room-temperature water with a mild cleanser, not in the dishwasher. Never microwave plastic containers, not even those labeled microwave-safe, such as frozen entrée trays. Instead, use a glass or ceramic container. Before putting hot soup or gravy into plastic containers to freeze, first allow it to cool. Throw out any plastic kitchenware that is scratched, chipped, or discolored — damaged plastic is most likely to leach chemicals.
- **Do not assume that plastics with no triangle-enclosed numeral are safe.** Dr. vom Saal cautions, "Manufacturers know that consumers are looking for BPA, so

they're taking identifying numbers off their products and packaging." Don't fall prey to such tricks.

Frederick S. vom Saal, PhD, curators' professor of biological sciences at the University of Missouri, Columbia. He is a leading researcher on the effects of BPA and has conducted dozens of studies on this topic.

Perhaps you wouldn't dream of microwaving plastic food containers, because you know that heating plastic can allow toxins to leach into your food. But you probably don't think twice before dunking your fancy mesh tea bag into boiling-hot water. Well, you may want to give that some thought right now.

Yes, those pyramid-shaped mesh sachets filled with pretty multihued leaves lend sophistication to your daily tea-drinking ritual.

But: Even though they're often called "silky," those bags aren't made from silk. Most are actually made from plastic, either polyethylene terephthalate (PET), polylactic acid (PLA, or corn plastic), or food-grade nylon (indeed, nylon is a plastic).

PET, PLA, and nylon are widely used for food packaging, and their safety as packaging materials has been tested. "However, when you subject plastics to stressors such as heat, the molecules begin to break down and they can leach — no matter whether it's a microwave oven or a cup of hot water that is warming the contents," says Sonya Lunder, MPH, a senior analyst at the Environmental Working Group, an environmental health research and advocacy organization. "So, is stuff leaching out of the plastic in the tea bag and getting into your beverage? The answer is yes."

Problems with plastics: No studies have looked specifically at leaching from plastic tea bags, so we don't yet know how much of any particular toxin might be getting into our tea. But past experience should teach us to be wary. After all, people used to think it was perfectly OK to microwave food in plastic containers — until we learned that certain plastics contain bisphenol A (BPA), an endocrine disruptor that has estrogen-like effects on the body and that has been linked to breast cancer, prostate cancer, diabetes, obesity, heart fertility, early puberty, and cognitive and behavioral problems in children!

The plastics used for tea bags don't contain BPA. But PET plastics can contain phthalates (not because these chemicals are used as ingredients in the plastic, but rather because they may originate from recycled content), and phthalates are another type of endocrine disruptor that has been linked to birth defects. There is also some concern that PET may leach antimony trioxide, a heavy metal. "We just don't know whether the amount of various substances in PET, PLA, and/or food-grade nylon might someday prove to have negative health effects," Lunder says. "As yet, there is no scientific consensus about what is too much, who is at risk, or what other health effects we may be seeing from plastic food packaging. But given the worrisome potential effects on our hormones, I advise that people avoid heating plastics at every opportunity."

It boils down to this: If you enjoy an occasional cup of tea made from a fancy "silky" tea bag, you probably don't need to worry too much — that once-in-a-while treat isn't likely to hurt your health. However, it's possible that your body may reach potentially harmful levels of various chemicals if you are drinking tea made from plastic tea bags multiple times each day — particularly if you try to be frugal by making a second cup from a single tea bag, given that repeated stress in the form of heat can make plastics leach even more.

What about good old paper tea bags? They might not be any better than plastic, because many are treated with epichlorohydrin, a compound that has been linked to cancer, infertility, and suppressed immune function.

Your best bet: Buy yourself a nice metal tea ball. They typically cost only a few dollars. When you want a cup of tea, fill the ball with your favorite organic loose-leaf tea, and let it steep in the mug. When the drink is as strong as you like, remove the strainer and enjoy your tea — worry-free.

Sonya Lunder, MPH, senior analyst, Environmental Working Group, Washington, DC. Lunder's research focuses on toxic chemicals in food, water, air, and consumer products. EWG.org.

WANT DIABETES? DRINK SODA

To prevent diabetes, we're often told by health experts what not to eat, such as too many refined carbohydrates from breads, pasta, and ice cream.

What not to drink may be just as important.

Latest finding: Researchers at the Harvard School of Public Health analyzed health data from 310,000 people who participated in eleven studies that explored the connection between sugar-sweetened beverages (SSBs) and diabetes.

Fact: SSBs include soda, fruit drinks (not 100 percent fruit juice), sweetened iced teas, energy drinks, and vitamin water drinks. And in the last few decades, the average daily intake of calories from SSBs in the United States has more than doubled, from 64 to 141. The beverages are now "the primary source of added sugars in the U.S. diet," wrote the Harvard researchers in *Diabetes Care.*

The researchers found:

• **Drinking one to two twelve-ounce servings of SSBs per day was linked to a 26 percent increased risk of type 2 diabetes,** compared with people who drink one or fewer SSBs per month.

The increased risk for diabetes among those drinking SSBs was true even for people who weren't overweight, a common risk factor for diabetes. The researchers concluded that while SSBs are a risk factor for overweight, they're also a risk factor for diabetes whether you gain weight or not.

"The association that we observed between sodas and risk of diabetes is likely a cause-and-effect relationship," says Frank Hu, PhD, professor of nutrition and epidemiology at the Harvard School of Public Health.

Theory: A typical twelve-ounce serving of soda delivers ten teaspoons of sugar. That big dose of quickly absorbed sugar drives up blood sugar (glucose) levels, in turn driving up blood levels of insulin, the hormone that moves glucose out of the bloodstream and into cells, leading to insulin resistance, with cells no longer responding to the hormone and blood sugar levels staying high, eventually leading to diabetes.

SSBs also increase C-reactive protein, a biomarker of chronic, low-grade inflammation, which is also linked to a higher risk for diabetes.

- **Cola-type beverages also contain high levels of advanced glycation end products,** a type of compound linked to diabetes, say the researchers.

And many SSBs are loaded with fructose, a type of sugar that can cause extra abdominal fat, another risk factor for diabetes.

Bottom line: "People should limit how much sugar-sweetened beverages they drink and replace them with healthy alternatives, such as water, to reduce the risk of diabetes, as well as obesity, gout, tooth decay, and cardiovascular disease," says Vasanti Malik, PhD, a study researcher.

Good-For-You Beverages
"I help many of my clients break the habit of regularly drinking soda, sweetened iced tea, and other sugary beverages," says Lora Krulak, a healthy foods chef and self-described "nutritional muse" in Miami, Florida. "I show them how to make other beverages that have natural sugar or are naturally sweetened, so they don't miss the sugary drinks."

One of her favorite thirst-quenching combinations:
- 2 to 3 liters of water (sparkling or still)
- Juice of 2 lemons
- Juice of 2 limes
- Small bunch of mint
- Pinch of salt
- 1 tablespoon of maple syrup, honey, or coconut sugar or stevia to taste (stevia is a natural, low-calorie sweetener)

1. Let the mixture steep for 30 minutes before drinking.

"It's good to make a lot of this drink, so it's

in your refrigerator and you can grab it any time," says Krulak. When leaving home, put some in a water bottle and carry it with you.

Cut Sugar Cravings
"If one of my patients is craving sugary drinks, it means his or her blood sugar levels aren't under control," says Ann Lee, ND, LAc, a naturopathic doctor and licensed acupuncturist in Lancaster, Pennsylvania.

To balance blood sugar levels and control sugar cravings, she recommends eating every three to four hours, emphasizing high-protein foods (lean meats, chicken, fish, eggs, nuts, and seeds), good fats (such as the monounsaturated fats found in avocados and olive oil), and high-fiber foods (such as beans, whole grains, and vegetables).

She also advises her clients to take nutritional supplements that strengthen the adrenal glands, which play a key role in regulating blood sugar levels.

Recommended: Daily B-complex supplement (B-50 or B-100) and vitamin C (2,000 to 5,000 mg daily, in three divided doses, with meals).

For healthy drinks, she recommends green tea sweetened with honey or stevia or a combination of three parts seltzer and one part fruit juice.

Frank B. Hu, MD, PhD, an epidemiologist, nutritional specialist, and professor of medicine at Harvard Medical School and the Harvard School of Public Health, both in Boston. He is codirector of Harvard's Program in Obesity Epidemiology and Prevention.

Vasanti Malik, research fellow in the Harvard School of Public Health.

Lora Krulak, healthy foods chef and "nutritional muse" in Miami, Florida. LoraKrulak.com.

Ann Lee, ND, LAc, naturopathic doctor and licensed acupuncturist in Lancaster, Pennsylvania. DoctorNaturalMedicine.com.

VITAMIN D MAY LOWER
RISK FOR DIABETES

Researchers in Germany have found that people with adequate blood levels of vitamin D had a lower risk for type 2 diabetes than those with low levels of vitamin D. Protection against diabetes, which is a chronic inflammatory condition, is believed to come from vitamin D's anti-inflammatory effect. People should have their vitamin D levels checked annually and ensure that they have blood levels of between 50 and 80 ng/ml. Older adults are at increased risk of developing vitamin D insufficiency in part because, as they age, skin cannot synthesize vitamin D as efficiently, they are likely to spend more time indoors, and they may have inadequate intakes of the vitamin, according to the Institute of Medicine (US) Committee to Review Dietary Reference Intakes for Vitamin D and Calcium.

C. Herder et al., "Effect of Serum 25-Hydroxy-vitamin D on Risk for Type 2 Diabetes May Be Partially Mediated by Subclinical Inflammation: Results from the MONICA/KORA Augsburg Study," *Diabetes Care* (2011).

HIDDEN GI PROBLEMS CAN CAUSE DIABETES AND MORE

If you have a stomachache, nausea, or some other digestive problem, you know that it stems from your gastrointestinal (GI) tract. But very few people think of the GI system when they have a health problem such as arthritis, depression, diabetes, asthma, or recurring infections.

Surprising: Tens of millions of Americans are believed to have digestive problems that may not even be recognizable but can cause or complicate many other medical conditions.

Latest development: There's now significant evidence showing just how crucial the digestive system is in maintaining your overall health. How could hidden GI problems be responsible for such a wide range of seemingly unrelated ills?

Here's how: If you can't digest and absorb food properly, your cells can't get the nourishment they need to function properly, and you can fall prey to a wide variety of ailments.

Good news: A holistically trained clinician can advise you on natural remedies (available at health-food stores unless otherwise noted) and lifestyle changes that can often correct hidden digestive problems.*

* Consult your doctor before trying these remedies — especially if you have a chronic medical condition or take any medication.

Low Levels of Stomach Acid

Stomach acid, which contains powerful, naturally occurring hydrochloric acid (HCl), can decrease due to age, stress, and/or food sensitivities.

Adequate stomach acid is a must for killing bacteria, fungi, and parasites and for the digestion of protein and minerals. Low levels can weaken immunity and, in turn, lead to problems that can cause or complicate many ailments, including diabetes, gallbladder disease, osteoporosis, rosacea, thyroid problems, and autoimmune disorders.

If you suspect that you have low stomach acid: You can be tested by a physician — or simply try the following natural remedies (adding one at a time each week until symptoms improve):

- **Use apple cider vinegar.** After meals, take one teaspoon in eight teaspoons of water.
- **Try bitters.** This traditional digestive remedy usually contains gentian and other herbs. Bitters, which also are used in mixed drinks, are believed to work by increasing saliva, HCl, pepsin, bile, and digestive enzymes. Use as directed on the label in capsule or liquid form.
- **Eat umeboshi plums.** These salted, pickled plums relieve indigestion. Eat them whole as an appetizer or dessert or use um-

eboshi vinegar to replace vinegar in salad dressings.

- **Take betaine HCl with pepsin with meals that contain protein.** The typical dosage is 350 mg. You must be supervised by a healthcare professional when using this supplement — it can damage the stomach if used inappropriately. If you still have symptoms, ask your doctor about adding digestive enzymes such as bromelain and/ or papain.

Too Much Bacteria

When HCl levels are low, it makes us vulnerable to small intestinal bacterial overgrowth (SIBO). This condition occurs when microbes are introduced into our bodies via our food and cause a low-grade infection or when bacteria from the large intestine migrate into the small intestine, where they don't belong. Left untreated, this bacterial overgrowth can lead to symptoms, such as bloating, gas, and changes in bowel movements, characteristic of irritable bowel syndrome (IBS). In fact, some research shows that 78 percent of people with IBS may actually have SIBO.

SIBO is also a frequent (and usually overlooked) cause of many other health problems, including Crohn's disease, scleroderma (an autoimmune disease of the connective tissue), and fibromyalgia.

SIBO can have a variety of causes, including low stomach acid, overuse of heartburn drugs called proton pump inhibitors (PPIs), and low levels of pancreatic enzymes. Adults over age sixty-five, who often produce less stomach acid, are at greatest risk for SIBO.

Important scientific finding: A study recently conducted by researchers at Washington University School of Medicine found that, for unknown reasons, people with restless legs syndrome are six times more likely to have SIBO than healthy people.

To diagnose: The best test for SIBO is a hydrogen breath test — you drink a sugary fluid, and breath samples are then collected. If hydrogen is overproduced, you may have SIBO. The test, often covered by insurance, is offered by gastroenterologists and labs that specialize in digestive tests. A home test is available at www.breathtests.com.

How to treat: The probiotic VSL 3, available at www.vsl3.com, can be tried. However, antibiotics are usually needed. Rifaximin is the antibiotic of choice because it works locally in the small intestine.

Leaky Gut Syndrome

The acids and churning action of the stomach blend food into a soupy liquid (chyme) that flows into the small intestine. There, the intestinal lining performs two crucial functions — absorbing nutrients and blocking unwanted substances from entering the bloodstream.

But many factors, such as chronic stress, poor diet, too much alcohol, lack of sleep, and use of antibiotics, prednisone, and certain other medications, can inflame and weaken the lining of the small intestine. This allows organisms, such as bacteria, fungi, and parasites, and toxic chemicals we encounter in our day-to-day activities to enter the blood. The problem, called increased intestinal permeability, or leaky gut syndrome, is bad news for the rest of your body.

What happens: The immune system reacts to the organisms and substances as foreign, triggering inflammation that contributes to or causes a wide range of problems, such as allergies, skin problems, muscle and joint pain, poor memory and concentration, and chronic fatigue syndrome.

To diagnose: A stool test that indicates the presence of parasites, yeast infections, or bacterial infection is a sign of leaky gut. So are clinical signs, such as food intolerances and allergies. However, the best test for leaky gut checks for urinary levels of the water-soluble sugars lactulose and mannitol — large amounts indicate a leaky gut.

How to treat: If you and your doctor believe that you have leaky gut, consider taking as many of the following steps as possible:

- **Chew your food slowly and completely to enhance digestion.**
- **Emphasize foods and beverages that can help heal the small intestine,** including foods in the cabbage family, such as kale, vegetable broths, fresh vegetable juices (such as cabbage juice), aloe vera juice, and slippery elm tea.
- **Take glutamine.** This amino acid is the main fuel for the small intestine — and a glutamine supplement is one of the best ways to repair a leaky gut. Start with 1 to 3 g daily, and gradually increase the dosage by a gram or two per week to up to 14 g daily. Becoming constipated is a sign that you're using too much.
- **Try the probiotic *L. plantarum*.** A supplement of this gut-friendly bacteria, such as Transformation Enzyme's Plantadophilus, can help heal the small intestine.
- **Add quercetin.** This antioxidant helps repair a leaky gut. In my practice, I've found that the products PERQUE Pain Guard and PERQUE Repair Guard work

better than other quercetin products.
Typical dosage: 1,000 mg daily.

• **Use digestive enzymes with meals to help ensure your food is completely digested.** Good brands include Enzymedica, Thorne, and Now.

Liz Lipski, PhD, CCN, a Duluth, Georgia–based nutritionist who is board-certified in clinical nutrition and holistic nutrition. She is author of several books, including *Digestive Wellness: Strengthen the Immune System and Prevent Disease Through Healthy Digestion.* InnovativeHealing.com.

WEIGHT LOSS: THE KEY TO DIABETES PREVENTION

Losing weight is the single most effective way to prevent diabetes.

Reason: Putting on even as little as ten pounds — especially around your middle — automatically increases insulin resistance. Losing just fifteen pounds reduces your risk of developing diabetes by more than half.

A simple, proven way to lose weight: Eat smaller portions. Use small (ten-inch) plates at home — and therefore serve smaller portions — since studies show that people tend to finish whatever is on their plates. Also, avoid fruit juices and soft drinks as well as white foods (white bread, baked potatoes and french fries, pasta, white rice), all of which cause sharp rises in blood sugar. Finally, make sure that every meal contains a mix of high-fiber fruits and vegetables and high-quality protein (fish or lean meat).

Another key: Do an hour of exercise at least five times a week. A good program for most people is forty-five minutes of aerobic exercise — such as walking, biking, or swimming — and fifteen minutes of light weight lifting.

Reason: Regular exercise encourages weight loss and increases your body's sensitivity to insulin. This effect only lasts a short time, however, which is why it's important to exercise often.

For many, these steps will be enough to prevent diabetes. If your body's ability to respond to insulin is 75 percent of normal and you can lower your insulin resistance by 25 percent through diet and exercise — a typical response — then your blood-sugar regulation will be brought back in balance.

Anne Peters, MD, professor of clinical medicine, Keck School of Medicine of the University of Southern California in Los Angeles, and director of the USC Westside Center for Diabetes. She is author of *Conquering Diabetes — A Cutting Edge, Comprehensive Program for Prevention and Treatment.*

STAND UP AND MOVE

Exercise is not enough to take off the pounds if you spend a lot of time sitting. When people sit for long periods — doing desk jobs, using computers, playing video games, watching television, or for other reasons — the enzymes that are responsible for burning fat shut down.

Result: People who sit too much have significantly greater risk for premature heart attack, diabetes, and death.

Self-defense: In addition to exercising, it is important to stand up and move around as much as possible throughout the day — walk around the office, go up and down stairs, take a break from the computer and go outdoors, or do something else to get out of a seated position.

Marc Hamilton, PhD, associate professor of biomedical sciences, University of Missouri-Columbia, and leader of a study of the physiological effects of sitting, published in *Diabetes.*

TOO MUCH SUGAR IN YOUR DIET CARRIES MORE RISK THAN WEIGHT GAIN

We all know that it's not good for our health to consume too much sugar. Excessive amounts of sugar in the diet are widely known to cause weight gain. But that's only part of the story.

Both table sugar and high-fructose corn syrup (HFCS) contain fructose, which recent research has shown can increase the risk for diabetes, fatty liver disease, high blood pressure, and chronic kidney disease when consumed in excessive amounts. Currently, most Americans consume way too much added sugar in their daily diets, putting them at risk for all these diseases.

What's the Trouble with Fructose?

Fructose is a simple sugar. It is found naturally in honey, fruits, and some vegetables. But a typical fruit contains only about 8 g of fructose, compared to about 20 g in a sugary soda. Unlike soda, fruits and vegetables contain nutrients and antioxidants that are beneficial to health.

The two main sources of fructose in the American diet are table sugar (which is squeezed from beet and cane plants) and HFCS (which is processed using enzymes that turn corn starch into glucose and fructose). Table sugar and HFCS are almost identical in their chemical composition — and both, consumed in excess, can contribute to health problems.

But few Americans are aware of just how much added sugar they are getting in their diets. That's because many added sugars are often listed as ingredients that are not recognizable as sugar and are found in unexpected food sources (see page 55 for a list of these terms). For example, added sugar is found in not only obvious places like soft drinks and other sweet beverages, but also in great abundance in many salad dressings, condiments (such as ketchup), cereals, crackers, and even bread.

Emerging Research on Fructose

While there are many studies being conducted on different types of added sugars, there is important research that now focuses on various forms of fructose. For example, recent research suggests that fructose is harmful because it increases levels of uric acid, a naturally occurring acid found in the urine. In crystalline form, uric acid can deposit in the joints and lead to gout.

Eating foods rich in a compound called purines (found in foods such as anchovies, beer, brewer's yeast supplements, clams, goose, gravy, herring, lobster, mackerel, meat extract, mincemeat, mussels, organ meats, oysters, sardines, scallops, and shrimp) can also produce high levels of uric acid.

Smart Ways to Limit Sugar

It's important to remove added sugar from your diet — with a special focus on fructose due to its unique potential risks that are now being discovered in new research.

To minimize the health risks associated with added sugars, try these steps:

- **Beware of "hidden" sugar.** When buying processed foods, remember that added sugars can appear on food labels in various ways. (See various names for sugar on page 55.)
- **Avoid any prepared or processed product that does not provide an ingredient list.**
- **Don't eat more than four fruits daily.** Even the naturally occurring fructose found in fruit counts toward your total daily intake of fructose. It's also important to limit your intake of fruit juice, which has been stripped of the nutritious fiber present in whole fruit and often contains added sugar.
- **Limit fructose intake to 25 to 35 g per day.** Consuming more than that amount could trigger the physiological changes that may lead to disease.

To learn the fructose content of specific foods, go to the USDA Food Database.

- **Take nutritional supplements.** Limiting fruit in your diet may lower your levels of important nutrients. To replace them, take a multivitamin plus an additional 250 mg of vitamin C daily.
- **Be cautious when eating in restaurants.** Limit restaurant meals and takeout food to menu items for which you know the ingredients.
- **Be prepared for sugar withdrawal.** In rare cases, you may develop withdrawal symptoms from sugar and fructose, such as headache, fatigue, and an intense craving for sweets. To help ease these symptoms, be sure to drink plenty of water (five to eight cups daily).

Sugar Aliases

Take this list to the supermarket with you to help you identify the various terms for added sugars:

- Beet sugar
- Brown sugar
- Cane sugar
- Corn sweetener
- Corn syrup
- Demerara sugar
- Fruit juice concentrate
- Granulated sugar
- High-fructose corn syrup
- Honey

- Invert sugar
- Maple syrup
- Molasses
- Muscovado sugar
- Raw sugar
- Sucrose
- Syrup
- Table sugar
- Tagatose
- Turbinado sugar

Richard J. Johnson, MD, professor and chief of the division of renal diseases and hypertension at the University of Colorado, Denver. He is author of *The Sugar Fix: The High-Fructose Fallout That Is Making You Sick.*

How a Quick Massage Can Help You Beat Diabetes

No one wants to be overweight, have diabetes, or grow old prematurely. Well, a new study shows that there's a simple strategy that may help prevent all three that is actually quite fun and relaxing.

A massage might do the trick!

We're not talking about an expensive, hour-long massage either — recent research shows that an inexpensive massage lasting just ten minutes can be beneficial.

Stop the Damage!

Mark Tarnopolsky, MD, PhD, a professor of medicine and head of neuromuscular and neurometabolic disease at McMaster University in Canada, explains that the researchers in this specific massage study found two very interesting differences in muscles that had been massaged after exercise.

A gene pathway that causes muscle inflammation was "dialed down" in these muscles both immediately after the massage and two and a half hours after the massage. (Specific genes can be present in our tissues but not always active.) Dr. Tarnopolsky says that this is helpful knowledge because muscle inflammation is a contributor to delayed-onset muscle soreness, so it confirms biologically what we've always believed through anecdotal observation — a postexercise massage can help relieve muscle soreness.

Conversely, another sort of gene was "turned on" by the massage — this is a gene that increases the activity of mitochondria in muscle cells. Mitochondria are considered the power packs of our muscles for their role in creating usable energy. Better mitochondrial functioning has been shown by other studies to help decrease insulin resistance (a key risk factor for type 2 diabetes) and obesity and even to slow aging. When Dr. Tarnopolsky was asked about whether it's a stretch to link postexercise massage to these benefits, he said that it's not unreasonable — there is a potential connection, and future research will need to be done to confirm it.

Treat Yourself to a Massage

The massage type that Dr. Tarnopolsky and his colleagues used was a standard combination of three techniques that are commonly used for postexercise massage — effleurage (light stroking), petrissage (firm compression and release), and stripping (repeated longitudinal strokes). It's easy to find massage therapists in spas, salons, fitness centers, and private practices who use these techniques. Or you could ask your spouse or a friend to try some of these moves on you (even if his or her technique isn't perfect), because there's a chance that it could provide the benefits, says Dr. Tarnopolsky — he just can't say for sure, since that wasn't studied.

Dr. Tarnopolsky studied massage only after exercise, so that's when he would recommend getting one, but it's possible that massaging any muscles at any time may have similar benefits — more research will need to be done to find out.

Remember, you don't have to break the bank on a prolonged sixty-minute massage — a simple ten- or twenty-minute rubdown can do the trick.

Mark Tarnopolsky, MD, PhD, division of neurology, department of pediatrics and medicine, McMaster University, Ontario, Canada.

2
Do You Have Diabetes?
Symptoms and Tests

You might think that you've come to an age where you would know if you had a disease or not — perhaps you're familiar with how your body works, keep in great shape, or visit the doctor on a regular basis. Just because you're being careful doesn't mean you should not get tested or read up on the warning signs.

For example, you could have prediabetes and not even know. And if you do, it means you are much more likely to develop full-blown diabetes. What about that strange rash on your skin? It might not be just a simple irritation, but rather a sign you should be looking closer at your blood sugar.

This section is not about fear but empowerment and the confidence as an older adult to ask the right questions of your doctor. We provide you with plenty of ideas for how to screen for diabetes and hopefully instill the confidence you need to recognize symptoms if they arise.

Do You Have Prediabetes?
What You Must Know
to Protect Yourself

As Americans continue to pack on the pounds, doctors are seeing a surge in weight-related health problems. An increasingly common condition that now affects about 40 percent of American adults is prediabetes, characterized by blood glucose (sugar) levels that are higher than normal but not yet at diabetic levels. People with prediabetes are five to fifteen times more likely to develop full-blown diabetes than people without this condition.

These are alarming statistics. Diabetes has serious potential consequences, including blindness, kidney failure, erectile dysfunction, heart failure, stroke, as well as nerve damage and circulation problems that can necessitate amputation.

Good news: Diabetes and its devastating consequences can often be prevented — by reversing prediabetes.

How the Disease Progresses

There are two main types of diabetes. With type 1 diabetes, the body's immune system attacks the pancreas, impairing or destroying its ability to produce insulin, the hormone that helps cells absorb glucose and convert it to energy. Prediabetes and body weight are generally only minor contributors to type 1 diabetes.

In contrast, the development of type 2 diabetes — which accounts for about 90 percent of all diabetes cases — is greatly influenced by prediabetes and excess weight. An obese person is eighty times more likely to develop type 2 diabetes than a person of normal weight. With type 2 diabetes, the pancreas usually does produce insulin, but the body's cells cannot use it properly. A person generally passes through several stages on the way to developing type 2 diabetes.

When we eat, the amount of glucose in our blood rises, alerting the pancreas that it needs to produce insulin. Excess fat, nutritional deficiencies, and the stress hormone cortisol interfere with cells' ability to accept and use insulin, leaving excess glucose in the blood. When this happens, a person is said to have insulin resistance.

Sensing that the insulin is not doing its job, the pancreas churns out even more. But since the cells cannot accept the excess insulin, it remains in the blood, along with the excess glucose. When blood glucose levels reach a certain point (as measured with blood tests), the condition qualifies as prediabetes, and if levels climb higher still, it qualifies as diabetes.

High blood glucose levels cause many of the complications of diabetes, including damage to the kidneys, nerves, and eyes. However, in the years during which prediabetes and diabetes are developing, a bigger problem is high blood insulin.

Reason: Insulin helps produce muscle — but when insulin levels get too high, the hormone instead promotes formation of visceral fat, which in turn makes insulin resistance even worse. Insulin elevations also increase production of triglycerides and cholesterol, which clog arteries; C-reactive protein, which promotes damaging inflammation; and cortisol, which contributes to various diseases.

What the Tests Should Tell Us

Too many doctors use antiquated guidelines for interpreting test results, then tell patients all is well when, in fact, the patients are at risk. I urge you to ask your doctor for the specific results of your tests and compare them with my guidelines below, which I have based on the most recent evidence. You may spot a warning sign that your doctor missed.

- **Fasting glucose test.** Routinely given at annual checkups, this test involves fasting for at least eight hours (optimally twelve hours), then having blood drawn to measure glucose levels.

Do You Have Prediabetes?

If you are age sixty-five or older, you are at increased risk for prediabetes regardless of the characteristics described below. For this reason, you should ask your doctor about receiving a fasting glucose test.

If you are under age sixty-five, answer the following questions. Speak to your doctor about receiving a fasting glucose test if you score 5 or higher.*

AGE	POINTS
20–27	0
28–35	1
36–44	2
45–64	4

SEX	
Male	3
Female	0

FAMILY HISTORY OF DIABETES	
No	0
Yes	1

* Source: Richelle J. Koopman et al., "Tool to Assess Likelihood of Fasting Glucose Impairment," *Annals of Family Medicine* 6, no. 6 (November 2008): 555–561.

HEARTRATE (beats per minute)	POINTS
Less than 60	0
60–69	0
70–79	1
80–89	2
90–99	2
Greater than 100	4

To determine your heart rate, place the tips of the first two fingers lightly over one of the blood vessels in your neck or the pulse spot inside your wrist just below the base of your thumb. Count your pulse for ten seconds and multiply that number by six.

HIGH BLOOD PRESSURE	
No	0
Yes	1

BODY MASS INDEX (BMI)	
Less than 25	0
25–29.9	2
30 or greater	3

To determine your BMI, consult the National Heart, Lung, and Blood Institute website, www .nhlbi.nih.gov (search BMI).

Problem: The range generally accepted as "normal" — from 65 to 99 mg/dL — is much too broad.

Evidence: A study published in the *New England Journal of Medicine* found that men with a fasting blood glucose level of 87 mg/dL had almost twice the risk of developing diabetes as did men whose level was 81 mg/dL or less. My guidelines:

▶ **Optimal** — 76 to 81 mg/dL
▶ **Normal** — 82 to 85 mg/dL
▶ **At risk** — 86 to 99 mg/dL
▶ **Prediabetic** — 100 to 125 mg/dL
▶ **Diabetic** — 126 mg/dL and above

Though most doctors do not order it routinely, you can ask your doctor to have your insulin levels checked as part of your fasting glucose test. These results are not used to officially diagnose diabetes, but they do provide additional information about your risk. Although the generally accepted guidelines put the normal range for blood insulin levels at 6 micro-international units per milliliter (mcU/ml) to 35 mcU/ml, I think this range is far too wide to be meaningful. My guidelines:

▶ **Optimal** — 7 mcU/ml or less
▶ **At risk** — 8 to 10 mcU/ml
▶ **Prediabetic** — 11 to 25 mcU/ml
▶ **Dangerous** — above 25 mcU/ml

- **Oral glucose tolerance test with glucose and insulin levels.** A more accurate way to measure blood insulin levels, this test requires fasting for twelve hours and having blood drawn, then drinking a glucose solution and having blood drawn again after one, two, and up to three hours. Many medical doctors fail to order this test because they are unaware that it dramatically improves the ability to identify prediabetic patients. I often order this test for patients who are overweight, have a strong family history of diabetes, or have a history of elevated fasting glucose levels — even if their most recent fasting glucose test results appeared normal. In this way, I have diagnosed type 2 diabetes in several patients whose fasting glucose results did not suggest any problems. My guidelines for blood drawn at the two-hour point:

  ▶ **Normal** — blood glucose below 140 mg/dL, or insulin levels at or below 55 mcU/ml.

  ▶ **Prediabetic** — blood glucose of 140 to 159 mg/dL, or an increase in glucose of 50 mg/dL or more within one hour, or insulin levels at 56 to 90 mcU/ml.

  ▶ **Dangerous** — blood glucose of 160 mg/dL or higher, or insulin levels above 90 mcU/ml.

- **Hemoglobin A1C (HbA1C).** This blood test indicates damage to blood proteins caused when glucose binds to the oxygen-carrying hemoglobin in red blood cells, creating free radicals (harmful negatively charged molecules). Results are expressed as a percentage. A British study involving 10,232 adults indicated that HbA1C results accurately predict health problems, including heart attacks (for which prediabetes and diabetes are risk factors). For each 1 percent rise in HbA1C, study participants' heart attack risk increased by 20 percent. My guidelines:
  - ▶ **Normal** — 4.5 to 4.9 percent
  - ▶ **At risk** — 5.0 to 5.6 percent
  - ▶ **Prediabetic** — 5.7 to 6.9 percent
  - ▶ **Diabetic** — 7.0 percent or higher

Steps to Take to Preempt Prediabetes

Fortunately, there is a lot you can do to prevent prediabetes — or even to reverse it if you have it.

- **Lose excess weight.** This is without question the most important step. To determine if you are at a healthful weight, calculate your body mass index (BMI), a ratio of your weight to the square of your height (for a free online BMI calculator, go to www.nhlbi.nih.gov and search "BMI calculator"). BMI of 30 or higher indicates obesity and a strong likelihood of developing pre-diabetes or diabetes; BMI between 25 and 29.9 puts you at risk for prediabetes. If necessary, a holistic doctor or nutritionist can help you devise a personal weight-loss plan.

- **Reduce body fat percentage.** Apart from its effect on weight, excess body fat increases prediabetes risk. I measure a patient's body fat percentage with bioelectrical impedance, a painless test that involves placing electrodes on your hand and foot. For women, an ideal range is 21 to 24 percent; anything above 31 percent is risky. For men, ideal is 14 to 17 percent; above 25 percent is risky.

Self-defense: Build muscle and banish excess fat by doing thirty minutes of aerobic exercise, such as brisk walking, five days a week, plus thirty minutes of strength training twice weekly.

- **Eat right.** Good dietary habits help to control weight; prevent spikes and drops in blood glucose levels; slow digestion, giving the pancreas time to produce insulin; boost energy, making it easier to exercise; and provide nutrients that optimize health.

  ► Eat three meals a day at regular times, keeping portions moderate. Never skip breakfast.

  ► Keep snacks small.

  Options: Nuts, seeds, low-sugar protein

drinks, vegetables, or fruit.

▶ Include a small portion of protein at every meal.

Good choices: One or two eggs, 1.5 ounces of nuts, or three ounces of fish, chicken, turkey, or lean meat.

▶ Eat at least one or two servings of whole grains daily. For variety, try quinoa, couscous, and bread made with spelt or kamut flour.

▶ Avoid sugary foods, processed foods, trans fats (found in some margarines, baked goods, and crackers), and saturated fats (in meats, dairy foods, and many vegetable oils).

▶ Have at least two servings of fruits and three or more servings of vegetables daily.

• **Take appropriate supplements.** Many manufacturers offer a "blood sugar control formula" that provides a combination of nutrients to help stabilize blood glucose and promote proper insulin function. Alternatively, you can follow the following guidelines.

If you are at risk for prediabetes, take:

▶ Chromium, a mineral, at 500 micrograms (mcg) daily.

▶ Pycnogenol (maritime pine extract) at 200 mg daily.

If you have been diagnosed with prediabetes, also take:

▶ Biotin (vitamin B-7) at 500 mcg daily.
▶ Alpha-lipoic acid, an antioxidant, at 300 mg daily.
▶ Magnesium at 400 mg daily.
▶ Vitamin D at 1,000 international units (IU) daily.

If you use diabetes medication, check with your doctor before taking these supplements — your medication dosage may need to be adjusted. These supplements are sold in health-food stores, are generally safe, rarely cause side effects, and can be taken indefinitely. Ideally, however, your improved diet and more healthful lifestyle will decrease your risk for prediabetes or reverse the condition, so the supplements will eventually no longer be necessary.

For a complete guide on prediabetes, I recommend *Stop Prediabetes Now,* by Jack Challem and Ron Hunninghake, MD, from which the following checklist has been adapted. Check off all the risk factors that apply to you. If you have five or more checks, see your doctor — you may be at high risk for prediabetes.

I have:

▶ A brother, sister, or parent with diabetes
▶ A personal history of gestational diabetes (diabetes during pregnancy)

► A waist measurement of more than thirty-five inches (women) or forty inches (men)

I have been diagnosed with:
► High blood sugar or insulin levels
► High blood pressure
► High cholesterol or high triglycerides (a type of fat in blood)
► Hypothyroidism (low thyroid hormone)
► Polycystic ovary syndrome
► Carpal tunnel syndrome, Bell's palsy, or gout (which may be linked to diabetes)

I often:
► Skip breakfast
► Breakfast only on coffee and/or something starchy (bagel, muffin)
► Feel tired after meals, especially lunch
► Nap during the day or early evening
► Have trouble falling asleep at night
► Have trouble getting up in the morning
► Crave sweets
► Crave starchy foods (pasta, pizza, bread)
► Snack late at night
► Drink nondiet soft drinks daily
► Have one or more sweet foods daily
► Lack energy
► Skip exercise
► Feel thirsty
► Urinate frequently
► Have trouble maintaining an erection

► Feel less interested in sex than I used to
► Feel stressed, irritable, or depressed

Mark A. Stengler, NMD, a naturopathic medical doctor and leading authority on the practice of alternative and integrated medicine. Dr. Stengler is author of the *Health Revelations* newsletter, *The Natural Physician's Healing Therapies,* and *Bottom Line's Prescription for Natural Cures.* He is also the founder and medical director of the Stengler Center for Integrative Medicine in Encinitas, California, and former adjunct associate clinical professor at the National College of Natural Medicine in Portland, Oregon. MarkStengler.com.

HIDDEN DIABETES — YOU CAN GET A CLEAN BILL OF HEALTH AND STILL BE AT RISK

With all the devastating complications of type 2 diabetes, such as heart disease, stroke, dementia, and blindness, you might assume that most doctors are doing everything possible to catch this disease in its earliest stages. Not so.

Problem: There are currently no national guidelines for screening and treating type 2 diabetes before it reaches a full-blown stage.

Research clearly shows that the damage caused by type 2 diabetes begins years — and sometimes decades — earlier, but standard medical practice has not yet caught up with the newest findings on this disease.

Fortunately, there are scientifically proven ways to identify and correct the root causes of diabetes so that you never develop the disease itself.

When the Problem Starts

Diabetes is diagnosed when fasting blood sugar (glucose) levels reach 126 mg/dL and above. Prediabetes is defined as blood sugar levels that are higher than normal but not high enough to indicate diabetes. Normal levels are less than 100 mg/dL.

What most people don't know: Although most doctors routinely test blood sugar to detect diabetes, it's quite common to have a normal level and still have "diabesity," a condition typically marked by obesity and other changes in the body that can lead to the same complications (such as heart disease, stroke, and cancer) as full-fledged diabetes.

Important: Even if you're not diabetic, having belly fat — for example, a waist circumference of more than thirty-five inches in women and more than forty inches in men — often has many of the same dangerous effects on the body as diabetes.

Important finding: In a landmark study in Europe, researchers looked at twenty-two thousand people and found that those with fasting blood sugar levels of just 95 mg/dL — a level that's generally considered healthy — already had significant risks for heart disease and other complications.

An Earlier Clue

Even though we've all been told that high blood sugar is the telltale sign of diabetes, insulin levels are, in fact, a more important hallmark that a person is in the early stages of the diabetes continuum.

High blood sugar is typically blamed on a lack of insulin — or insulin that doesn't work efficiently. However, too much insulin is actually the best marker of the stages leading up to prediabetes and diabetes.

Why is high insulin so important? In most

cases, it means that you have insulin resistance, a condition in which your body's cells aren't responding to insulin's effects. As a result, your body churns out more insulin than it normally would.

Once you have insulin resistance, you've set the stage to develop abdominal obesity, artery-damaging inflammation, and other conditions that increasingly raise your risk for prediabetes and diabetes.

A Better Approach

Because doctors focus on prediabetes and diabetes — conditions detected with a blood sugar test — they tend to miss the earlier signs of diabesity. A better approach:

• **Test insulin as well.** The standard diabetes test is to measure blood sugar after fasting for eight or more hours. The problem with this method is that blood sugar is the last thing to rise. Insulin rises first when you have diabesity.

My advice: Ask your doctor for a two-hour glucose tolerance test. With this test, your glucose levels are measured before and after consuming a sugary drink — but ask your doctor to also measure your insulin levels before and after consuming the drink.

What to look for: Your fasting blood sugar should be less than 80 mg/dL; two hours later, it shouldn't be higher than 120 mg/dL.

Your fasting insulin should be 2 to 5 IU/dL — anything higher indicates that you might have diabesity. Two hours later, your insulin should be less than 30 IU/dL.

Cost: fifty to one hundred dollars (usually covered by insurance). I advise all patients to have this test every three to five years and annually for a person who is trying to reverse diabetes.

Steps to Beat Obesity

With the correct lifestyle changes, most people can naturally reduce insulin as well as risk for diabesity-related complications, such as heart disease.

Example: The well-respected Diabetes Prevention Program sponsored by the National Institutes of Health found that overweight people who improved their diets and walked just twenty to thirty minutes a day lost modest amounts of weight and were 58 percent less likely to develop diabetes. You can reduce your risk even more by following these steps:

• **Manage your glycemic load.** The glycemic index measures how quickly different foods elevate blood sugar and insulin. A high-glycemic slice of white bread, for example, triggers a very rapid insulin response, which in turn promotes abdominal weight gain and the risk for diabesity.

My advice: Look at your overall diet and try to balance higher-glycemic foods with lower-glycemic foods. In general, foods that are minimally processed — fresh vegetables, legumes, fish, etc. — are lower on the glycemic index. These foods are ideal because they cause only gradual rises in blood sugar and insulin.

- **Eat nonwheat grains.** Many people try to improve their diets by eating whole-wheat rather than processed white bread or pasta. It doesn't help.

    Fact: Two slices of whole wheat bread will raise blood sugar more than two tablespoons of white sugar. If you already have diabetes, two slices of white or whole wheat bread will raise your blood sugar by 70 to 120 mg/dL. Wheat also causes inflammation, stimulates the storage of abdominal fat, and increases the risk for liver damage.

    These ill effects occur because the wheat that's produced today is different from the natural grain. With selective breeding and hybridization, today's wheat is high in amylopectin A, which is naturally fattening. It also contains an inflammatory form of gluten along with short forms of protein, known as exorphins, which are literally addictive.

    Best: Instead of white or whole-wheat bread and pasta, switch to nonwheat grains such as brown or black rice, quinoa, buckwheat, or amaranth. They're easy to cook, taste good, and they don't have any of the negative effects. Small red russet potatoes are also acceptable.

- **Give up liquid calories.** The average American gets 175 calories a day from sugar-sweetened beverages. Because these calories are in addition to calories from solid food, they can potentially cause weight gain of eighteen pounds a year. The Harvard Nurses' Health Study found that women who drank one sugar-sweetened soft drink a day had an 82 percent increased risk of developing diabetes within four years.

  Moderation rarely works with soft drinks because sugar is addictive. It activates the same brain receptors that are stimulated by heroin.

  My advice: Switch completely to water. A cup of unsweetened coffee or tea daily is acceptable, but water should be your main source of fluids.

  Bonus: People who are trying to lose weight can lose 44 percent more in twelve weeks just by drinking a glass of water before meals.

  Important: Diet soda isn't a good substitute for water — the artificial sweeteners that are used increase sugar cravings and slow metabolism. Studies have found a 67 percent increase in diabetes risk in people who use artificial sweeteners.

Mark Hyman, MD, founder and medical director of the UltraWellness Center in Lenox, Massachusetts. A leading expert in whole-systems medicine that addresses the root causes of chronic illness, he is chairman of the Institute for Functional Medicine in Gig Harbor, Washington. Dr. Hyman is also the author of several books, including *The Blood Sugar Solution: The UltraHealthy Program for Losing Weight, Preventing Disease,* and *Feeling Great Now!* DrHyman .com.

WHAT IS TYPE 1.5 DIABETES?

How does type 1.5 diabetes differ from other types of diabetes?

Type 1 diabetes is an autoimmune disorder in which the body's own immune system destroys the insulin-producing cells of the pancreas. As a result, the body does not produce enough of the hormone insulin to control blood sugar levels.

Type 2 diabetes is characterized by insulin resistance — the body responds to insulin inefficiently and fails to keep blood sugar at a normal level. The vast majority of people with diabetes have type 2.

A person who shows attributes of both type 1 and type 2 is said to have type 1.5 diabetes. What initially appeared to be type 2 diabetes is actually slowly evolving into type 1 diabetes. Type 1.5 diabetes is also called slow-onset type 1 or latent autoimmune diabetes in adults (LADA). It is diagnosed through a blood test for antibodies. Diet, exercise, and some oral medications may help keep the condition under control, but many type 1.5 patients require insulin within ten years of diagnosis.

Anne Peters, MD, professor of clinical medicine, Keck School of Medicine, University of Southern California, Los Angeles, and director of the USC Westside Center for Diabetes. She is author of *Conquering Diabetes: A Complete Program for Prevention and Treatment.*

IS IT A RASH . . . OR DIABETES?

We all know that we should keep an eye on moles and any other skin changes that might be a sign of skin cancer.

But there's another reason to look closely at your skin: it can point to — or sometimes even predict — internal diseases that you might not be aware of.

Many internal diseases are accompanied by skin symptoms. The yellowish skin tint (jaundice) caused by hepatitis is a common one — but there are other serious health problems that most people don't associate with skin changes.

Skin symptoms: Rash or pimple-like eruptions (sometimes containing pus) under the breasts, between the buttocks, or in other skinfolds.

Possible underlying cause: Candidiasis, a fungal infection that commonly affects people with diabetes. This infection can also lead to whitish spots on the tongue or inner cheeks.

Candidiasis of the skin or mucous membranes that is chronic or difficult to control can be a red flag for poor blood sugar control — and it can occur in patients who haven't yet been diagnosed with diabetes. People with poor blood sugar control often have impaired immunity, increasing their risk for infections such as candidiasis.

Next step: Most candidiasis infections are easily treated with topical antifungal preparations. People with persistent/severe cases may need an oral medication, such as over-the-counter clotrimazole or prescription fluconazole.

Also: Dark patches of skin that feel velvety and thicker than normal (especially on the neck and under the arms) could be due to acanthosis nigricans, a sign of insulin resistance, a condition that often precedes diabetes. The skin may also smell bad or itch.

Acanthosis nigricans often will improve without treatment when you get your blood sugar under control, so get tested for insulin resistance and glucose tolerance.

Cindy Owen, MD, an assistant professor of dermatology and associate program director at the University of Louisville School of Medicine, where she practices medical and inpatient dermatology with a focus on the skin signs of internal disease and drug reactions. She has published many articles in medical journals such as the *Archives of Dermatology* and *Journal of Cutaneous Pathology.*

THIS DIY TEST FOR DIABETES COULD SAVE YOUR LIFE

If you're conscientious about your health, you probably see your doctor for an annual physical or perhaps even more often if you have a chronic condition or get sick.

But if you'd like to keep tabs on your health between your doctor visits, there's an easy, do-it-yourself test that can give you valuable information about your body.

Here's a self-test for diabetes — repeat it once every few months, and keep track of the results. *See your doctor if you don't "pass" this "Pencil Test."* *

Why this test? It checks the nerve function in your feet — if abnormal, this could indicate diabetes, certain types of infections, or autoimmune disease.

The prop you'll need: A pencil that is freshly sharpened at one end with a flat eraser on the other end, and a friend to help.

What to do: Sit down so that all sides of your bare feet are accessible. Close your eyes, and keep them closed throughout the test.

Have your friend lightly touch your foot with either the sharp end or the eraser end of the pencil. With each touch, say which end of the pencil you think was used.

* This self-test is not a substitute for a thorough physical exam from your doctor. Use it only as a way to identify potential problem areas to discuss with your physician.

Ask your friend to repeat the test in at least three different locations on the tops and bottoms of both feet (twelve locations total). Have your friend keep track of your right and wrong answers.

Watch out: Most people can easily tell the difference between sharp and dull sensations on their sensitive feet. If you give the wrong answer for more than two or three locations on your feet, have your doctor repeat the test to determine whether you have nerve damage (neuropathy).

Beware: Neuropathy is a common sign of diabetes, certain autoimmune disorders, including lupus and Sjögren's syndrome, infection, such as Lyme disease, shingles, or hepatitis C, or excessive exposure to toxins, such as pesticides or heavy metals (mercury or lead).

David L. Katz, MD, MPH, an internist and preventive medicine specialist. He is co-founder and director of the Yale-Griffin Prevention Research Center in Derby, Connecticut, and clinical instructor at the Yale School of Medicine in New Haven, Connecticut. Dr. Katz is also president of the American College of Lifestyle Medicine and author of *Disease-Proof: Slash Your Risk of Heart Disease, Cancer, Diabetes, and More — by 80 Percent.*

WHAT YOUR URINE
SAYS ABOUT YOUR HEALTH

You would be surprised by how much information can be gleaned from the urine that you produce each day (one to two quarts, on average). For example, the simple "dipstick" urine test that doctors often use to check for a urinary tract infection can also help them diagnose kidney disease, diabetes, cancer, and other conditions. But there is more.

What you may not realize: If you know what to look for, you can tell a lot about your health just by being aware of the physical characteristics of your urine — such as color, smell, and frequency.

Color

When you're healthy and drinking enough water, your urine should be mainly clear or straw-colored with just a hint of yellow. The yellow color comes from urochrome, a pigment produced by the breakdown of a protein in red blood cells.

Urine is naturally darker in the morning because you don't drink water while you sleep. If a color change persists, however, it could be a problem. For example:

• **Brown or dark brown.** Pay attention if your urine is dark for more than a week.
  What this usually means: Liver disease. The liver normally breaks down and ex-

169

cretes bilirubin, a pigment that's produced by the turnover of red blood cells. Patients with liver disease accumulate bilirubin. This will initially cause jaundice, a yellowing of the skin or the whites of the eyes. As more bilirubin accumulates, it can cause the urine to become brown. A combination of dark-colored urine and jaundice means that liver disease might be getting worse. See your doctor right away.

Dark-colored urine can also be a side effect of some antibiotics, laxatives, and muscle relaxants. Eating large amounts of fava beans, rhubarb, or aloe can cause brown urine as well. In some cases, dark-colored urine can signal kidney failure.

• **Red or pink.** Urine that's tinged with red or pink could simply mean that you have been eating beets. (The medical term for beet-induced urine changes is beeturia). Or it could mean that you're urinating blood.

The amount of blood will affect the color. If the urine resembles cabernet wine, you're bleeding a lot; urine that's pinkish or just slightly red contains only traces of blood. A microscopic amount of blood won't be visible — it can be detected only with a laboratory test.

What this usually means: Blood in the urine is always a problem. Make an appointment to see your doctor. If you see blood and it also hurts when you urinate, you could have an infection in the urethra, bladder, or kidney or even a malignancy in the bladder. Bleeding without pain can also indicate these conditions.

- **Green.** Though rare, a person's urine can turn a greenish color.

   What this usually means: Green urine can appear when you've consumed a chemical dye — from food coloring, for example, or from taking medications such as amitriptyline, an antidepressant, or indomethacin, a nonsteroidal anti-inflammatory drug. In some cases, urine with a greenish tint can signal a urinary tract infection with certain bacteria (such as *Pseudomonas*) that affect the color.

   If your urine is greenish, increase fluid intake to see if it clears. If it doesn't in two days, see your doctor or a urologist.

Odor

If you're healthy, your urine should be highly diluted, consisting of about 95 percent water, with only small amounts of dissolved chemical compounds and metabolic byproducts. It typically has no — or only a faint — odor.

Of course, everyone is familiar with the effect that asparagus and some other foods, such as onions or fish, have on the smell of one's urine. This strong "rotten" smell is due to the chemical compounds in certain foods, particularly molecules that are not completely broken down by the body. The smell usually disappears within a day or so.

Some other less common urine smells include:

- **Ammonia-like.** If your urine is concentrated, with a larger-than-normal amount of urea (a chemical compound in urine), you might smell an aroma that resembles ammonia. Or you might just notice that it has a stronger smell than usual.

  What this usually means: Dehydration. The less water you drink, the higher the concentration of urea and other substances — and the stronger the smell. You can diagnose this yourself by drinking, say, one extra glass of water an hour for several hours to add water to your urine. The strong urine smell will probably disappear within a few hours. If it does not, see your doctor.

- **Foul-smelling.** If your urine smells foul or unusual in any way for more than a few days, pay attention to the odor.

  What this usually means: If it's not caused by a food that you've eaten, it could signal an infection in the bladder or kidneys. Less often, it's due to a metabolic disorder that reduces the body's ability to fully break down foods during digestion.

  Uncontrolled diabetes can cause an abnormally sweet odor, and penicillin can cause a distinctive medicinal odor.

  Even if you have no other symptoms, such

as pain while urinating, if your urine continues to have an unusually strong smell for more than a couple of days, talk to your doctor.

Foamy or Bubbly

It's natural to see foam in the toilet when you really have to go and have a heavy stream. But urine that's consistently foamy or bubbly could mean that you're losing protein.

What this usually means: Kidney disease. Large amounts of protein in the urine is one of the main signs of chronic kidney disease. See your doctor right away.

Mucus or Cloudy

Mucus in urine could indicate inflammation in the urinary tract.

What this usually means: Urinary tract infection. See your doctor.

Cloudy urine can also be related to infection but is often just an indication that your urine is alkaline, which is harmless at low levels.

Volume and Frequency

The average adult typically urinates four to eight times in twenty-four hours. A change in the frequency of your urinary habits, including getting up more than twice a night to urinate or an increase or decrease in the amount that you urinate, warrants attention.

173

What this usually means: An increase in the frequency of urination, along with an increase in volume, is one of the telltale signs of diabetes.

If the amount of urine seems the same but you're urinating more often, you could have a urinary tract infection. If this is the case, you'll probably have very strong urges to urinate even when just a small amount comes out.

Frequency of urination and/or urinary urgency in the absence of a urinary tract infection can indicate an overactive bladder.

In men, enlargement of the prostate gland can trigger urinary urgency. Patients with neurological conditions, such as multiple sclerosis, can also have this symptom.

Don't worry if there's been a decrease in the amount or frequency of urination. You probably just need to drink more water. If this doesn't help, see your doctor.

Jonathan M. Vapnek, MD, a urologist and clinical associate professor of urology at Mount Sinai School of Medicine in New York City. A member of the American Urological Association, he was named by *New York Magazine* as one of New York City's best urologists. Dr. Vapnek has authored or coauthored more than thirty-five papers on urological topics.

GET THAT EYE EXAM

You may know that a good eye exam can reveal more than just your eye health. But did you know that it can detect signs of multiple sclerosis, diabetes, high blood pressure, rheumatoid arthritis, high cholesterol, and Crohn's disease? In a study of insurance claims, 6 percent of these conditions were first detected by eye doctors.

Why: The eyes contain blood vessels, nerves, and other structures that can be affected by chronic illness. If you're over age forty, get an eye exam at least every two years.

Linda Chous, OD, chief eye-care officer, UnitedHealthcare Vision, Minneapolis.

Put yourself on a weight-loss diet, and you can measure your success with a bathroom scale. If fitness is your goal, you can track your improvement by charting how fast you can run or walk a mile.

But how can you tell if your brain is as fit as the rest of you?

If you're having memory problems, that's an obvious red flag. But even if you're basically healthy (or are being treated for a chronic condition such as high blood pressure), a routine medical exam can tell a lot about your brain health — if you know what the seemingly basic tests may mean, according to former U.S. Surgeon General Richard Carmona, MD. A physical checkup reveals information about your brain — and the additional tests you may need.

Lay It All Out

Doctors aren't mind readers — they don't know what you're worried about unless you tell them. At your physical, tell your doctor about any changes in your health (even if you think they sound trivial).

Where most people get tripped up: There's always that routine question about medications you're taking. Don't assume that your doctor knows everything he/she has prescribed — include every medication and supplement you're taking.

Many common prescription or over-the-counter drugs — alone or in combination — can affect your brain. The following types of drugs are among the most commonly associated with dizziness, fuzzy thinking, and/or memory problems. All drugs within each class can addle a person's brain, not only the specific drug examples given.

• Allergy medications (e.g., antihistamines)
• Antianxiety medications
• Antibiotics
• Antidepressants
• Blood pressure medications
• Sleep aids

If you are taking one of these types of medications and are experiencing cognitive problems, ask your physician about switching to a different drug.

Fortunately, the fuzzy thinking and/ or problems with memory usually go away when the drug is discontinued. And because everyone responds differently to individual medications, you may be able to safely take a different drug that's within the same class.

Clues from Your Physical

Even if you're not having cognitive problems, your physical can give you a measure of key markers of brain health. For example, most people know that high blood pressure is linked to increased risk for certain types of dementia (normal blood pressure is 120/80 or below). But low blood pressure (lower than 90/60) may make you dizzy, fatigued, and unable to think clearly. Other important brain-health markers include:

- **Eyes.** When your doctor shines that bright light in your eyes, he is looking at the retina, the light-sensitive tissue at the back of the eye that is connected directly to the optic nerve leading to the brain. Blood vessels in the retina reflect vascular health in the whole body — including the brain.
- **Hearing, balance, and coordination.** While many diseases can cause problems with hearing, balance, or coordination, one possibility is dysfunction of the eighth cranial nerve, which connects directly to the brain. Ears have fluid-filled canals that relay information to the brain via the eighth cranial nerve and act as a kind of gyroscope, giving us our sense of orientation in space. When we change position, the fluid moves, and the brain adjusts our balance and coordination. With some inner-ear disorders, such as Ménière's disease or labyrinthitis, people are dizzy, lose hearing, or fall frequently due to loss of balance and coordination.
- **Reflexes.** A tap on your knee with a tiny hammer sends an electrical impulse to the

spinal cord, which then sends a signal back to the foot, triggering a kick. A weak or delayed response could indicate a problem with the nervous system or brain.

- **Sensation.** All of the senses are housed in the brain, including the sense of touch. Any change in sensation — tingling hands or feet, weak hands, and/ or numbness anywhere in the body — could signal a problem in the brain.

Digging Deeper

If your memory is failing or you're having other cognitive problems, such as difficulty making decisions or planning activities, your doctor may want to run tests for:

- **Inflammation.** A blood test for C-reactive protein (CRP) measures general levels of inflammation in the body. High levels of CRP (above 3.0 mg/L) could be due to a simple infection, cardiovascular disease that may also be putting your brain at risk, or an autoimmune disease, such as lupus or multiple sclerosis, which can cause problems with memory and thinking as well as physical symptoms.
- **Vitamin deficiencies.** A vitamin B-12 deficiency can lead to memory loss, fatigue, and light-headedness. Other common nutrient deficiencies that can affect thinking include vitamin D and omega-3 fatty acids — there are tests for both.

- **Diabetes and glucose tolerance.** Left untreated, diabetes can dramatically increase one's risk for dementia. If your doctor suspects you have diabetes (or it runs in your family), get your blood glucose level tested (following an overnight fast).

  Useful: An HbA1C test, which gives a broader picture of your glucose level over the previous six to twelve weeks. While most people, especially after age forty-five, should get glucose testing at least every three years, it's particularly important for those having cognitive symptoms.
- **Tick-borne illness.** Lyme disease and Rocky Mountain spotted fever can cause mental fuzziness.

Also helpful: Liver function tests, including new genomic tests, may also be ordered to assess your liver's ability to remove toxins. If the body doesn't clear toxins, this can alter brain metabolism, possibly leading to cognitive decline.

Richard Carmona, MD, FACS, MPH, president of the Tucson, Arizona–based Canyon Ranch Institute and vice chairman of Canyon Ranch, a health resort, spa, and wellness retreat. He served as U.S. Surgeon General from 2002 to 2006 and is author of *Canyon Ranch's 30 Days to a Better Brain*.

ARE YOU GETTING THE MOST FROM YOUR BLOOD TESTS? EVEN DOCTORS MAY MISS SIGNS OF HEALTH PROBLEMS

Unless your doctor tells you there's a problem, you may not give much thought to the blood tests that you receive periodically.

But standard blood tests and certain other blood tests that you may request from your doctor can offer valuable — even lifesaving — clues about your health, including explanations for such vexing conditions as short-term memory loss and fatigue.

What you may not realize: If your doctor says that your test results are "normal," this is not the same as "optimal" or even "good."

For example, a total cholesterol reading of 200 mg/dL is considered normal, even though the risk of developing heart disease is sometimes higher at this level than it would be if your numbers were lower. Always ask your doctor what your target should be.

Blood test results that you should definitely make note of — and certain tests you may want to request:*

• **Low potassium.** Low potassium (hypokalemia) is worrisome because it can cause fatigue, constipation, and general weakness,

* These blood tests are typically covered by health insurance.

along with heart palpitations.

Causes: An imbalance of the hormone insulin often causes low potassium. It can also be due to problems with the adrenal glands or a loss of fluids from vomiting and/or diarrhea. A magnesium deficiency or a high-sodium diet can lead to low potassium too. It is also a common side effect of certain medications, including diuretics, such as hydrochlorothiazide; laxatives; and some asthma drugs, such as albuterol.

▶ *Normal potassium:* 3.6 to 5.2 mEq/L.

▶ *Optimal potassium:* 4.5 to 5.2 mEq/L.

What to do: If your potassium is not optimal, your doctor will probably recommend that you eat more potassium-rich foods, such as fruits (bananas, oranges, cantaloupe), vegetables (tomatoes, sweet potatoes), and whole grains (quinoa, buckwheat). You'll also be advised to reduce your sodium intake to less than 2,300 mg daily — high sodium depletes potassium from the body. Additionally, you may be advised to take a magnesium and potassium supplement.

Also: Keep your stress level low. Chronic stress can lead to a high level of the hormone cortisol — this can overwhelm the adrenal glands and lead to low potassium.

• **"Normal" glucose.** Most people know

that high fasting blood glucose (126 mg/dL or above) is a warning sign of diabetes. But you may not be aware that slight increases in blood sugar — even when it is still within the so-called normal range — also put you at greater risk.

Surprising: Among forty-six thousand people who were tracked for ten years, for every one-point rise in fasting blood glucose over 84 mg/dL, the risk of developing diabetes increased by about 6 percent. Vascular and kidney damage may begin when glucose reaches 90 mg/dL — a level that's within the normal range.

Causes: High blood glucose usually occurs when the body's cells become resistant to the hormone insulin and/or when the pancreas doesn't produce enough insulin. Obesity and genetic factors are among the main causes.

▶ *Normal glucose:* 65 to 99 mg/dL.
▶ *Optimal glucose:* 70 to 84 mg/dL.

What to do: If your fasting glucose isn't optimal or if tests show that it's rising, try to get the numbers down with regular exercise, weight loss, and a healthier diet.

Powerful spice: Add one-quarter teaspoon of cinnamon to your food each day. People who take this small dose can lower their blood glucose by 18 to 29 percent.

Alternative: A standardized cinnamon

extract in capsule form (125 to 250 mg, two to three times daily).

- **High homocysteine.** Most doctors recommend a homocysteine test only for patients with existing heart problems. Everyone should get it. High homocysteine may damage arteries and increase the risk for heart disease and stroke.

Causes: Homocysteine rises if you don't get enough B-complex vitamins or if you're unable to properly metabolize methionine, an amino acid that's mainly found in meat, fish, and dairy. Vegetarians tend to have higher homocysteine levels. Other causes include a lack of exercise, chronic stress, smoking, and too much caffeine.

▶ *Normal homocysteine:* Less than 15 umol/L.

▶ *Optimal homocysteine:* 8 umol/L or below.

What to do: If your homocysteine level isn't optimal, take a daily B-complex vitamin supplement that has at least 50 mg of vitamin B-6.

Also helpful: A fish oil supplement to reduce inflammation and protect the arteries. Take 1,000 mg, two to three times daily.*

* Check with your doctor before using fish oil, especially if you take a blood thinner — fish oil can interact with it and certain other medications.

- **Low DHEA.** This is a hormone that's used by the body to manufacture both testosterone and estrogen. It's also an antioxidant that supports the immune system and increases insulin sensitivity and the body's ability to metabolize fats. DHEA is not usually measured in standard blood tests, but all adults should request that their levels be tested.

Low DHEA is a common cause of fatigue, weight gain, depression, and decreased libido in men and women of all ages. Over time, it can damage the hippocampus, the memory center of the brain.

Causes: It's normal for DHEA to slightly decrease with age. Larger deficiencies can indicate an autoimmune disease (such as rheumatoid arthritis) or chronic stress.

▶ *Normal DHEA:* Levels of this hormone peak in one's late twenties. Normal levels vary widely with age and sex.

▶ *Optimal DHEA:* The high end of the normal range is optimal — it reflects a reserve of DHEA.

Examples: 200 to 270 mcg/dL for men, and 120 to 180 mcg/dL for women.

What to do: If your DHEA level isn't optimal, managing emotional stress is critical. Get at least eight hours of sleep every night, exercise aerobically for about thirty minutes, three to four times a week, and practice relaxation techniques, such as yoga and meditation.

Also helpful: A daily supplement (25 to 50 mg) of DHEA. If you take this supplement, do so only under a doctor's supervision — you'll need regular blood tests to ensure that your DHEA level doesn't get too high.

• **High LDL-P (LDL particle number).** Traditional cholesterol tests look only at triglycerides and total LDL and HDL cholesterol. I advise patients to get a fractionated cholesterol test for a more detailed picture.

Important: Patients with a large number of small LDL particles have an elevated risk for a heart attack even if their overall LDL level is normal. The greater the number of these cholesterol particles, the more likely they are to lodge in the lining of blood vessels and eventually trigger a heart attack.

Causes: Genetics is partly responsible for high LDL and LDL-P. A poor reading can be due to metabolic syndrome, a group of factors that includes abdominal obesity, elevated triglycerides, and high blood pressure. A diet high in animal fats and processed foods can also cause an increase in LDL-P.

▶ *Normal LDL-P:* Less than 1,300 nmol/L.

▶ *Optimal LDL-P:* Below 1,000 nmol/L on an NMR lipoprofile (this test is the most accurate).

What to do: If your LDL-P level is not optimal (and you have not had a heart attack or other coronary event), I recommend exercise, weight loss, blood pressure and blood sugar management, more antioxidant-rich foods such as vegetables, berries, and legumes, and three to five cups of green tea daily — it's a potent antioxidant that minimizes the oxidation of cholesterol molecules, which is important for reducing heart attacks.

Also: Daily supplements of bergamot extract, which has been shown to change the size of cholesterol particles (Earl Grey tea, which is flavored with oil of bergamot, provides a less potent dose), and aged garlic extract, which has a beneficial effect on multiple cardiovascular risk factors. If these steps do not sufficiently improve your LDL-P level, talk to your doctor about taking a statin and/or niacin.

James B. LaValle, RPh, CCN, a clinical pharmacist, nutritionist, and founder of Progressive Medical Center, Orange County, California. He is the author of *Your Blood Never Lies: How to Read a Blood Test for a Longer, Healthier Life.* Jim LaValle.com.

3
FOODS THAT FIGHT DIABETES

One of mankind's favorite reasons for living is good food and drink. Holidays are usually surrounded by delicious treats, communities come together over comforting feasts, and recipes become legacies, passed down generation to generation. However, sometimes that traditional apple pie can be a danger, and for diabetics (and those trying to prevent diabetes) looking after their weight and blood sugar, it's especially important to be diligent and healthy. Adult men and women over a certain age gain weight more easily, and it can be difficult to break old habits and treasured traditions.

Happily, there are many ways to fight diabetes through food. From spices to fruits to meat alternatives, you can still experience great taste and variety while fending off diabetes.

BEANS FOR YOUR BLOOD SUGAR

A humble everyday food is amazingly good at helping to control diabetes and prevent the complications of this deadly disease — yet many diabetes patients ban it from their diets.

I'm talking about legumes — beans, chickpeas, lentils — which truly are close to magical when it comes to their health effects, particularly for folks with type 2 diabetes.

So if you're among the crowd of bean holdouts, you should try to give beans and other legumes a place of honor in your daily diet. Your life could depend on it!

Beans and Your Blood Sugar

For diabetes patients, keeping blood sugar levels as close to normal as possible is crucial, but controlling those fluctuating levels can be a real challenge. Many patients take antihyperglycemic drugs for this purpose, yet diet remains a major factor in diabetes management.

A lot of people with diabetes focus on high-fiber foods such as whole grains to help avoid problems like heart disease. And fiber does help (though the exact mechanism is unknown). But now a new Canadian study shows that beans and other legumes do the job even better.

The secret behind legumes' awesome power lies in their low glycemic index (GI) status. The GI is a scale from 0 to 100 that ranks foods based on their immediate effects on blood glucose levels. The lower its GI, the less of a blood sugar spike a particular food causes.

Beans Best the Competition

The study included 121 men and women with type 2 diabetes. Participants were divided into two groups and assigned to follow one of two healthful diets that were fairly equal in total calories, fat, protein, and carbohydrates consumed.

As part of their diet, the first group was told to consume about 190 grams (two half-cup servings) of beans or other legumes each day. The second group's diet included an equal amount of whole grains, such as whole-wheat cereals and breads and brown rice. Each group also avoided the alternate food — in other words, the bean group avoided whole grains and the whole-grain group avoided beans.

After three months: The whole-grain group did benefit from their diet — but the bean eaters benefited even more.

Hemoglobin A1C values — indicated by a blood test that measures average blood glucose levels for the previous three-month period — dropped significantly more in the legume group than in the whole-grain group.

Using an equation that calculates risk for coronary heart disease (CHD), researchers found that the legume group's CHD risk score fell from 10.7 to 9.6. This was largely the result of the legume eaters' decrease in systolic blood pressure (the top number of a blood pressure reading) from 122 to 118. In contrast, in the whole-grain group, neither the CHD risk score nor blood pressure decreased significantly.

Also: In the legume group, the average weight loss and waist-size reduction slightly exceeded those of the whole-grain group.

Give a High Five for Low GI

The study's lead author, David Jenkins, MD, PhD, DSc, says that his team purposely chose study participants who already had reasonably good diets. "We wanted to see how people doing well could make further improvements," he explains.

And in fact, both the legume group and the whole-grain group did improve. On the hemoglobin A1C test, for instance, both groups got their levels down below 7.0 — a benchmark that often allows patients to eventually decrease their diabetes medication.

Still, the legumes came out ahead for several reasons. Unlike whole grains, beans are a very good source of protein — and protein does not cause blood sugar to fluctuate the way carbs can. Beans also provide plentiful potassium, which may reduce blood pressure by counteracting the effects of sodium. But the primary factor in beans' favor, Dr. Jenkins says, is that they are among the lowest-GI foods, because their complex carbohydrates are digested slowly.

Who Should Give a Hill of Beans?

Legumes are particularly good for diabetes patients, but just about everyone can benefit from better blood sugar control. Are you hesitant because you don't care for the taste or texture? There are many types of beans and other legumes to choose from — so keep experimenting until you find some you enjoy!

It's easy to incorporate one cup of these potent orbs into your daily diet since they are so versatile.

Tasty suggestions: Add white beans to vegetable soups and meat stews; use black or kidney beans plus tofu as the basis for chili; top salads with edamame (boiled green soy beans); serve lentils as a side dish or salad; enjoy the many varieties of hummus, made from chickpeas; or purée any type of bean to make dip, adding what tastes good to you — olive oil, pepper, and/or other spices you love.

And don't worry about gas. Despite the "musical" reputation of beans, the study participants registered few complaints in this department. However, if you are concerned about bloating or flatulence, Dr. Jenkins advises starting with just one-half cup per day and increasing gradually over several weeks to give your digestive system time to adjust.

David Jenkins, MD, PhD, DSc, professor, department of nutritional science, and Canada Research Chair in Nutrition and Metabolism, University of Toronto, Canada. He is also director of the Risk Factor Modification Centre, St. Michael's Hospital, Toronto, and lead author of a study on legumes and diabetes control published in *Archives of Internal Medicine.*

CONTROL BLOOD SUGAR AND KEEP FIT WITH PREBIOTIC SUNCHOKES

The sunchoke looks like the love child of a potato and a piece of ginger. But this gnarled and knobby root vegetable has its own irresistible flavor — slightly nutty, crisp like jicama or water chestnut, with a hint of artichoke flavor that becomes more intense when cooked. If you're a veg-head, it's a fun addition to your daily menu.

Although nutritionists know that the sunchoke — a root vegetable also known as the Jerusalem artichoke — is great for glucose control, scientific studies to back up this idea have been few and far between. Now, a team of researchers from Japan has demonstrated that sunchokes may help prevent type 2 diabetes and fatty liver disease (a condition that often goes with diabetes and that can lead to life-threatening liver cirrhosis and hepatitis). But even if the researchers' claim is too ambitious, there are plenty of reasons to get familiar with sunchokes, their many health benefits, and delicious recipes.

Lessons from Fat Rats

The Japanese researchers fed rats a diet that was either 60 percent fructose (fruit sugar) or 60 percent fructose and 10 percent sunchoke powder to see whether sunchokes could prevent diabetes in the rodents. That is, they regularly fed the rats lots of sugar to get their blood sugar levels to spike (hyperglycemia) and their innate blood sugar controller — their insulin-producing pancreas — to malfunction. After four weeks of these diets, the blood and livers of the rats showed that, although signs of diabetes and fatty livers developed in all of them from all that fructose, the effects were milder in the rats that were also eating sunchokes. The sunchoke eaters did so much better, in fact, that the researchers suggested that at least 10 percent of the daily diet of people at risk for diabetes and fatty liver disease should consist of sunchokes.

A 10 percent-sunchoke-per-day diet seems a bit much. Tamara Duker Freuman, RD, CDN, registered dietitian and clinical preceptor for the Dietetic Internship Program at Columbia University's Teacher's College, agrees, noting that similar tests would need to be performed in humans to really know whether eating sunchokes could similarly lessen risk of diabetes in people, and if so, how much would be needed to cut off diabetes at the pass. Besides, rather than overloading your diet with sunchokes in quest of glucose control, it would be more reasonable to simply add them, in moderation, to the list of healthful nondrug food and remedies that you already know help prevent diabetes.

"Sunchokes have a low glycemic index, which is why they are considered to be a great food choice if you have diabetes — they don't cause blood sugar to spike. The new research from Japan, however, is suggesting that sunchokes work on a metabolic level to help prevent diabetes and fatty liver disease," Freuman explains. "That's an ambitious claim." Until human studies can confirm the findings of these Japanese researchers, Freuman offers these health-boosting reasons to enjoy the little tubers.

A Prebiotic Power Food

Sunchokes are the tuberous root of a type of sunflower that's native to North America. They provide generous amounts of iron and potassium and help the body absorb certain minerals, such as calcium, and they are rich in fiber, which helps prevent certain types of cancer, such as colon cancer.

In fact, sunchokes are packed with an important type of fiber called inulin, which is a prebiotic. "Inulin is a carbohydrate, but because your body can't digest it, it doesn't affect your blood sugar," says Freuman. This characteristic gives the sunchoke its low glycemic effect. But even though you can't digest inulin, the healthful probiotic bacteria in your gut feast on it and, in fact, need it to provide their health benefits to you, explains Freuman.

But inulin does have one unfortunate downside — which also puts a crimp in the advice of the Japanese researchers to load your daily diet with sunchokes. Eating too much inulin — more than ten grams a day — can make you gassy. Since one-half cup of sunchokes has eighteen grams of inulin in it, Freuman suggests eating no more than one-quarter cup at a time if you are new to this root vegetable but want to add it to your diet. Within six to eight hours — the amount of time it takes for the sunchokes to travel from your mouth to your colon — you'll know whether your body tolerates the inulin well or not. As your body gets used to this new food, you may be able to increase how much you eat without the gassy side effect.

Delicious Ways to Eat Sunchokes

Freuman also finds that cooking sunchokes, rather than eating them raw, lessens the inulin's gassy effect. So instead of chomping on your first chokes raw, try some of these ways to prepare them (no need to peel the sunchokes — just scrub them well):

- **Roasted sunchokes.** Roughly cut sunchokes into one-inch chunks, and toss them in olive oil and salt. Roast at 400°F for about forty minutes until they are tender and golden brown.
- **Sunchoke chips.** Slice the chokes thinly using a mandoline or sharp knife. Toss the slices in oil, salt, pepper, and any of your

favorite spices — these are especially yummy with garlic powder and thyme — and spread them in a single layer on a baking sheet. Bake at 400°F for fifteen minutes, flip them over, and bake for another ten to fifteen minutes or until crisp. These chips are addictive, so don't dive into a giant batch until you've made friends with inulin!

- **Sunchoke mash.** Steam or boil sunchokes as you would potatoes, and season them with butter, salt, and pepper. Or boil and mash them with potatoes to add a new taste sensation to an old standard.
- **Sunchoke soup.** After roasting sunchokes, simmer them in a saucepan with onions and garlic sautéed in olive oil along with broth or water. Season with thyme or rosemary. Stir in one-quarter cup of milk, cream, or yogurt. Then purée.
- **Sunchoke salads and snacks.** Slice or shave raw sunchokes, and add to salads (toss them in lemon juice or vinegar first, since the cut sides will discolor), or just eat out of hand.

So certainly, if you are looking for new healthy foods to keep your blood sugar on an even keel as well as optimize the health of your friendly gut bacteria, look for sunchokes at farmers' markets and your grocery store (they are in season from late fall to early spring).

Tamara Duker Freuman, RD, CDN, a registered dietitian in private practice and a clinical preceptor for the Dietetic Internship Program at Columbia University's Teacher's College, both in New York City. Tamara Duker.com.

CINNAMON — CHEAP, SAFE, AND VERY EFFECTIVE

Insulin is the hormone that controls blood sugar levels. Cinnamon is its twin. Says Richard Anderson, PhD, a researcher at the Beltsville Human Nutrition Research Center in Maryland and the coauthor of more than twenty scientific papers on cinnamon and diabetes, "Cinnamon stimulates insulin receptors on fat and muscle cells the same way insulin does, allowing excess sugar to move out of the blood and into the cells."

Several studies provide proof of cinnamon's effectiveness in preventing and controlling diabetes:

- **Stopping diabetes before it starts.** In Britain, researchers studied healthy men — one group received three grams of cinnamon a day and the other a placebo.

  After two weeks, the men taking the cinnamon supplement had a much improved glucose tolerance test — the ability of the body to process and store glucose. They also had better insulin sensitivity — the ability of the insulin hormone to usher glucose out of the bloodstream and into cells.

- **Long-term management of diabetes.** In a study by a doctor in Nevada, 109 people with type 2 diabetes were divided into two groups, with one receiving one gram of cinnamon a day and one receiving a placebo. After three months, those taking the cinnamon had a 0.83 percent decrease in A1C, a measure of long-term blood sugar control. Those taking the placebo had a 0.37 percent decrease. (A decrease of 0.5 percent to 1.0 percent is considered a significant improvement in the disease.)

"We used standard, off-the-shelf cinnamon capsules that patients would find at their local stores or on the internet," says Paul Crawford, MD, the study's author, in the *Journal of the American Board of Family Medicine.*

Important: He points out that the drop in A1C seen his study would decrease the risk of many diabetic complications — heart disease and stroke by 16 percent; eye problems (diabetic retinopathy) by 17 to 21 percent; and kidney disease (nephropathy) by 24 to 33 percent.

• **After a bad night's sleep, include cinnamon in your breakfast.** Several recent studies show that sleep deprivation increases the risk of diabetes.

Solution: Writing in the *Journal of Medicinal Food,* researchers in the Human Performance Laboratory at Baylor University recommended the use of cinnamon to reverse insulin resistance and glucose intolerance after sleep loss.

- **Oxidation under control.** Oxidation — a kind of biochemical rust — is one of the processes behind the development of diabetes. In a study by French researchers in the *Journal of the American College of Nutrition* of twenty-two people with prediabetes, three months of supplementation with a cinnamon extract dramatically reduced oxidation — and the lower the level of oxidation, the better the blood sugar control.

One Teaspoon Daily

"Try to get one-quarter to one teaspoon of cinnamon daily," says Dr. Anderson. Sprinkle it in hot cereals, yogurt, or applesauce. Use it to accent sweet potatoes, winter squash, or yams. Try it with lamb, beef stew, or chilies. It even goes great with grains such as couscous and barley and legumes such as lentils and split peas.

Or you can use a cinnamon supplement. Consider taking one to three grams per day, says Dr. Anderson, which is the dosage range used in many studies that show the spice's effectiveness.

Best: Cinnulin PF — a specially prepared water extract of cinnamon — is a supplement used in many studies showing the spice's effectiveness in supplement form. It is widely available in many brands, such as Swanson and Doctor's Best.

The dosage of Cinnulin PF used in studies is typically 250 mg, twice a day.

Richard Anderson, PhD, lead researcher at the Beltsville Human Nutrition Research Center, U.S. Department of Agriculture, Maryland.

EAT WALNUTS ...
PREVENT DIABETES

We've been losing the fight against diabetes — the prevalence of this deadly disease has increased by more than 175 percent since 1980.

Good news: There's an easy and economical way to help guard against type 2 diabetes. Just eat a particular type of nut — the walnut.

The news comes from a huge Harvard study that looked at data on nearly 138,000 women.

Every two years, participants answered detailed questions about their health and lifestyle. Every four years, they completed lengthy questionnaires about their diets, indicating how often they consumed each of more than 130 foods, with answers ranging from "never or less than once per month" to "six or more times per day."

At the start of the study, none of the women had diabetes. By the end of the ten-year follow-up, nearly six thousand had developed the disease.

The researchers performed a careful analysis that adjusted for age, body mass index, family history of diabetes, smoking, menopausal status, and other factors that affect diabetes risk. They also adjusted for consumption of various unhealthful foods (such as sugar-sweetened drinks and processed meats) and healthful foods (whole grains, fish, fruits, vegetables, and various types of nuts).

What they found: Women who ate two or more ounces of walnuts per week, on average, had a 24 percent lower risk for type 2 diabetes. Those who ate just one ounce of walnuts per week had a 13 percent lower risk.

Other types of nuts conferred some benefits, but mainly through weight control, the researchers say. The walnut, however, has a number of properties that make it a winner in the fight against diabetes.

For one thing, of all the common tree nuts, walnuts are highest in polyunsaturated fats, containing 47 percent of these fats by weight — and there is good evidence that polyunsaturated fats have favorable effects on how the body uses insulin. Walnuts are also the richest of all nuts in a particular type of healthful polyunsaturated fat called alpha-linolenic acid. What's more, walnuts are high in fiber and plant protein and have been shown to decrease total cholesterol and LDL "bad" cholesterol. These nuts are also loaded with vitamin E and polyphenols that have antioxidant properties.

Bonus: Even though walnuts (like other nuts) are high in calories, they don't seem to cause weight gain in a balanced diet —

perhaps because they are so filling and satisfying.

Do men get similar protection against diabetes from eating walnuts? Research will have to prove it, but odds are good that they would.

Going nuts: The best part is that walnuts aren't some specialty product you have to go out of your way to buy, and you don't have to drown yourself in walnuts to get the benefits. Two ounces is only twenty-eight walnut halves per week. That's just four halves per day.

Walnuts are a great snack to have on the road or at work because they don't need to be refrigerated (though if you're going to store them for a while, putting them in the fridge or freezer will keep them fresher longer). While this new study did not look at whether the participants ate their walnuts raw, roasted, or otherwise cooked, you can certainly use them in cooking if you like, because heat won't significantly affect their health benefits.

To increase your intake, try adding chopped walnuts to cereal, salad, rice, or soup, stirring ground walnuts into a smoothie or yogurt, and spreading walnut butter on celery sticks or apple slices.

Frank Hu, MD, PhD, professor of medicine, Harvard Medical School and Channing Division of Network Medicine, Brigham and Women's Hospital, and professor of nutrition and epidemiology, Harvard School of Public Health, all in Boston. His study was published in *Journal of Nutrition*.

ONIONS — BIG FLAVOR, BIGGER BENEFIT

Chances are you eat onions all the time without giving them a second thought. What you might not realize about this vegetable (yes, onions are vegetables) is that they offer much more than flavor. Onions are rich in antioxidants, which have anti-inflammatory properties. Even the onion's famous eye-watering effect is the result of volatile gases, many of which are also antioxidants. Raw onions provide slightly more health benefits than cooked onions, but cooked onions are nothing to sniff at. Find out what onions can do for your health:

• **Provide cancer protection.** An *American Journal of Clinical Nutrition* study found that people who eat a lot of onions (more than one cup of onions daily) have an 80 percent lower risk of developing prostate cancer than those who eat very few onions. Eating onions frequently was also found to provide protection against colorectal, laryngeal, and ovarian cancers.

• **Reduce blood sugar.** Within four hours of eating three-quarters of a cup of chopped onion, study participants with diabetes had reduced blood sugar levels, according to a study by Sudanese researchers published in *Environmental Health Insights.*

- **Minimize scars and ease bug bite itch.** Onion extracts may reduce scar formation on the skin. In a study conducted by Korean researchers, the antioxidants in onions were found to reduce scarring by increasing the activity of an anti-inflammatory enzyme. Creams containing onion extract, such as Mederma (sold at most pharmacies), can reduce scarring. You can also slice an onion in half and rub it on a bug bite to relieve the itch.

In the Kitchen

Add onions as an ingredient in omelets, salads, and sauces — or let them take center stage, as in the delicious side dish described below. It features sumac, a Middle Eastern spice, available in the spice section of some grocery stores and online.

Sautéed Onions in Sumac

Chop two large red or sweet onions. Sauté in olive oil until soft. Sprinkle with sumac, a mild spice with a lemony flavor.

Mark A. Stengler, NMD, a naturopathic medical doctor and leading authority on the practice of alternative and integrated medicine. Dr. Stengler is author of the *Health Revelations* newsletter, *The Natural Physician's Healing Therapies,* and *Bottom Line's Prescription for Natural Cures.* He is also the founder and medical director of the Stengler Center for Integrative Medicine in Encinitas, California, and former adjunct associate clinical professor at the National College of Natural Medicine in Portland, Oregon. MarkStengler.com.

VINEGAR FOR WEIGHT LOSS
(AND IT LOWERS BLOOD SUGAR!)

We tend to think of vinegar mostly for salad dressing, but it actually has a long history as a folk medicine to ease such conditions as headaches and indigestion. Now, several studies highlight vinegar's benefit for weight management and blood sugar control. Mark Stengler, NMD, a naturopathic medical doctor and founder and medical director of the Stengler Center for Integrative Medicine in Encinitas, California, tells why this common product is so uncommonly helpful — and how to use it for better health.

Researchers believe that it is the acetic acid in any type of vinegar (apple cider, balsamic, white or red wine) that produces the health effect, interfering with enzymes involved in the digestion of carbohydrates and those that alter glucose metabolism (so that insulin does not spike).

One study found that mice fed a high-fat diet and given acetic acid developed up to 10 percent less body fat than those not given acetic acid. Another study found that having small amounts of vinegar at bedtime seemed to reduce waking blood glucose levels in people.

Adding vinegar to a meal slows the glycemic response — the rate at which carbohydrates are absorbed into the bloodstream —

by 20 percent.

Reason: Again, the acetic acid in vinegar seems to slow the emptying of the stomach, which reduces risk for hyperglycemia (high blood sugar), a risk factor for heart disease, and helps people with type 2 diabetes manage their condition.

Ways to add vinegar to meals: Use malt vinegar on thick-cut oven fries; marinate sliced tomatoes and onions in red wine vinegar before adding the vegetables to a sandwich; mix two parts red wine vinegar with one part olive oil, and use two tablespoons on a green salad; mix a tablespoon or two with soy sauce, olive oil, garlic, and herbs for a meat marinade.

For blood sugar balance (for those with diabetes or on diabetes medication) or for weight loss, dilute one to two tablespoons (some people start with teaspoons) in an equal amount of water, and drink it at the beginning of a meal.

Mark A. Stengler, NMD, a naturopathic medical doctor and leading authority on the practice of alternative and integrated medicine. Dr. Stengler is author of the *Health Revelations* newsletter, *The Natural Physician's Healing Therapies,* and *Bottom Line's Prescription for Natural Cures.* He is also the founder and medical director of the Stengler Center for Integrative Medicine in Encinitas, California, and former adjunct associate clinical professor at the National College of Natural Medicine in Portland, Oregon. MarkStengler.com.

Carol S. Johnston, PhD, RD, associate director, nutrition program, Arizona State University, Mesa, and coauthor of a study published in *Diabetes Care.*

GREAT "WHEY" TO
CONTROL BLOOD SUGAR

For people with type 2 diabetes, eating isn't the problem. It's what happens after eating that can be dangerous. Glucose accumulates in the bloodstream, where levels go way up after a meal. This phenomenon, called spiking, irritates blood vessels and throws your metabolism out of whack, increasing risk for cardiovascular disease, eye and kidney damage, and possibly Alzheimer's disease and cancer too.

A short, brisk exercise session before meals helps prevent postmeal blood glucose spiking. Here's another, even easier (and surprising) trick for keeping your blood sugar where it should be — it involves using whey.

Whey to Go!

It turns out that whey protein — yes, that stuff you see sold in giant tubs in the bodybuilder and sports section of health-food stores — is a great premeal tonic for glucose control. Whey protein products are powdered, concentrated milk protein — made from the watery stuff that accumulates and rises to the surface of containers of cottage cheese and yogurt that you probably drain off. Studies have shown that beginning a meal with a whey protein drink helps get postmeal insulin secretion into action, which, in turn, helps reduce glucose spiking.

This effect was recently confirmed in a small international study that also pinpointed how whey protein does its magic. The study took fifteen people with type 2 diabetes, divided them into two groups, and fed them a sugary breakfast — with the difference being that one group drank 50 g (about three and a half tablespoons) of whey protein dissolved in water before eating breakfast, and the other group drank just plain water. Each group took a turn at drinking the whey protein on different days so that the effect could be gauged on every participant.

Results: When participants drank whey protein before breakfast, they accumulated an average 28 percent less blood glucose after the meal. And the whey had a strong and protective impact — insulin levels nearly doubled in whey drinkers within the first half hour after eating and remained high. This happened because, in the whey drinkers, an insulin-stimulating hormone called glucagon-like peptide-1 (GLP-1) didn't degrade as quickly as it normally would. The presence of additional GLP-1 gave insulin a better chance of doing its job.

Here's the kicker: The researchers pointed out that the effect of whey on glucose control and insulin secretion was better than what would be expected from using diabetes drugs such as glipizide, glyburide, and nateglinide.

Whereas the side effects of diabetes drugs

can include headaches, joint aches, nasal congestion, back pain, and flu-like symptoms, whey protein is well-tolerated in doses of up to 50 g per day.

Whey for You

Although 50 g per day taken before breakfast was looked at in the research study, how much daily whey protein do you need in an ordinary life setting to control blood sugar spiking? Naturopath Andrew L. Rubman, ND, founder and director of the Southbury Clinic for Traditional Medicines in Southbury, Connecticut, recommends using up to 800 mg per kilogram of body weight. That's a daily dosage of about 44 g for a 120-pound person, 54 g for a 150-pound person, and 91 g for a 250-pound person. These dosages refer to products that are whey isolate, not whey concentrate. Whey isolate provides more protein and significantly less lactose than whey concentrate, Dr. Rubman says.

The daily dosage should be adjusted so that you are taking the least amount you need to best control symptoms associated with blood sugar spiking — and this will differ from one person to another, says Dr. Rubman. People who have chronic kidney problems should seek medical supervision before supplementing their diets with any dose of whey protein.

Side effects of whey were not reported in the study, but high doses of more than 50 g per day, particularly of whey concentrate, can cause digestive troubles such as increased bowel movements, nausea, thirst, bloating, cramps, and lack of appetite, says Dr. Rubman. These effects are mostly caused by the lactose in whey products. Other possible side effects include tiredness and headache, low blood pressure, and low blood sugar. So everything in moderation if you decide to include a whey protein supplement in your diet.

Also, people with allergies to milk should avoid whey (it is milk protein, after all). It can also interfere with certain drugs, such as levodopa for Parkinson's disease, alendronate for osteoporosis, and quinolone antibiotics and tetracycline antibiotics such as doxycycline — so if you take any such drug, speak with your doctor or pharmacist for guidance on whether (and when) you can safely take whey protein and at what dosage.

Study titled "Incretin, Insulinotropic, and Glucose-Lowering Effects of Whey Protein Pre-Load in Type 2 Diabetics: A Randomized Clinical Trial," published in *Diabetologia*.

THE "NEW" SUPERFOOD:
PRUNES . . . YES, PRUNES

Prunes are amazingly good for us. They are nutrient-rich and inexpensive, they can satisfy a sweet tooth without the horrid effects of processed sugar, and they can even help you get going with a healthy, slimming diet. But there's a lot more to this simple, inexpensive superfood — yes, superfood — that could make you healthier and get you thinking about prunes in a whole new way.

A Magic Ingredient

"Prunes have a unique combination of nutrients that aren't found in other foods, not even other dried fruits," Maria Stacewicz-Sapuntzakis, PhD, says. She would know. She's been dedicated to research on the health benefits of prunes since 2000 and has authored two scholarly reviews on research done on them. Prunes are very high in a sugar alcohol called sorbitol, which is the key magic ingredient to the prune's health benefits, she says.

On its own, too much dietary sorbitol can cause gas and unwanted laxative effects, and 50 g or more a day is considered excessive. In fact, the FDA makes companies add warning labels about the laxative effect of sorbitol to food products that contain it. But you'd have to eat more than half a pound of prunes in one sitting to total 50 g — and if you do try that at home, you sure will be "sitting." Dr. Stacewicz-Sapuntzakis goes on to explain that five prunes contain a modest 7 g of sorbitol and that the sorbitol in prunes combines with other nutrients in the fruit to pump up its nutritional and health-enhancing powers.

According to Dr. Stacewicz-Sapuntzakis, two daily servings of prunes (that's ten to twelve) can help your body do the following:

- **Lose weight.** Despite the fact that they average twenty-five calories each, snacking on prunes can help you lose weight. Research recently reported at the European Congress on Obesity found that dieters who ate prunes lost more pounds and more inches and felt fuller longer than dieters who didn't eat them. The finding on satiety matched earlier research that found that eating prunes as a midmorning snack can help you eat less at lunchtime.

- **Regulate blood sugar.** Although prunes are sweet, they rate relatively low on the glycemic index scale, which measures how fast and how much a certain food raises blood sugar levels. This makes prunes a good food choice for folks with hyperglycemia or diabetes. Sorbitol itself has a low glycemic value, which may explain why something that tastes so much like candy keeps blood sugar levels on an even keel instead of making them spike.

- **Strengthen bones.** Prunes contain several nutrients, including boron, copper, vitamin K, and, as mentioned, potassium, that help prevent bone loss. Plus, sorbitol — that secret ingredient — increases absorption of calcium from prunes and other foods.
- **Prevent or slow arteriosclerosis.** Studies in animals and humans suggest that compounds in prunes can lower blood levels of cholesterol and thereby prevent or slow the progression of arteriosclerosis — or hardening of the arteries — caused by buildup of cholesterol and other debris on artery walls.
- **Prevent colon cancer.** The fiber, phenolic compounds (which are antioxidant substances found in fruits), and sorbitol help prunes move waste through the colon quickly enough to keep bile acid byproducts from injuring the lining of the colon, which can be cancer causing.

The Best Ways to Eat Prunes

Is drinking prune juice just as good as eating prunes? Dr. Stacewicz-Sapuntzakis recommends the latter. "If you eat the whole fruit, you get the benefits of all the great nutritional compounds in prunes. Some of these compounds become lost in prune juice," she says. But if you have never eaten prunes and now have an interest in adding them to your diet, start slowly with four or five a day, Dr. Stacewicz-Sapuntzakis recommends. Once you're sure that your body can tolerate them without an unwanted laxative effect, work up to ten to twelve each day. That racks up 240 calories, but you'll feel full longer than if you ate the same amount of calories in the form of, say, bread and cheese.

And prunes can be a lot more than wrinkled things you pluck from a box. Consider these tasty ways to enjoy them:

- **Homemade no-bake energy bars.** Place a handful of prunes in a food processor along with any combination of your favorite nuts and seeds, such as almonds, walnuts, and sesame, sunflower, or pumpkin seeds. You can add some shredded coconut too, maybe even sprinkle in some unsweetened cacao to sate a chocolate craving. Process the ingredients into a paste, and then press the mixture into a baking dish. Chill until firm, and cut into squares for a perfect on-the-go energy boost and healthy sweet-tooth satisfier.
- **Prunes in a blanket.** Wrap individual prunes in paper-thin slices of prosciutto — or do the same using turkey bacon if you prefer — then roast at 400°F until crisp on the outside, sweet and gooey inside. Bet you can't eat just one!
- **Spicy Moroccan-style stew.** Simmer prunes with lamb, beef, or chicken and aromatic Moroccan spices, such as ginger,

saffron, cinnamon, and pepper, to serve up a traditional Moroccan stew called tagine. Bon appétit and healthy eating with prunes!

Maria Stacewicz-Sapuntzakis, PhD, professor emerita, department of kinesiology and nutrition, University of Illinois at Chicago.

THE FRUIT THAT FIGHTS
HYPOGLYCEMIA

Hypoglycemia is a dangerous condition commonly associated with diabetes in which blood sugar levels fall below 70 mg/dL. It can happen periodically to some people with diabetes when the drugs used to treat the condition, such as insulin, work too well and cause an excessive drop in blood sugar.

Best food: Apricots. Seven to eight dried apricot halves provide 15 g of a fast-acting carbohydrate when you have a crash in blood sugar. Fresh apricots will also help, but the carbohydrates (sugars) aren't as concentrated. And dried apricots are easy to store and take with you.

What to do: Eat seven or eight dried apricot halves as soon as you notice the symptoms of hypoglycemia, such as fatigue, dizziness, sweating, and irritability.

Also helpful: Anything sugary, including a small amount of jelly beans. When your blood sugar is crashing, you need sugar immediately. Toby Smithson, RD, LDN, a nutritionist who has had diabetes for forty years, always carries jelly beans. They're even mentioned on the American Diabetes Association website.

Other sources of fast-acting sugars include honey and fruit juices.

David Grotto, RD, LDN, a registered dietitian and founder and president of Nutrition Housecall, LLC, a Chicago-based nutrition consulting firm that provides nutrition communications, lecturing, and consulting services, along with personalized, at-home dietary services. He is author of *The Best Things You Can Eat.*

How Full Fat Helps Diabetes

Surprise! According to a study from Harvard published in *Annals Internal Medicine,* people with the highest circulating levels of a type of fatty acid that is found only in whole-fat dairy are one-third as likely to get diabetes as those with the lowest circulating levels. Higher levels of the fatty acid — called trans-palmitoleic acid — were also associated with lower body mass index (BMI), smaller waist circumference, lower triglycerides (potentially harmful blood fats), higher levels of HDL "good" cholesterol, less insulin resistance, and lower levels of C-reactive protein, a marker for general inflammation.

How the study was done: At the study's start, researchers began with baseline measurements of glucose, insulin, inflammatory markers, circulating fatty acids, and blood lipids (such as triglycerides and cholesterol) from stored 1992 blood samples of 3,736 participants in the National Heart, Lung, and Blood Institute–funded Cardiovascular Health Study. Those data were compared with the same participants' dietary records and recorded health outcomes (including the incidence of diabetes) over the following ten years. During this period, 304 new cases of diabetes were recorded. When the participants were grouped according to their circulating levels of trans-palmitoleic acid, the researchers discovered that those with higher levels had the lowest rates of diabetes.

How Much Dairy?

While other studies have suggested a similar phenomenon with dairy consumption, this is the first to have used objective chemical markers in the blood to determine the relationship between this specific fatty acid and the onset of diabetes. The participants with the highest levels averaged about two servings of whole-fat dairy foods a day.

This is not a license to indulge yourself in a daily serving of strawberry shortcake with extra whipped cream or a giant ice cream from Cold Stone Creamery, but you might want to consider switching from skim milk to whole milk with your morning cereal and selecting full-fat yogurt over low-fat or nonfat. The difference in calories isn't great — and you may be getting some real metabolic and cardio-vascular benefits.

Dariush Mozaffarian, MD, DrPH, associate professor, division of cardiovascular medicine, Brigham and Women's Hospital and Harvard Medical School, department of epidemiology, Harvard School of Public Health, Boston.

BETTER THAN MEAT! HERE ARE OTHER PROTEINS YOU SHOULD TRY

When it comes to getting enough muscle-building protein, most people do just fine by having a juicy steak, a generous chicken breast, or a tasty fish fillet a few times a week.

The problem is, most Americans need to get more protein from other foods and a little less from animals, since research suggests a more plant-based diet decreases risk for diabetes, as well as other chronic health problems like heart disease and obesity. Balancing animal protein with protein from plants and other foods is one of the simplest ways to improve your diet. Of course, you don't have to be a vegetarian or vegan to enjoy meat-free protein foods.*

For Breakfast

If you want protein in the morning, here are alternatives to eggs and sausage:

• **Quinoa.** Often used as a dinner side dish, quinoa can also be eaten as a great nutty-tasting grain for breakfast. Technically a seed, quinoa has 8 g of protein per cooked

---

* Adults over age nineteen should consume 0.37 g of protein per pound of body weight, according to the Institute of Medicine (IOM). Example: If you weigh 150 pounds, you need about 55 g of protein daily.

cup. It's also naturally gluten-free.

For a great protein-packed breakfast: Have a bowl of quinoa with chopped fruit and nuts, or top it with sautéed spinach and a poached egg.

- **Cottage cheese.** It is not a plant-based food, but it's an excellent source of protein. In fact, you may be surprised to find out that a half cup of 1 percent milk fat cottage cheese contains more than twice as much protein (14 g) as an egg.

  Caution: Most cottage cheese is high in sodium, so be sure to stick to the low-sodium variety if you are on a low-sodium diet.

  Not a fan of curds? Puree it. Make "whipped cottage cheese" in your blender, and flavor it with cinnamon for a delicious spread to smear on apple slices, or add chives and basil for a veggie dip.

For Lunch or Dinner

Want a quick and easy protein for lunch or dinner? Tofu or beans are excellent choices, but you may want to try something new. Here's what I suggest:

- **Split peas.** Dried peas have four times more protein than brown rice — and four times more fiber. If you don't want to cook your own split pea soup, certain prepared varieties are worth trying.

- **Spinach.** Most people don't realize that cooked spinach — at 4 g per half cup — offers more protein than most other vegetables. It also contains antioxidant vitamins A, C, and E and is a rich plant source of iron and calcium.

  To get a lot of spinach, buy it frozen. Since frozen spinach is precooked, it's easier to eat more than if you are downing it raw in, say, a salad. Toss it into soups, pasta sauce, bean burritos, or lasagna. Frozen spinach is picked at peak season before freezing, so it retains its nutrients for months. And it's a great value!

Dawn Jackson Blatner, RD, a registered dietitian in private practice in Chicago. She is author of *The Flexitarian Diet: The Mostly Vegetarian Way to Lose Weight, Be Healthier, Prevent Disease, and Add Years to Your Life* and the nutrition consultant for the Chicago Cubs. As a flexitarian expert, she gets most of her protein from plants. DawnJacksonBlatner.com.

BEYOND BROCCOLI: HEALTHY (WEIRD) FOODS THAT CAN STOP DIABETES AND MORE

Have you ever heard of bilberry? Enoki? What about noni or goji berry? When it comes to being loaded with nutrients and healthful phytochemicals, these unheard-of foods stand side-by-side with the likes of blueberries and broccoli. Here's a list of seven unfamiliar foods that are worth knowing about:

Bilberry

Bilberries are high in phytochemicals, including a class of compounds known as anthocyanins. A 2010 laboratory study published in *Journal of Medicinal Foods* found that bilberry extract inhibited the growth of breast cancer cells. The berries may also improve blood glucose levels, helping to prevent diabetes. During World War II, British pilots who ate bilberries before evening bombing raids noticed improvements in their night vision. Some compounds in bilberries may help prevent macular degeneration, a common cause of blindness.

Helpful: You can substitute fresh bilberries for blueberries. Or look for bilberry juice. It won't provide the fiber that you would get from fresh berries, but it still has the phytochemicals. Bilberries are available online and in health-food stores.

Trout

Salmon gets all the publicity, but like salmon, trout is a fatty fish with large amounts of omega-3 fatty acids. These good fats have been linked to a reduced risk for heart disease, rheumatoid arthritis, dementia, and other chronic conditions. In 2009, scientists discovered that a peptide (short strands of amino acids) in trout reduced both cholesterol and triglycerides in rats. It may do the same in humans. Trout is also high in vitamins B-6 and B-12, selenium, thiamine, and riboflavin.

Helpful: Trout is just as easy to prepare as salmon, because the fat keeps it tender, making it less likely to suffer from overcooking than a leaner fish.

One delicious recipe: Combine the juice of three lemons (about six tablespoons of bottled lemon juice) with three tablespoons of olive oil, one-quarter cup of chopped parsley, and ground pepper to taste. Dip trout fillets in the mixture, place them on a baking sheet, and bake at 400°F for about fifteen minutes.

Bitter Melon

Also known as goya, bitter melon is a fruit that is often combined with pork or other meats and used in stir-fries in Asian restaurants. Many people love it, but its bitter taste takes some getting used to. The payoff is worth it. A report in *Nutrition Review* noted that a diet high in bitter melon (three or more servings per week) helps reduce insulin resistance, a condition that can progress to type 2 diabetes. Also, bitter melon is high in antiviral compounds, which can keep you healthier in cold and flu season. And bitter melon is among the best sources of vitamin C, with about 60 mg in a one-cup serving, about the same amount as in one orange. It is available in Asian grocery stores.

Helpful: The bitterness can be tempered by adding sweetness to a recipe. For example, you could add dried cranberries or one tablespoon of apricot jam to a bitter melon stir-fry.

Jicama

This crunchy, juicy vegetable (the *j* is pronounced like an *h*) is as popular throughout Mexico and Central and South America as iceberg lettuce is in the United States. In 2002, researchers in Thailand identified antiviral activity in jicama. It is rich in vitamin C and potassium and also high in fiber, with 5.9 g supplying 24 percent of the recommended daily amount.

Helpful: Jicama is usually eaten raw — it's the best way to preserve the vitamin C content. You can add slices or cubes to a garden salad or serve it alone, drizzled with lime juice (and chili powder if you like), as a tangy counterpoint to richer dishes.

Enoki

Unlike the standard white button mushrooms sold in every American supermarket, enoki mushrooms have long, threadlike stalks, each topped by a delicate white dome. A Singapore-based study found that enoki contains a protein that boosts immune function. It's also a powerful antioxidant that can suppress free radicals, important for reducing inflammation in arteries, joints, and other parts of the body.

Helpful: The mushrooms have a mild, almost fruity taste. In Japan, they're added to miso soup. Or you can eat them raw, sprinkled on salads or in side dishes. They are available in Asian grocery and specialty stores.

Noni

This is not a fruit that you want to take a bite out of — in its unadulterated form, it has a singularly nasty taste. (Its nickname is "vomit fruit.") It's usually juiced and then combined with other fruit juices. After it's blended, it adds a sharp but not unpleasant taste, similar to the taste of unripened pomegranate. Noni is rich in many phytochemicals, including some with potent antioxidant effects. A 2010 animal study found that noni may help to lower blood pressure. It also appears to inhibit the growth of melanoma, a deadly form of skin cancer.

Helpful: In health-food stores, look for a product that is 100 percent pure noni juice. Then mix one to two ounces of noni juice with other fruit juices, such as apple or pear juice. Experiment to determine what tastes best to you.

Goji Berry

Dried goji berries are popular in Australia and Asia, where they are enjoyed as a slightly tangy-sweet snack. Goji can also be used to make juice or a fruity spread. Gojis are high in antioxidants. In a 2009 study published in *Nutrition Research,* participants who drank four ounces of goji juice daily for thirty days had significantly reduced free radical activity in the blood. The berries are also thought to help protect against diabetes and atherosclerosis. And they're high in fiber, with 3 g in one-quarter cup. They are available online and in some health-food stores.

Helpful: Munch them as a snack, or add them to muffins or other baked goods.

Caution: If you're taking a blood-thinning medication such as warfarin, talk to your doctor before eating goji berries. They may change the drug's effects.

Unless otherwise noted, these foods are available at most supermarkets.

Tonia Reinhard, RD, a registered dietitian, professor at Wayne State University in Detroit, and author of *Superfoods: The Healthiest Foods on the Planet.*

CALLING ALL CARNIVORES:
YOU CAN BECOME A VEGGIE LOVER

Let's say you are given the choice of a thick, juicy steak for dinner or a heaping plate of yellow squash, spinach, and other brightly colored vegetables. What will it be?

If you're a hard-core meat eater, there's no contest. But if you don't like vegetables, the sad truth is that you are depriving yourself of proven health-promoting nutrients that help fight everything from heart disease to cancer.

Surprising: Even though nutritionists recommend that we eat three to five servings of vegetables each day, only 21 percent of men are meeting that goal. And the average woman isn't doing much better — just 31 percent consume that many veggies in their daily diets, and that's largely because women tend to eat more salads (mostly lettuce) than men do.

Why don't we eat more vegetables? Americans have traditionally been big meat eaters with vegetables thrown in only as side dishes. And some people just don't like the taste of vegetables. Fortunately, there's a way to conquer one's aversion to veggies — and gain the amazing nutritional benefits of these foods.

A Taste Explosion!

It's old news that boiling vegetables is not the way to go — too often, you end up with veggies that are limp, mushy, and relatively tasteless.

What's a better choice? Steaming brings out the natural flavor of fresh vegetables and gives them the kind of crunch and texture that greatly increases their mouth appeal.

But there's an even better alternative that gives vegetables the meaty texture that meat lovers crave. And by choosing ingredients carefully, you can also make the veggies more aromatic and flavorful. Try these ideas to make veggies more appealing.

Roasting or Grilling

If you roast or grill your veggies, their natural sugars will caramelize, which kicks up the flavor. For roasting, in particular, it helps to toss them in an aromatic oil such as pumpkin oil (this oil provides a hearty, full flavor that appeals to most meat lovers).

Good choices for roasting or grilling: Carrots, leeks, onions, butternut squash, potatoes (whole or wedged), peppers (sweet and hot), turnips and other root vegetables, and tomatoes, eggplant, and other vine-grown veggies.

What to do: Mix two cups of coarsely chopped veggie chunks with one tablespoon of cooking oil, such as pumpkin oil. You can place veggies on cookie sheets or racks lined with aluminum foil for easy cleanup. For root vegetables, roast at 400°F for about forty to forty-five minutes, stirring at the halfway point. For the last five to ten minutes, you can add more fragile vegetables, such as thin asparagus or cherry tomatoes.

If grilling, use a veggie grill basket or wrap vegetables in foil packets. Start with four to five minutes of direct heat. Add another four to five minutes if needed.

Spice It Up!

Herbs (preferably fresh to provide maximum flavor) and spices are great ways to not only make vegetables taste delicious but also add even more disease-fighting nutrients.

Flavorful, health-promoting herbs: Rosemary, sage, tarragon, and basil.

Best spices to try: Cinnamon, cumin, and peppercorns.

For the die-hard meat lover, you can also add a saucy, bold flavor to your veggies by using condiments that are commonly associated with meat — for example, try some Worcestershire sauce on mushrooms such as baby portabellas.

Other good condiments: Horseradish, Pickapeppa sauce, or any hot sauce of choice.

Where to Shop

One of the best ways to boost your veggie quota is to shop at local food co-ops, farmers' markets, or pick-your-own farms for a wide selection of in-season locally grown vegetables and fruit.

Resource: To find a farmers' market near you, check the USDA's website at www.usdalocalfooddirectories.com.

Irresistible Quesadillas

Black bean quesadillas are a great way to slip in veggies.

What to do: Spread refried black beans (or canned black beans that have been rinsed and drained) on a whole-wheat tortilla. Cover with onion and/or green/red bell peppers, salsa, and shredded cheddar cheese, and top with another tortilla. Heat flat in a skillet until hot, turn over, and heat again until the cheese has melted. Cut into wedges, and serve with guacamole.

Helpful: Add a little chili powder or cumin to the beans to perk up the flavor!

Susan Mitchell, PhD, RD, a registered dietitian and licensed nutritionist based in Winter Park, Florida. The coauthor of three books, including *Fat Is Not Your Fate,* she speaks nationally on nutrition, health, and wellness issues. She also hosts the podcast "Straight Talk About Eating Smart" at www.GrowingBolder.com.

MAGNESIUM-RICH FOODS PROTECT AGAINST TYPE 2 DIABETES

When researchers studied 4,497 healthy adults' diets for twenty years, those who consumed the most magnesium (about 200 mg per one thousand calories) were 47 percent less likely to develop diabetes than those who consumed the least (about 100 mg per one thousand calories).

Theory: Magnesium enhances enzymes that help the body process blood sugar.

Self-defense: Eat more magnesium-rich whole grains, nuts, legumes, and green leafy vegetables to reach the recommended dietary allowance of 320 mg for women and 420 mg for men.

Examples: One-quarter cup of wheat bran contains 89 mg of magnesium; one ounce of dry-roasted almonds contains 80 mg; one-half cup of cooked frozen spinach, 78 mg; one ounce of dry-roasted cashews, 74 mg; three-quarters cup of bran flakes cereal, 64 mg; one cup of instant fortified oatmeal, prepared with water, 61 mg.

Ka He, MD, chair and professor, epidemiology and biostatistics, Indiana University, Bloomington. Environmental Nutrition. EnvironmentalNutrition.com.

How to Juice for Healing Power

Juice has gotten a bad rap. We're often advised to eat whole fruits and vegetables — for the fiber and because they are lower in calories than an equal amount of juice. But for the many Americans who don't eat the recommended three to five servings of vegetables and two to three servings of fruit daily, juice can be a lifesaver — literally. Juice is loaded with nutrients that protect against heart disease, cancer, diabetes, arthritis, Alzheimer's, and other chronic conditions.

We can pack in a day's worth of fruits and vegetables in just twelve to sixteen ounces of juice. How to do it right:

- **Opt for fresh juice, not packaged.** Packaged juices, whether in a can, bottle, carton, or frozen, are lower in nutrients. And packaged juices have been pasteurized, which destroys health-giving compounds.

  Example: Fresh apple juice contains ellagic acid, an anticancer nutrient that shields chromosomes from damage and blocks the tumor-causing action of many pollutants. In contrast, commercial apple juice contains almost no ellagic acid.

- **Use a quality juicer.** If you juice once or twice a week, try a high-speed centrifugal juicer. They're relatively inexpensive, starting at one hundred dollars or so. (Examples: Juice Fountain Duo or Juice Fountain Elite, both from Breville.)

- **If you juice more frequently,** consider investing in a "slow juicer" (three hundred dollars and up) that typically operates at 80 revolutions per minute (RPM), compared with the 1,000 to 24,000 RPM of a centrifugal model. (I use the Hurom Juicer.) A slow juicer expels significantly more juice and better preserves delicate nutrients. And because the damaged compounds produced by a centrifugal juicer taste a little bitter, a slow juicer provides better-tasting juice.

  Follow this basic juice recipe: Use four unpeeled carrots and two unpeeled, cored apples cut into wedges as a base for creating other juice blends by adding such things as a handful of kale, spinach, radishes, and/or beets. Ideally, use organic fruits and vegetables. If not, be sure to wash them thoroughly.

- **Keep blood sugar balanced.** Fruit and vegetable juices can deliver too much natural sugar, spiking blood sugar levels, a risk factor for diabetes.

  What you need to know: The metabolic impact of the sugar in a particular food can be measured using the glycemic index (GI) — how quickly a carbohydrate turns into glucose (blood sugar). But a more accurate way to measure this impact is with the glycemic load (GL) — a relatively new calculation that uses the GI but also takes into account the amount of carbohydrate in a specific food. Beets, for example, have a high GI but a low GL. Charts providing the GI and the GL are available on the internet. I like those at www.mendosa.com.

Bottom line: Limit the intake of higher-GL juices such as orange, cherry, pineapple, and mango. You can use them to add flavor to lower-GL choices such as kale, spinach, celery, and beets.

Michael T. Murray, ND, a naturopathic physician and leading authority on natural medicine. He is author of *The Complete Book of Juicing: Your Delicious Guide to Youthful Vitality.* DoctorMurray.com.

FIVE CUPS OF COFFEE A DAY CAN BE GOOD FOR YOU!

Even coffee drinkers find it hard to believe that their favorite pick-me-up is healthful, but it seems to be true. People who drink coffee regularly are less likely to have a stroke or get diabetes or Parkinson's disease than those who don't drink it. There's even some evidence that coffee can help prevent cancer, although the link between coffee and various cancers is preliminary and still being investigated.

For Lower Diabetes Risk

More than twenty studies have found that coffee drinkers are less likely to get diabetes than those who don't drink coffee. When we analyzed the data from nine previous studies, which included a total of more than 193,000 people, we found that those who drank more than six or seven cups of coffee daily were 35 percent less likely to have type 2 diabetes (the most common form) than those who drank two cups or less. Those who consumed four to six cups daily had a 28 percent lower risk for diabetes.

Some of the studies were conducted in Europe, where people who drink a lot of coffee — up to ten cups daily — are the ones least likely to have diabetes.

Both decaf and regular coffee seem to be protective against diabetes. This suggests that the antioxidants in coffee — not the caffeine — are the active agents. It's possible that these compounds protect insulin-producing cells in the pancreas. The minerals in coffee, such as chromium and magnesium, have been shown to improve insulin sensitivity.

Caution

Some caveats about coffee:

- **Moderation matters.** Some people get the jitters or have insomnia when they drink coffee. In rare cases, the caffeine causes a dramatic rise in blood pressure. It's fine for most people to have three, four, or five cups of coffee a day — or even more. But pay attention to how you feel. If you get jittery or anxious when you drink a certain amount, cut back. Or drink decaf some of the time.
- **Hold the milk and sugar.** Some of the coffee beverages at Starbucks and other coffee shops have more calories than a sweet dessert. Coffee may be good for you, but limit the add-ons.
- **Use a paper filter.** Boiled coffee, coffee made with a French press, or coffee that drips through a metal filter has high levels of oils that can significantly raise levels of LDL, the dangerous form of cholesterol.

  Better: A drip machine that uses a paper filter. It traps the oils and eliminates this risk.

Frank B. Hu, MD, PhD, an epidemiologist, nutritional specialist, and professor of medicine at Harvard Medical School and the Harvard School of Public Health, both in Boston. He is codirector of Harvard's Program in Obesity Epidemiology and Prevention.

GREEN TEA FIGHTS DIABETES

Green tea has remarkable powers to combat disease. I think we all should include green tea in our daily health regimen.

The leaves of the evergreen shrub *Camellia sinensis* are used to make green, black, and oolong tea — but green tea contains the most epigallocatechin gallate (EGCG). EGCG (a type of plant compound called a polyphenol, flavonoid, or catechin) is a powerful anti-inflammatory and antioxidant. Research shows that chronic low-grade inflammation (produced by an immune system in over-drive) and oxidation (a kind of internal rust that damages cells) are the two processes that trigger and advance most chronic diseases. Evidence shows that green tea can prevent and treat many of these diseases.

Type 2 Diabetes

Type 2 diabetes is a major risk factor for cardiovascular disease and can lead to many other disastrous health problems, including kidney failure, blindness, and lower-limb amputation.

In a study of sixty people with diabetes, those who took a daily supplement of green tea extract for two months significantly reduced hemoglobin A1C — a biomarker of blood sugar levels.

How it works: People with diabetes who drank green tea for twelve weeks boosted their levels of insulin (the hormone that helps move sugar out of the blood and into muscle cells) — and decreased their levels of A1C.

The Right Amount

To guarantee a sufficient intake of EGCG, I recommend one or more of the following strategies. You can safely do all three.

- **Drink green tea.** Five to ten eight-ounce cups a day of regular or decaf.
  Best: For maximum intake of EGCG, use whole-leaf loose tea rather than a teabag, using one teaspoon per cup. Steep the tea for at least five minutes.
- **Take a supplement of green tea extract.**
  Minimum: 400 mg a day of a supplement standardized to 90 percent EGCG.
- **Add a drop of green tea liquid extract to green tea or another beverage.** Look for a product that is standardized to a high level (at least 50 percent) of EGCG, and follow the dosage recommendation on the label.
  Example: HerbaGreen from HerbaSway, at 90 percent polyphenols, 50 percent from EGCG.

Safe Use

Talk to your doctor if you use:
- **An antiplatelet drug (blood thinner),** such as warfarin, because green tea also

thins the blood.

- **A bronchodilator for asthma or chronic obstructive pulmonary disease,** because green tea can increase its potency.
- **An antacid,** because green tea can decrease the effect.

Patrick M. Fratellone, MD, executive medical director of Fratellone Medical Associates in New York City, attending physician at St. Luke's Hospital, Roosevelt Hospital, and Beth Israel Hospital in New York City, former chief of medicine and director of cardiology at Atkins Center for Complementary Medicine, and coauthor of a comprehensive review article on the health benefits of green tea in *Explore.* FratelloneMedical .com.

GOOD NEWS! EVEN MORE HEALTH BENEFITS FROM DARK CHOCOLATE

About twenty-nine million Americans, including one in four people over the age of sixty-five, have diabetes or chronically high blood sugar — a disease that raises the risk of dying from heart disease by 70 percent. Long-term complications can include kidney failure and blindness. Studies show that chocolate can prevent diabetes and help prevent complications in those who have the disease.

In a recent study of nearly eight thousand people published in *Clinical Nutrition,* those who ate one ounce of chocolate two to six times weekly had a 34 percent lower risk of being diagnosed with diabetes than people who ate chocolate less than once a month.

Prevention of diabetic complications: In a study of ninety-three postmenopausal women with type 2 diabetes published in *Diabetes Care,* those women who ate flavanol-rich chocolate every day for one year not only had better blood sugar control, they also had an eleven times lower risk of developing heart disease, compared with women who ate low-flavanol chocolate.

More research: Cellular and animal studies show that cocoa flavanols can protect the insulin-producing beta cells of the pancreas (insulin is the hormone that ushers blood sugar out of the bloodstream and into cells), the kidneys (diabetes is the cause of nearly half of all cases of kidney failure), and the retina (nearly 30 percent of people with diabetes have diabetic retinopathy, a cause of vision loss and blindness).

Which Chocolate Is Best?

Nearly every client in my health-coaching practice gets a recommendation to consume a daily dose of about 400 mg of cocoa flavanols — the amount used in many of the studies that show a therapeutic effect.

Important: Higher doses don't produce better results.

And the healthiest way to get those flavanols is with unsweetened cocoa powder that delivers all the flavanols of dark chocolate without burdening your daily diet with extra calories and sugar. Using cocoa powder also helps you control your intake — it's notoriously easy to consume an entire three-ounce bar of chocolate even though your optimal daily "dose" is only one ounce.

Red flag: Do not use "Dutch" cocoa powder, which is treated with an alkalizing agent for a richer color and milder taste — a process that strips cocoa of 98 percent of its epicatechin.

My advice: Mix one tablespoon of unsweetened cocoa powder in an eight-to-twelve-ounce mug of hot water or milk (nondairy milks such as coconut, almond, soy, and rice milk are delicious alternatives) and add a no-calorie natural sweetener, such as stevia.

Good products: I recommend Cocoa Via, the powder developed by Mars, Incorporated. The Mars Center for Cocoa Health Science has conducted extensive scientific research on cocoa flavanols for two decades, and one stick of its powder reliably delivers 375 mg of cocoa flavanols, standardized for epicatechin. You can mix it with cold or warm milk, coffee drinks, smoothies, yogurt, or oatmeal. Another high-quality cocoa powder is Cocoa Well from Reserveage.

Dark chocolate bars don't reliably deliver a therapeutic dose of cocoa flavanols. But if you prefer to eat dark chocolate, look for a bar with 70 percent or more cocoa, and consume about one ounce (28 g) per day. According to a report from www.Consumer Lab.com, dark chocolate brands with high levels of flavanols (about one-quarter to one-half the amount in the best brands of cocoa powder) include Endangered Species, Ghirardelli, and Lindt.

Bill Gottlieb, CHC, founder and president of Good For You Health Coaching. He is author of *HealthDefense: How to Stay Vibrantly Healthy in a Toxic World* and *The Every-Other-Day Diet: The Diet That Lets You Eat All You Want (Half the Time) and Keep the Weight Off,* with Krista Varady, PhD. BillGottliebHealth.com.

Spirulina Slows Aging and Prevents Chronic Disease

When you think of a superfood, you probably think of salmon or blueberries — not the algae that floats on the surfaces of lakes, ponds, and reservoirs.

But there's a type of blue-green algae that has been used for food and medicine in developing countries for centuries, that NASA has recommended as an ideal food for long-term space missions, that is loaded with health-giving nutrients, and that might be a key component in a diet aimed at staying healthy, reversing chronic disease, and slowing the aging process.

That Algae Is Spirulina

Spirulina grows mainly in subtropical and tropical countries, where there is year-round heat and sunlight. It is high in protein (up to 70 percent), rich in antioxidants, and loaded with vitamins and minerals, particularly iron and vitamin B-12. And it has no cellulose — the cell wall of green plants — so its nutrients are easy for the body to digest and absorb.

Green Medicine

Dried into a powder, spirulina can be added to food or taken as a tablet or capsule. And ingested regularly, spirulina can do you a lot of good. Scientific research shows there are many health problems that spirulina might help prevent or treat:

- **Anemia.** Researchers from the University of California at Davis studied forty people age fifty and older who had been diagnosed with anemia (iron deficiency), giving them a spirulina supplement every day for three months. The study participants had a steady rise in levels of hemoglobin, the iron-carrying component of red blood cells, along with several other factors that indicated increased levels of iron.
- **Weakened immunity.** In the UC Davis study mentioned above, most of the participants ages sixty-one to seventy also had increases in infection-fighting white blood cells and in an enzyme that is a marker for increased immune activity, in effect, reversing immunosenescence, the age-related weakening of the immune system. Immunosenescence is linked not only to a higher risk for infectious diseases such as the flu, but also to chronic diseases with an inflammatory component, such as heart disease, Alzheimer's, and cancer.
- **Allergies.** Spirulina has anti-inflammatory properties and can prevent the release of histamine and other inflammatory factors that trigger and worsen allergic symptoms. Studies also show that spirulina can boost levels of IgA, an antibody that defends against allergic reactions. In one study,

people with allergies who took spirulina had less nasal discharge, sneezing, nasal congestion, and itching.

- **Cataracts and age-related macular degeneration.** Taking spirulina can double blood levels of zeaxanthin, an antioxidant linked to a reduced risk for cataracts and age-related macular degeneration, reported researchers in *BMJ.*
- **Diabetes.** In several studies, researchers found that adding spirulina to the diets of people with type 2 diabetes significantly decreased blood sugar levels.

  Caution: Spirulina has not been approved by the FDA for treating diabetes, so consult your doctor before taking it.
- **Lack of endurance.** In a small study, men who took spirulina for one month were able to run more than 30 percent longer on a treadmill before having to stop because of fatigue, reported Greek researchers in *Medicine & Science in Sports & Exercise.*
- **Heart disease.** Nearly a dozen studies have looked at the effect of spirulina intake on risk factors for heart disease, both in healthy people and people with heart disease. Most of the studies found significant decreases in negative factors (such as LDL "bad" cholesterol, total cholesterol, triglycerides, apolipoprotein B, and blood pressure) and increases in positive factors (such

as HDL "good" cholesterol and apolipoprotein A1).

Ideal Dose

A preventive daily dose of spirulina is one
teaspoon. A therapeutic dose, to control or
reverse disease, is about one tablespoon.

Spirulina has been on the market for more
than a decade, and it's among the substances
listed by the FDA as "Generally Recognized
as Safe" (GRAS).

Caution: If you have an autoimmune disease, such as multiple sclerosis, rheumatoid
arthritis, or lupus, talk to your doctor. Spirulina could stimulate the immune system,
making the condition worse.

Best Products

Like many products, the quality of spirulina
varies. Look for the following:

- **Clean taste.** Top-quality spirulina tastes
  fresh. If spirulina tastes fishy or "swampy"
  or has a lingering aftertaste, it's probably
  not a good product.
- **Bright color.** Spirulina should have a
  vibrant, bright blue-green appearance
  (more green than blue). If spirulina is olive-
  green, it's probably inferior.
- **Cost.** You get what you pay for — and good
  spirulina can be somewhat pricey.

Example: Spirulina Pacifica, from Nutrex Hawaii — grown on the Kona coast of Hawaii since 1984 and regarded by many health experts as one of the most nutritious and purest spirulina products on the market — costs fifty dollars for 360 1,000-mg tablets. Store it in the refrigerator.

- **Growing location.** The best spirulina is grown in clean water in a nonindustrialized setting, as far away as possible from an urban, polluted environment. If you can, find out the growing location of the product you're considering buying.

How to Add It to Food

There are many ways to include spirulina in your daily diet, including the following:

- **Put it in smoothies.** Add between one teaspoon and one tablespoon to any smoothie or shake.
- **Add to juice.** Add one teaspoon or tablespoon to an eight-ounce glass of juice or water, shake it up, and drink it.
- **Sprinkle it on food.** Try spirulina popcorn, for instance — a great conversation starter at a potluck. To a bowl of popcorn, add one to two tablespoons of spirulina powder, three to four tablespoons of grated Parmesan cheese, two or three tablespoons of olive oil, one-half teaspoon of salt, and one-eighth teaspoon of cayenne pepper.

- **Add it to condiments.** Put one-quarter teaspoon in a small jar of ketchup, barbecue sauce, mustard, or salad dressing. This way, you'll get a little each time you use these products.

Jennifer Adler, MS, CN, a certified nutritionist, natural foods chef, and adjunct faculty member at Bastyr University, Kenmore, Washington. She is the founder and owner of Passionate Nutrition, a nutrition practice with offices throughout the Northwest, and cofounder of the International Eating Disorders Institute. PassionateNutrition.com.

4
DELICIOUS DIABETES-FRIENDLY RECIPES

Living with diabetes doesn't mean you have to sacrifice taste. True, there are some challenges when eating healthy, but all are easily overcome with a bit of creativity. You might even find that your favorite luxuries are still on the menu!

There are some basic principles and facts to remember as you plan your cooking. Diabetics who eat small, consistent amounts of carbohydrates with every meal or snack have better control of their blood sugar levels and body weight. However, a woman who has prediabetes or diabetes should moderate carb intake to about 45 g per meal, and men should have no more than about 60 g per meal, according to the American Diabetes Association. (A health-care provider can help adjust amounts based on your individual needs and age.) As a rule, stay away from anything excessive!

Fiber — especially the soluble kind — can also be a secret weapon! It takes longer to metabolize than other carbs, so it improves blood sugar control and lowers insulin resistance in both people who have diabetes and those who don't. Consistently getting the right amount of fiber can even lessen (or in some instances, eliminate) the need for diabetes medication. The American Diabetes Association recommends that women consume at least 25 g of fiber per day; men should get a minimum of 38 g daily. Reap the health benefits above by eating foods naturally high in fiber — whole grains, beans, fruits, and vegetables. Aim for eight servings a day of fruits and veggies, with a heavier focus on your vegetables. While fruit is indeed a great source of fiber and nutrients, it is also high in sugar, even if it is naturally occurring.

Finally, don't forget healthy fats. Replacing saturated fats and trans fats with monounsaturated fatty acids (MUFAs), such as olive oil, canola oil, peanut oil, nuts, nut butters, and avocado, helps lower total and LDL "bad" cholesterol levels, improves the function of blood vessels, and benefits insulin levels and blood sugar control.

The following are recipes packed full of flavor, but also approved by Bottom Line experts for those trying to prevent or better manage diabetes. They should give you a solid jumping-off point on your way to eating deliciously (and consciously).

SUPER VEGETABLE SOUP

This soup is bursting with nutrients from all of the vegetables.

- 12 ounces low-sodium vegetable stock
- 1/4 cup chopped carrots
- 1/4 cup chopped leeks
- 1/4 cup chopped zucchini
- 1/4 cup chopped shredded cabbage
- 1 (14-ounce) can cannellini beans, drained and rinsed

1. Combine all ingredients and simmer 10 minutes. Serve chunky or puréed.

Source: Lisa R. Young, PhD, RD, adjunct professor of nutrition at New York University and a registered dietitian in private practice, both in New York City. She is the author of *The Portion Teller Plan*. PortionTeller.com.

MINESTRONE WITH FRENCH LENTILS

Generally speaking, the more intense the color, the richer the antioxidant content of a vegetable, fruit, or legume, which is why this recipe features ingredients such as squash, green lentils, and escarole. Exceptions: Onions and garlic, although white, provide high levels of antioxidant flavonoids.

- 1/4 cup olive oil
- 3 garlic cloves, sliced thin or chopped fine

261

- 1 medium yellow onion, diced
- 1 cup French green lentils
- 2 celery stalks, cut into 1/2-inch pieces
- 8 cups low-sodium chicken or vegetable stock
- 1 (28-ounce) can chopped tomatoes
- 2 small yellow squash, diced
- 1/4 pound trimmed green beans, cut into 1/2-inch pieces
- 4 cups escarole (cut leaves across in 1-inch strips)
- 2 medium zucchini, diced
- Salt and pepper to taste

1. In a large soup pot, heat the olive oil on a medium setting. Put in garlic, onion, lentils, and celery, and stir. Add stock and tomatoes, and simmer for 40 minutes. Then place squash, green beans, escarole, and zucchini in the pot. Season with salt and pepper, and return to a boil. Lower heat, and simmer for 10 minutes.
Serves six to eight.

Source: Patti Tveit Milligan, RD, CNS, a natural foods nutritionist and a registered dietitian in Fountain Hills, Arizona, and Gregory Anne Cox, a chef in Hampton Bays, New York.

RED LENTIL AND APRICOT SOUP

Lentils are loaded with nutrients and come in a variety of colors, tastes, and textures. They cook faster than other legumes and don't need to be soaked. They are great either as the main ingredient in soups and salads or combined with other foods in vegetarian or meat dishes.

Like beans, their legume cousins, lentils pack a nutritional punch. One-half cup of cooked lentils has about 9 g of protein and 8 to 10 g of fiber. They are also a good source of folate, iron, manganese, and phosphorus. Lentils contain valuable antioxidant phytonutrients, particularly catechins and proanthocyanidins.

Fiber-rich and cholesterol-free, lentils slow the absorption of sugars into the bloodstream and help prevent type 2 diabetes. They protect the heart by reducing blood lipid levels. Their high fiber content helps you feel full, making it easier to practice portion control and watch calories.

- 1 cup dried red lentils
- 1 cup finely chopped onion
- 1 cup canned diced tomatoes
- 1/2 cup chopped Turkish dried apricots
- 2 teaspoons grated fresh ginger
- 1 garlic clove, finely chopped
- 1/2 teaspoon ground cumin
- 1/2 teaspoon ground turmeric
- 1/4 teaspoon ground cinnamon
- 1/8 teaspoon ground black pepper

- 1/2 cup cilantro leaves, chopped
- 4 tablespoons pomegranate juice

1. Place the lentils in a mixing bowl. Fill the bowl with cool water, covering the lentils by two inches. Using your hand, swish the lentils until the water is cloudy. Carefully pour out the water. Repeat this two to three times, until the water stays almost clear. The lentils will be stuck together in a lump after the last draining. Push them into a large, deep saucepan.
2. Add to the pot the onions, tomatoes, apricots, ginger, garlic, cumin, turmeric, cinnamon, and pepper. Add four cups water. Bring the liquid to a boil, then reduce the heat and simmer the soup, covered, until the lentils are soft, about 30 minutes. Turn off the heat, mix in the cilantro, and season the soup to taste with salt.
3. To serve, divide the soup among four deep soup bowls. Drizzle one-fourth of the pomegranate juice in a swirl in the center of each bowl. Serve immediately.
Serves four.

Source: Dana Jacobi, a New York City–based recipe developer and cookbook author. Her cookbooks include *The Essential Best Foods Cookbook* and *12 Best Foods Cookbook*. DanasMarketBasket.com.

HERBED CHICKEN BREAST

Because diabetics are at a greater risk for life-threatening complications such as hypertension, heart disease, and stroke, it's particularly important that they keep blood glucose in control while maintaining normal levels of blood pressure and blood lipids (cholesterol). It can be challenging to do all that while still preparing food that is flavorful and appealing. Liven up your meals with garden-fresh herbs, many of which are available year-round, even in supermarkets. Fresh herbs are densely packed with flavor. You can use herbs in a variety of ways throughout the seasons, such as this simple chicken recipe.

- 4 chicken breasts
- 1 tablespoon extra-virgin olive oil
- 1 teaspoon dried rosemary
- 1 teaspoon poultry seasoning
- 1 teaspoon salt-free lemon pepper
- 1 tablespoon minced garlic
- 1/2 teaspoon red pepper flakes
- Cooking spray

1. In medium bowl, combine olive oil, rosemary, poultry seasoning, lemon pepper, garlic, and red pepper flakes. Add chicken breasts and turn to coat. Cover and refrigerate 1 hour.
2. Preheat oven to 375°F.
3. Preheat sauté pan to medium-high heat.

Spray pan with cooking spray. Add chicken breasts to pan and sear to desired color, about 10 seconds, then turn over and sear other side.

4. When both sides are seared, remove chicken from pan and place in a baking dish or on a cookie sheet. Do not cover. Place in oven. Cook meat until it is done, at 165°F internal temperature. When chicken is done, remove from oven and let rest for two to four minutes.
Serves four.

Source: Chris Smith, the Diabetic Chef, an executive chef working in the healthcare field. A graduate of the prestigious Culinary Institute of America, Smith has also worked as a chef at the four-star Le Cirque restaurant in Manhattan. He is author of two cookbooks, *Cooking with the Diabetic Chef* and *The Diabetic Chef's Year-Round Cookbook.* He lectures widely about cooking for people with diabetes.

SWEET POTATO SPAGHETTI AND MODERN MINI MEATBALLS

How do you "healthy up" a truly classic favorite dish like spaghetti and meatballs? Instead of pasta, this substitutes spiralized sweet potatoes. The meatballs call for a smaller amount of leaner beef, enhanced with oats and mush-

rooms. *The sauce starts with a low-calorie marinara, then adds beets and red peppers for more flavor and nutrition.*

For meatballs:
- 1/4 cup rolled oats, uncooked
- 2 tablespoons fresh thyme leaves
- 8 ounces cremini mushrooms, cleaned and stems trimmed
- 1/2 medium yellow onion, finely chopped
- 2 teaspoons extra-virgin olive oil
- 1/8 teaspoon salt
- 1/4 teaspoon freshly ground pepper
- 1/2 pound lean ground beef (10 percent fat)
- 1 large egg, lightly beaten

For sauce:
- 1 2/3 cups low-sodium, low-fat, low-sugar marinara sauce
- 1 medium beet, peeled and grated
- 1 red bell pepper, very finely chopped
- 2 tablespoons fresh thyme leaves, minced
- 1/4 teaspoon salt
- 1/4 teaspoon freshly ground pepper

For sweet potato spaghetti:
- 4 cups spiral-cut sweet potato
- Additional thyme leaves and freshly ground pepper for garnish

1. *Prepare meatballs:* Process oats and thyme

267

leaves in a food processor until finely ground, about 30 to 40 seconds. Transfer to a large bowl.

2. Place mushrooms in food processor, and pulse until very finely minced, 12 to 15 pulses. Scrape mushrooms onto a plate. Place onion pieces in food processor, and pulse until very finely chopped, about 10 pulses. Add to mushrooms.

3. Heat a large skillet over medium heat. Add olive oil, then onion, and cook, stirring frequently, until evenly browned, about 6 minutes. Add mushrooms, and sprinkle with a pinch of salt. Reduce heat to medium-low and cook, stirring frequently, until mushrooms and onions are dry, about 7 minutes. Scrape into the oat mixture, and let cool completely.

4. When the oat/mushroom mixture is cool, add the salt and pepper and toss to mix. Add ground beef and egg, and mix well. Roll slightly rounded tablespoons of the meatball mixture into 20 mini meatballs, placing them on a plate. Cover and refrigerate 30 minutes.

1. *Prepare sauce:* Combine the marinara sauce, beet, bell pepper, and thyme in the skillet, and bring to a simmer over medium heat. Cover, reduce heat, and simmer 15 minutes, stirring frequently, until vegetables are tender. Cool and process until smooth in food processor. (If you prefer a chunkier

sauce, skip the processor.) Wipe the skillet clean.

1. *Prepare the noodles:* You can cook the noodles by placing them in a baking dish and roasting for 10 minutes at 400°F, or place them in a pan of boiling water and blanch for 30 seconds, or combine the noodles with two tablespoons of water in a large glass bowl and microwave at high power for 1 minute or until softened. Drain and arrange sweet potato noodles on platter.

2. Place the skillet over medium heat, and coat with cooking spray. Add one-third (or one-half, if your skillet is at least 8 inches in diameter) of the meatballs and cook, carefully turning the meatballs frequently with 2 soup spoons to keep their shape, until well browned all over and cooked through, 8 to 9 minutes. Reduce heat as necessary to keep from overbrowning. Transfer to a plate. Cook the remaining meatballs, adding them to the plate. Pour the marinara sauce into the skillet — if the sauce is too thick, add up to 3 to 4 tablespoons of water. Cook, stirring, just until hot, about 1 minute. Add the meatballs to the sauce, turning to coat. Serve over sweet potato noodles.
Serves four.

Source: Debby Maugans, food writer based

in Asheville, North Carolina, and author of *Small-Batch Baking, Small-Batch Baking for Chocolate Lovers,* and *Farmer & Chef Asheville.*

PECAN-CRUSTED ARCTIC CHAR

The pecan crust contrasts nicely with clean-tasting arctic char, a salmon cousin with a milder taste. If you cannot find arctic char, substitute freshwater trout, sea trout, pompano, halibut, or mahi mahi.

- 4 fillets arctic char, about 6 ounces each
- 2/3 cup finely chopped pecans
- 3 tablespoons whole-wheat panko (Japanese-style breadcrumbs)
- 1 tablespoon Dijon mustard
- 1 tablespoon mayonnaise
- Freshly ground black pepper
- Olive oil, for drizzling
- Lemon wedges, for serving

1. Preheat the broiler.
2. Place fish skin side down in an oiled shallow baking dish or on a broiler pan. Mix pecans and panko. Mix mustard and mayonnaise, and smear onto the fish. Season with black pepper. Press the pecan-panko blend onto the fillets. Drizzle with a little olive oil.
3. Cook under the broiler until the topping has browned and the fish is cooked through,

about six or seven minutes.

4. Transfer the fillets to dinner plates with a spatula and serve with lemon wedges. *Serves four.*

Source: Susan Stuck, food writer and editor specializing in nutrition, sustainable foods, traditional preserving techniques, and French and Italian cooking, based in Burlington, Vermont, and author or coauthor of several cookbooks including *The Taste for Living World Cookbook: More of Mike Milken's Favorite Recipes for Fighting Cancer and Heart Disease.*

COCOA AND TOASTED-ALMOND–CRUSTED SALMON

Derived from the dried seed of the cacao tree, pure cocoa powder delivers a powerful dose of natural flavanols that have been found to prevent clogged arteries, improve circulation, and reduce blood pressure.

- 1 tablespoon unsweetened cocoa powder
- 3/4 cup almonds, toasted and chopped
- 2 1/4 teaspoons olive oil
- 8 six-ounce portions center-cut salmon fillets
- 1/2 teaspoon salt
- 1/4 teaspoon black pepper

1. Combine cocoa powder, almonds, and olive oil, and mix well. Season salmon fillets with salt and pepper. Heat cooking oil in a large sauté pan over medium-high heat. Place four fillets in the pan, flesh side down. Sauté salmon for about 1 to 2 minutes, or until the flesh side is golden brown. Place fillets on greased sheet pan, seared side up. Repeat for other fillets.
2. Place sheet pan in preheated 375°F oven for four minutes. Remove from oven. Spread 1 1/2 tablespoons of crust mixture over each portion. Return to 375°F oven for one to two minutes or until desired doneness.

Source: Chef Ken Gladysz, executive chef at Hotel Hershey in Hershey, Pennsylvania.

CURRIED GRAINS AND CAULIFLOWER, CHARD, EGGS, AND CUCUMBER RAITA

Combine eggs with just the right proportion of healthy whole grains and vegetables, and voila! — nutritious, filling, and inexpensive lunches and dinners.

- 1 small (pickling) cucumber, peeled, halved lengthwise, and seeded
- 1 clove garlic, peeled and finely chopped
- 2/3 cup plain low-fat yogurt (one 8-ounce container)
- 5 large eggs

- 1 1/2 teaspoons curry powder, divided
- Salt and freshly ground pepper
- 2 teaspoons olive oil
- 1 1/2 cups small cauliflowerets (single florets)
- 1 1/2 cups chopped Swiss chard
- 2 cups hot, cooked multigrain whole-grain pilaf
- 2 tablespoons each sliced green onion, ground red pepper, for garnish

1. Grate cucumber on large holes of a grater. Place in a fine-mesh sieve, and press to remove liquid. Mash garlic and 1/8 teaspoon salt on cutting board with the flat side of a knife blade. Combine cucumber, garlic mixture, and yogurt in a small bowl and stir well.
2. Combine eggs, 1/2 teaspoon curry powder, and 1/4 teaspoon each salt and pepper in a medium bowl and whisk to blend.
3. Spray a large, nonstick skillet with cooking spray, add one teaspoon olive oil, and heat over medium-high heat. Add cauliflower, and sauté until lightly browned, two to three minutes. Sprinkle remaining curry powder over cauliflower, and toss well. Add 1/4 cup water, cover, reduce heat to medium, and cook until cauliflower is just tender, three to four minutes. Add chard, tossing just until it begins to wilt, about one minute. Stir in whole-grain pilaf, cover,

and cook until hot, stirring frequently. Divide into serving bowls.

4. Wipe skillet clean, spray with cooking spray, and place over medium-low heat. Add remaining one teaspoon of olive oil. Whisk the egg mixture just until it begins to froth. Pour egg mixture into heated skillet, and cook until eggs begin to set on the bottom, 30 to 60 seconds. Using a heat-proof spatula, push the eggs across the skillet with sweeping motions, tilting the skillet a little to spread any uncooked egg onto the bottom of the skillet. Continue until the eggs appear set but moist. Remove from heat, and divide on tops of grains. Scatter eggs with green onion, and sprinkle with ground red pepper, if desired. Top with cucumber mixture, dividing evenly.
Serves three.

Source: Debby Maugans, food writer based in Asheville, North Carolina, and author of *Small-Batch Baking, Small-Batch Baking for Chocolate Lovers,* and *Farmer & Chef Asheville.*

CUBAN-STYLE BLACK BEANS AND PLANTAINS OVER OATMEAL
Research continues to accumulate that regular consumption of whole grains — at least three servings a day — can reduce cholesterol and

blood sugar levels, lower the risk of type 2 diabetes and cardiovascular disease, as well as boost immunity and improve your digestion and bowel function. And because they're chock-full of fiber and make you feel full longer, they can also help you lose weight.

The main ingredient here is steel-cut oats, which are more flavorful, chewier (in a good way), and less processed than rolled oats. Many people who don't like rolled oats find that they love steel-cut oats — so give these a try.

- 1 cup steel-cut oats
- 2 tablespoons olive oil
- 2 firm, ripe plantains, peeled and sliced lengthwise into 2-inch pieces
- 1 large onion, diced
- 1 green pepper, diced
- 1/2 cup chicken broth or stock
- 2 (15-ounce) cans black beans, drained and rinsed
- 1 teaspoon cumin
- 1 pinch salt and pepper to taste
- Fresh cilantro leaves (optional)
- Fresh sliced avocado (optional)
- Queso fresco cheese (optional)

1. Cook the oats according to the package directions, and set aside — but keep warm.
2. Heat 1 tablespoon of olive oil in a medium skillet over medium heat, and sauté the sliced plantains in it for four to five minutes

until they are golden and slightly browned.

3. Remove them from the pan, and then heat the remaining tablespoon of olive oil and sauté the diced onion and green pepper for five to seven minutes until the onion is translucent and beginning to brown.

4. Add the chicken stock, beans, cumin, salt, and pepper to the pan, and cook for another five to eight minutes until the beans are heated.

5. Divide the oatmeal into four servings, and top with the black beans and the plantains. If desired, garnish the dish with fresh cilantro, sliced avocado, and cheese.
Serves four.

Source: Sam Stephens, Quaker Oats chief creative oatmeal officer and owner of Oat-Meals Restaurant in New York City.

LIME AND CHICKEN CHILI
WITH AVOCADO

This Mexican-inspired chili gets a tart kick from limes. Tomatoes, beans, and yellow corn add protective fiber and phytonutrients.

• 2 tablespoons extra-virgin olive oil
• 1 large yellow onion, chopped
• 3 stalks celery, thinly sliced
• 1 jalapeño pepper, seeded and diced
• 5 garlic cloves, minced

- 1 pound whole boneless, skinless chicken breasts
- 1 cup frozen corn
- 1 (14.5-ounce) can no-salt diced tomatoes
- 1 (16-ounce) can cannellini beans, drained and rinsed
- 4 cups reduced-sodium chicken broth
- 1 1/2 teaspoons Italian seasoning
- 1 teaspoon oregano
- 1/4 teaspoon of cumin
- 2 whole limes
- 1/2 bunch cilantro, rinsed and chopped
- 1 medium avocado, cubed

1. In a soup pot, heat the extra-virgin olive oil over medium-high heat. Sauté the onion, celery, jalapeño pepper, and garlic cloves until tender — about six minutes. Then add the whole chicken breasts, corn, tomatoes, cannellini beans, chicken broth, Italian seasoning, oregano, and cumin to the pot. Stir the ingredients. Bring to a boil, then reduce heat, cover, and simmer for 55 minutes. Transfer the chicken breasts to a large platter, shred them with two forks, and return the chicken meat to the pot. Before serving, stir in the juice from one of the limes and the cilantro. Ladle the chili into bowls and garnish each serving with cubed avocado and a wedge from the remaining lime.
Serves six.

Source: Alice Bender, MS, RDN, head of nutrition programs for the American Institute for Cancer Research, a Washington, DC–based nonprofit devoted to research and education related to the role of nutrition in reducing cancer risk. Bender is also coauthor of the "Nutrition and Cancer Prevention" chapter in the reference book *Oncology Nutrition for Clinical Practice.*

NO-NOODLE EGGPLANT LASAGNA

The eggplant is sautéed and used in place of noodles. Use two large skillets to speed up the sauté time.

- 1 medium eggplant (about 3/4 pound)
- 1 tablespoon olive oil, divided
- Salt and freshly ground black pepper
- 1/2 cup sliced onion
- 2 garlic cloves, crushed
- 2 cups sliced mushrooms
- 1 1/2 cups ricotta cheese
- 1 cup shredded mozzarella cheese
- 1/2 cup freshly grated Parmesan cheese
- 1 cup basil leaves, in bite-size pieces
- 1 egg
- 1 cup pasta sauce

1. Preheat the oven to 350°F. Slice the eggplant into quarter-inch rounds. Heat 1/2 tablespoon of the olive oil in each of two skillets over medium-high heat. Add the

eggplant slices, and sauté two to three minutes per side or until they are soft. Remove the eggplant to a plate. Sprinkle with salt and pepper to taste.

2. Add the remaining 1/2 tablespoon of olive oil to one skillet over medium-high heat. Sauté the onion, garlic, and mushrooms together until the onion is transparent, about five minutes.

3. Mix the ricotta, mozzarella, and Parmesan together. Add the basil and egg.

4. To assemble, spoon a thin layer of pasta sauce over the bottom of a lasagna dish. Place a layer of eggplant slices over sauce. Spread about one-third of the pasta sauce over the eggplant. Spread one-third of the ricotta mixture over the pasta sauce. Spoon one-half of the mushroom mixture over the ricotta. Place a second layer of eggplant slices over the mushrooms. Spread another third of the ricotta mixture over the eggplant. Spread the remaining mushroom mixture over the ricotta. Spread another third of the remaining pasta sauce over the mushrooms. Place a third layer of eggplant slices over the pasta sauce. Spoon the rest of the pasta sauce over the eggplant. Spread the remaining ricotta mixture as the last layer.

5. Bake for 40 minutes. Remove, and let rest for 15 minutes. Cut into squares.
Serves four.

Source: Linda Gassenheimer, an award-winning author of numerous cookbooks, including *Delicious One-Pot Dishes: Quick, Healthy, Diabetes-Friendly Recipes.* Based in Florida, she writes the syndicated newspaper column "Dinner in Minutes." DinnerIn-Minutes.com.

LIME-SCENTED QUINOA WITH BLACK BEANS, TOMATO, AND CILANTRO

- 3 cups chicken or vegetable stock
- 1 1/2 cups uncooked quinoa
- 1/4 cup olive oil
- 1/4 cup fresh lime juice
- 1/4 cup finely chopped cilantro or flat-leaf parsley
- Salt and pepper to taste
- Zest of one lime
- 1 tablespoon hot sauce
- 1 (15-ounce) can black beans, drained and rinsed
- 1 cup diced red or yellow tomatoes
- 1 cup diced red bell pepper

1. Bring stock to a boil, and add quinoa. Stir, and bring back to a simmer. Cover, and cook for 12 to 14 minutes or until the quinoa is fluffy and tender. Strain and let cool. In a small bowl, whisk the oil, lime juice, cilantro, salt and pepper, zest, and hot sauce. Place quinoa, beans, tomatoes, and

red pepper in a medium bowl. Add the olive oil mixture, and toss. *Suggestion:* Serve with sautéed kale or spinach lightly tossed with olive oil and garlic.
Serves four.

Source: Patti Tveit Milligan, RD, CNS, a natural foods nutritionist in Fountain Hills, Arizona. She developed these recipes with Gregory Anne Cox, a chef in Hampton Bays, New York.

QUINOA WITH ROASTED WALNUTS, LEEKS, AND APPLES

- 2 cups chicken or vegetable stock (water may be used instead, but stock adds more flavor)
- 1 cup uncooked quinoa
- 2 tablespoons walnut oil
- 2 tablespoons olive oil
- 1 cup thinly sliced cleaned leeks, white part only
- 1 cup chopped green or red apple with peel
- 1/2 cup chopped roasted walnuts
- Salt and pepper to taste

1. Bring stock (or water) to a boil, and add quinoa. Stir, and bring to a simmer. Cover, and cook for 12 to 14 minutes or until the quinoa is fluffy and tender. Strain, and let cool. Heat a medium-sized sauté pan, and

add the oils. When oil is fragrant, add leeks, apple, and walnuts, and sauté until leeks are tender. Mix all ingredients. Can be served warm or chilled.
Serves four to six as a side dish.

Source: Patti Tveit Milligan, RD, CNS, a natural foods nutritionist in Fountain Hills, Arizona. She developed these recipes with Gregory Anne Cox, a chef in Hampton Bays, New York.

CREAMY MASHED POTATOES
Instead of mashed potatoes loaded with saturated fat from butter, enjoy these mashed potatoes made with yogurt and a surprise ingredient.

The addition of cauliflower is a sneaky-but-healthy nutrition hack — cauliflower delivers more fiber than potatoes while cutting the carb content of this dish in half! Plus, a 2014 study in BMJ offered further proof that diets high in produce are associated with lower risk for death, particularly cardiovascular mortality. Olive oil is a great source of MUFAs, and the yogurt adds creaminess and even a little protein while curbing carbs.

- 1 pound russet (baking) potatoes, peeled and halved
- 1 small head cauliflower, cut into florets
- 2 tablespoons olive oil

- 1 cup vegetable broth
- 1/2 cup plain nonfat Greek yogurt
- Garlic (optional)
- Rosemary (optional)

1. In a large pot, combine potatoes (leave the peels on for extra fiber and nutrients) and cauliflower. Cover with water, bring to a boil, then reduce heat to medium, and simmer for 20 minutes, or until the potatoes and cauliflower are easily pierced with a fork. Drain, and place in a large bowl with the olive oil and vegetable broth. Using an electric mixer on medium speed, beat until creamy. Add yogurt, and beat until just blended. Add garlic or rosemary if you desire.
Serves six.

Source: Laura Cipullo, RD, CDE, a registered dietitian and certified diabetes educator in private practice in New York City. Cipullo is author of *The Diabetes Comfort Food Diet* and is president of the New York chapter of the International Association of Eating Disorder Professionals.

BROCCOLI PENNE
Instead of white, blood sugar–spiking pasta with high-fat alfredo sauce, have this healthful broccoli pasta dish with mozzarella.

- 6 ounces multigrain penne pasta
- 2 cups fresh broccoli florets
- 1 cup halved grape tomatoes
- 6 ounces fresh, part-skim mozzarella cheese, cubed
- 1/4 cup pesto sauce
- 1 tablespoon lemon juice

1. Cook pasta in boiling water, and add broccoli florets to the pot during the last two minutes of cooking. Drain the pasta and broccoli, reserving 1/2 cup of the water. In a large bowl, place the pasta, broccoli, grape tomatoes, mozzarella cheese, pesto sauce, and lemon juice. Add the reserved pasta water to the bowl, one tablespoon at a time, stirring gently until the ingredients are combined.
Serves four.

Source: Laura Cipullo, RD, CDE, a registered dietitian and certified diabetes educator in private practice in New York City. Cipullo is author of *The Diabetes Comfort Food Diet* and is president of the New York chapter of the International Association of Eating Disorder Professionals.

QUINOA TABBOULEH
Parsley often is used by traditional healers as a diuretic to reduce water retention. It has a higher vitamin C content than citrus fruits, and

it contains oils that can block the effects of some carcinogens, including those produced when grilling meats. The chlorophyll in parsley is a natural breath freshener that is particularly effective at countering the odor of garlic.

Curly leaf parsley has a milder taste than flat leaf. Chefs often keep a bunch of parsley with its stem tips in a jar of water on the counter. They snip it with scissors, which is easier than chopping. Parsley with the stems in water will last about two to three days at room temperature or a few days longer in the fridge.

Quinoa has more protein and iron and fewer carbohydrates than any other grain. It's rich in lysine, an amino acid that aids in tissue growth and repair (and helps prevent and treat cold sores from the herpes virus). Quinoa is also rich in magnesium, a mineral that reduces the risk for heart attack and stroke.

- 4 cups cooked quinoa
- 1 cup minced parsley
- 3 green onions, chopped
- 1 cup seeded, chopped plum tomatoes
- 1 clove garlic, minced
- 1/4 cup olive oil
- Juice of one lemon
- Sea salt

1. Combine quinoa, parsley, green onions, and tomatoes. In a small bowl, whisk garlic with olive oil, lemon juice, and sea salt to

taste. Add the dressing to the quinoa mixture, and toss well.

Source: Delia Quigley, certified nutritional counselor (CNC) and creator of the Body Rejuvenation Cleanse, a five-week detoxification program. She teaches whole-foods preparation in Blairstown, New Jersey, and is author of *The Everything Superfoods Book*. DeliaQuigley.com.

SWEET POTATO HUMMUS

This starchy root vegetable is, to be honest, not the most attractive food — with its odd shape, imperfect skin, and dusting of dirt. But don't let the appearance stop you from incorporating sweet potatoes into your meals. Chock-full of vital nutrients, including vitamin A, vitamin C, beta-carotene, potassium, folate, fiber, B vitamins, and manganese, the sweet potato is one of the healthiest complex carbs around.

Change up your basic hummus by making it sweet or spicy, depending on your taste preference.

- 1 medium sweet potato, washed
- 1 (15-ounce) can garbanzo beans, drained and rinsed
- 2 tablespoons extra-virgin olive oil
- 1 tablespoon tahini (optional)
- *Sweet spices:* 1 teaspoon cinnamon and 1 teaspoon pumpkin spice

- *Spicy spices:* 1/2 teaspoon cayenne pepper, 1/2 teaspoon paprika, 1 teaspoon cumin

1. Preheat oven to 400°F. With a fork, poke holes in the sweet potato all over (both sides). Place the sweet potato on a baking sheet, and bake for 45 to 60 minutes (until you can squeeze it). Once cooked, remove the skin, and chop the potato into pieces. Add the chopped sweet potato and the other hummus ingredients into a blender, and mix until it makes a smooth consistency with no visible pieces of sweet potato. Add either sweet or spicy spices. Taste and add more spices, if needed.

Source: Janet Bond Brill, PhD, RDN, FAND, is a registered dietitian/nutritionist, a fellow of the Academy of Nutrition and Dietetics, and a nationally recognized nutrition, health, and fitness expert who specializes in cardiovascular disease prevention. Based in Hellertown, Pennsylvania, Dr. Brill is author of *Blood Pressure Down: The 10-Step Plan to Lower Your Blood Pressure in 4 Weeks — Without Prescription Drugs, Prevent a Second Heart Attack: 8 Foods, 8 Weeks to Reverse Heart Disease,* and *Cholesterol Down: 10 Simple Steps to Lower Your Cholesterol in 4 Weeks — Without Prescription Drugs.* DrJanet.com.

BROCCOLI-WALNUT FARRO CAKES

This muffin pan recipe combines familiar broccoli, red peppers, feta cheese, and toasted walnuts with a different kind of grain — farro. It's an ancient form of wheat with a chewy texture and nutty taste that's a good source of protein, fiber, iron, vitamin B-3, and zinc. Look for whole-grain versions, and follow cooking directions on the package.

Serve these cakes with a salad of arugula or watercress drizzled with our garlicky yogurt sauce, and you'll enjoy a nutritious bounty of flavors, textures, and colors. It's a meal in a bowl!

For yogurt sauce:
- 3/4 cup plain yogurt (can be whole, low-fat, or nonfat)
- 1 tablespoon extra-virgin olive oil
- 2 teaspoons fresh lemon juice
- 1 small clove garlic, crushed with 1/8 teaspoon sea salt

For cakes:
- 1/2 cup finely chopped red bell pepper
- 2 cups broccoli florets
- 1 cup drained, cooked farro
- 3/4 cup finely crumbled feta cheese
- 1/4 cup chopped walnuts, toasted
- 1/4 cup whole wheat panko
- 1 large egg, beaten

- 1/4 teaspoon sea salt
- 1/2 teaspoon freshly ground pepper

For salad:
- 3 cups fresh arugula or watercress leaves
- 2 teaspoons fresh lemon juice
- 2 teaspoons extra-virgin olive oil

1. Preheat oven to 350°F. Spray a six-cup muffin tin with cooking spray. Line the bottoms with circles of parchment paper cut to fit.
2. For the sauce, combine yogurt, olive oil, lemon juice, and crushed garlic, and mix well. Cover and refrigerate up to two hours ahead.
3. Place red bell pepper in a large bowl. Steam broccoli until just tender, about four minutes. Drain, and let cool. Chop broccoli florets into half-inch pieces, then add to bell pepper.
4. Add farro, cheese, walnuts, panko, egg, salt, and pepper to broccoli and bell pepper, and mix thoroughly. Divide evenly among muffin cups, then press down lightly with back of spoon to even the thicknesses. Cover with foil, and bake until set, about 15 minutes. Let cool 10 minutes in pan before removing.
5. Meanwhile, toss arugula or watercress with lemon juice and olive oil. Divide arugula on six serving plates. Place a warm cake on

top of each salad and drizzle with yogurt sauce.
Serves six.

Source: Debby Maugans, food writer based in Asheville, North Carolina, and author of *Small-Batch Baking, Small-Batch Baking for Chocolate Lovers,* and *Farmer & Chef Asheville.*

KALE BRUSCHETTA

With its sweet, nutty undertone, kale is a nutrition powerhouse, with vitamins A and C, calcium, magnesium, and iron.

- 1 cup kale, steamed
- Olive oil for sautéing
- 3 cloves garlic, finely chopped
- 1 (14-ounce) can cannellini beans, drained and rinsed
- Ground black pepper

1. Sauté kale in olive oil with garlic. Add beans, partially mashing them, and black pepper. Serve spooned onto toasted slices of whole-wheat Italian bread.

Source: Nevia No is the owner of Bodhitree Farm in Burlington County, New Jersey. She sells her produce at farmers' markets in New York City. BodhitreeFarm.com.

ROASTED BABY BRUSSELS SPROUTS AND BACON

Look for baby Brussels sprouts. The roasted sprouts will be crisp on the outside and tender inside, and the bacon adds a delectable smoky taste. If you don't like bacon, you can sprinkle a little smoked paprika over them.

- 1 tablespoon olive oil
- 1 pound frozen small Brussels sprouts (about 4 cups)
- Salt and freshly ground black pepper
- 4 bacon slices, diced into 1/2-inch pieces

1. Preheat the oven to 400°F. Line a baking sheet with foil. Add the oil, and roll the Brussels sprouts in the oil, making sure all sides are covered. Sprinkle with salt and pepper to taste, and toss well. Spread them in one layer on the sheet. Place the diced bacon over the Brussels sprouts. Roast 20 minutes. Remove from oven, and turn sprouts over. Roast another 10 minutes. **Serves four.**

Source: Linda Gassenheimer, an award-winning author of numerous cookbooks, including *Delicious One-Pot Dishes: Quick, Healthy, Diabetes-Friendly Recipes.* Based in Florida, she writes the syndicated newspaper column "Dinner in Minutes." DinnerIn Minutes.com.

Roasted Red Beets with Lemon Vinaigrette

Beets are delicious, easy to cook, and very effective for lowering blood pressure. They make a delicious side dish when roasted, peeled, and topped with a lemon vinaigrette and fresh parsley.

- 6 medium-sized beets, washed and trimmed of greens and roots
- 2 tablespoons extra-virgin olive oil
- 2 teaspoons fresh lemon juice
- 1 garlic clove, peeled and minced
- 1 teaspoon Dijon mustard
- 1/4 teaspoon kosher salt
- 1/4 teaspoon freshly ground black pepper
- 1/4 cup chopped fresh flat-leaf Italian parsley

1. Preheat the oven to 400°F. Spray a baking dish with nonstick cooking spray. Place the beets in the dish, and cover tightly with foil. Bake the beets for about one hour or until they are tender when pierced with a fork or thin knife. Remove from the oven, and allow to cool to the touch.
2. Meanwhile, in a small bowl, whisk together the olive oil, lemon juice, garlic, mustard, salt, and pepper for the dressing. When the beets are cool enough to handle, peel and slice the beets, arranging the slices on a platter. Drizzle with vinaigrette, and garnish

with parsley.
Serves six.

Source: Janet Bond Brill, PhD, RDN, FAND, is a registered dietitian/nutritionist, a fellow of the Academy of Nutrition and Dietetics, and a nationally recognized nutrition, health, and fitness expert who specializes in cardiovascular disease prevention. Based in Hellertown, Pennsylvania, Dr. Brill is author of *Blood Pressure Down: The 10-Step Plan to Lower Your Blood Pressure in 4 Weeks — Without Prescription Drugs, Prevent a Second Heart Attack: 8 Foods, 8 Weeks to Reverse Heart Disease,* and *Cholesterol Down: 10 Simple Steps to Lower Your Cholesterol in 4 Weeks — Without Prescription Drugs.* DrJanet.com.

ARAME RICE

Better known as seaweed, sea vegetables are among the most nutrient-rich foods on the planet. Many Americans are now familiar with nori (used to prepare sushi rolls) and wakame (added to miso soup). There are many other types of sea vegetables, including arame, which is high in iodine, iron, and calcium. It helps to lower blood pressure, strengthens bones and teeth, and is beneficial for the thyroid.

Many varieties of sea vegetables are sold in dried sheets, which can be used as wraps or sliced and added to salads, soups, and stews.

- 1/2 cup pine nuts
- 1/4 cup dried arame
- 3 cups cooked brown rice
- 1 cup cooked wild rice
- 2 green onions, minced
- 1/2 cup fresh parsley, minced
- 1/2 cup fresh mint, minced
- 1 teaspoon fresh thyme
- 3 tablespoons extra-virgin olive oil
- 2 tablespoons red wine vinegar
- 1 teaspoon ume plum vinegar

1. Toast pine nuts in a dry skillet until evenly browned. Set aside.
2. Soak dried arame in water for 10 minutes. Drain, then cover with water and simmer in a small saucepan for 10 minutes. Drain again.
3. In a large bowl, combine the arame with brown rice, wild rice, green onions, parsley, mint, and thyme.
4. In a separate bowl, whisk together olive oil and the two vinegars. Add the dressing and pine nuts to the arame mixture. Toss well.

Source: Delia Quigley, certified nutritional counselor (CNC) and creator of the Body Rejuvenation Cleanse, a five-week detoxification program. She teaches whole-foods preparation in Blairstown, New Jersey, and is author of *The Everything Superfoods Book*. DeliaQuigley.com.

ZAATAR FOR EVERYONE!

Zaatar (pronounced ZAH-tahr) is a spice-and-herb blend from the Middle East. It has an amazing and unique flavor that is aromatic, nutty, and tangy all at the same time — with three main ingredients that all are good for you.

Zaatar is used throughout the Middle East — it is sprinkled on hummus or grilled chicken, mixed in with feta cheese, or combined with sliced tomato and onions. You can also add it to couscous, salads, grilled chicken or fish, or cooked beans. Combined with oil, it makes a tasty paste for dipping. For the two variations below, simply mix all ingredients together.

Aromatic and Tart Zaatar
- 1/3 cup dried thyme
- 3 tablespoons sumac
- 1 1/2 teaspoons sesame seeds

Nutty and Crunchy Zaatar
- 1/4 cup dried thyme
- 2 tablespoons sumac
- 1 tablespoon sesame seeds

Source: Paula Wolfert, a California-based expert on Mediterranean and Middle Eastern food and cooking. She is an award-winning author of numerous cookbooks, including *The Food of Morocco*. Paula-Wolfert.com.

EVEN-BETTER-THAN-PEANUT WALNUT BUTTER

This is so delicious that it can entice even the most resolute peanut butter devotee. This recipe uses a mixture of raw and toasted walnuts, a little salt, and a teaspoon of honey to smooth out any residual bitter taste from tannins in traces of walnut peel that may cling to the nut after shelling. Toasting the walnuts adds texture and aroma too.

- 2 cups chopped raw walnuts
- 1 teaspoon honey
- 1/4 teaspoon salt

1. Preheat oven to 350°F. Spread one cup of the walnuts on a baking sheet and bake until fragrant, 8 to 10 minutes. Let cool completely. Place remaining raw nuts and the toasted and cooled walnuts in a food processor. Process until the mixture is a coarse paste, about 30 seconds. Add honey and salt, and process until smooth, 20 to 30 additional seconds. Scrape bowl as needed.
2. Store in a covered jar in the refrigerator. *Makes about one cup.*

Source: Debby Maugans, food writer based in Asheville, North Carolina, and author of *Small-Batch Baking, Small-Batch Baking for Chocolate Lovers,* and *Farmer & Chef Asheville.*

PUMPKIN PIE

Even if you have diabetes, you can enjoy this traditional favorite. For a scrumptious, reduced-carb pumpkin pie, try this easy recipe, with a tasty, whole-grain crust (and a dollop of whipped cream, if you like). *

- 1 Flaky Oat Piecrust (see following recipe)
- 1 1/2 cups canned or cooked mashed pumpkin
- 1/4 cup honey
- Sugar substitute equal to 1/2 cup sugar (check the label)
- 2 to 2 1/2 teaspoons pumpkin pie spice
- 1/8 teaspoon sea salt
- 1 1/2 teaspoons vanilla extract
- 1 1/4 cups evaporated nonfat or low-fat milk
- 1/2 cup fat-free egg substitute or two large eggs, beaten

1. Preheat the oven to 400°F. Prick several holes in the crust with a fork, and bake for five minutes. Remove from the oven, and set aside.

2. Place the pumpkin, honey, sugar substitute, pumpkin pie spice, salt, and vanilla in a large bowl, and stir with a wire whisk to mix well. Whisk in the evaporated milk and then the egg substitute or eggs.

3. Pour filling into the crust, and bake for 15 minutes. Reduce heat to 350°F, and bake

* Consult your doctor for advice on your recommended daily carbohydrate intake.

for about 35 minutes more or until a sharp knife inserted near the center of the pie comes out clean. Cool to room temperature, and refrigerate until ready to serve.

Flaky Oat Piecrust

- 3/4 cup whole-wheat pastry flour
- 1/2 cup quick-cooking (one-minute) oats
- 3/4 teaspoon baking powder
- 1/8 teaspoon sea salt
- 1/4 cup canola oil
- 2 tablespoons nonfat or low-fat milk

1. Place the flour, oats, baking powder, and salt in a medium bowl, and stir to mix well. Add the oil and milk, and stir until the mixture is moist and crumbly and holds together when pinched. Add a little more milk if needed. Set aside.
2. Place a 12-inch square of waxed paper on a flat surface. Shape the dough into a ball, and then pat into a 7-inch circle. Top with another 12-inch square of waxed paper, and use a rolling pin to roll the dough into a roughly 10-inch circle.
3. Coat a 9-inch pie pan with cooking spray. Carefully peel off the top sheet of waxed paper, and place the other sheet, crust side down, over the pie pan. Peel away the waxed paper, and press the crust into the pan.
4. If you'd like to add whipped cream to your pumpkin pie, canned "real" whipped cream is a convenient choice. Most brands have

only 15 calories and 1 g of carbohydrate per serving (two tablespoons).

Source: Sandra Woodruff, RD, LD/N, a registered dietitian and nutritionist based in Tallahassee, Florida. She is a past president of the Florida Dietetic Association and the author of several books, including *Secrets of Good-Carb/Low-Carb Living* and *Diabetic Dream Desserts.*

CHIA VANILLA PUDDING
Yes, these are the same seeds that cause Chia Pets to sprout, but these tiny black seeds are packed with cholesterol-lowering fiber — nearly 10 g per ounce. Chia seeds are also a good source of calcium. And it gets even better. A Canadian study found that regular consumption of chia seeds helps lower blood sugar levels — an important bonus for people with diabetes.

- 1/4 cup almonds
- 1/4 cup dates
- 3/4 cup water
- 2 tablespoons chia seeds
- 1 teaspoon vanilla extract
- 1/2 teaspoon ground cinnamon
- 1/4 cup raisins

1. In a blender, combine almonds, dates, and water until the mixture is smooth and creamy like pudding. Stir in chia seeds,

vanilla extract, cinnamon, and raisins. Refrigerate for an hour, allowing the seeds to absorb the liquid. Water makes the seeds soft and gel-like — it will remind you of tapioca pudding. Sprinkle with toppings such as chopped nuts or fresh berries. **_Serves two to four._**

Source: Emily von Euw, a raw food recipe creator and author of *Rawsome Vegan Baking.* She lives in Vancouver, British Columbia, Canada. ThisRawsomeVeganLife.com.

5
Natural Treatments for Diabetes

If you have a preexisting condition, it can sometimes be intimidating to add another medication or treatment to your routine. You should always heed your doctor's instructions; however, there is also no harm in at least exploring alternative remedies if they provide a gentler, easier solution to the problem. Mother Nature has been around for a long time, so she knows a thing or two.

Supplements, extracts, and even some psychical exercises can help in the fight against diabetes. Certain foods, as discussed in the last chapter, are another natural way to kick back against low blood sugar or obesity. Take some time within these pages to open your mind and think outside the box with natural treatments that could help your diabetes.

FIGHT DIABETES NATURALLY — THREE PROVEN NONDRUG REMEDIES

Scientific research and the experience of doctors and other health professionals show that supplements and superfoods can be even more effective than drugs when it comes to preventing and treating diabetes. I reviewed thousands of scientific studies and talked to more than sixty health professionals about these glucose-controlling natural remedies. One is magnesium. Studies show that magnesium significantly reduces the risk for diabetes. (Note: High doses of magnesium can cause diarrhea.)

Here are three more standout natural remedies.

Caution: If you are taking insulin or other medications to control diabetes, talk to your doctor before taking any supplement or changing your diet.

Gymnema

Gymnema sylvestre has been the standard antidiabetes recommendation for the past two thousand years from practitioners of Ayurveda, the ancient system of natural healing from India. Derived from a vine-like plant found in the tropical forests of southern and central India, the herb also is called gurmar, or "sugar destroyer" — if you chew on the leaf of the plant, you temporarily will lose your ability to taste sweets.

Modern science has figured out the molecular interactions underlying this strange phenomenon. The gymnemic acids in the herb have a structure similar to glucose molecules, filling up glucose receptor sites on the taste buds. They also fill up sugar receptors in the intestine, blocking the absorption of glucose.

And gymnemic acids stimulate (and even may regenerate) the cells of the pancreas that manufacture insulin, the hormone that ushers glucose out of the bloodstream and into cells.

Standout research: Studies published in *Journal of Ethnopharmacology* showed that three months of using a unique gymnema extract, formulated over several decades by two Indian scientists, reduced fasting blood glucose (a blood sample taken after an overnight fast) by 23 percent in people with type 2 diabetes (defined as fasting blood sugar levels of 126 mg/dL or higher). People with prediabetes (defined as those with blood sugar levels of 100 to 125 mg/dL) had a 30 percent reduction.

Important: The newest (and more powerful) version of this extract is called ProBeta, which is available at www.pharmaterra.com. A naturopathic physician who uses ProBeta with his patients told me that the supplement can lower fasting glucose in the 200s down to the 120s or 130s after five to six months of use.

Typical daily dose: ProBeta — two capsules, two to three times a day. Other types of gymnema — 400 mg, three times a day.

Apple Cider Vinegar

Numerous studies have proven that apple cider vinegar works to control type 2 diabetes. Several of the studies were conducted by Carol Johnston, PhD, RD, a professor of nutrition at Arizona State University.

Standout scientific research: Dr. Johnston's studies showed that an intake of apple cider vinegar with a meal lowered insulin resistance (the inability of cells to use insulin) by an average of 64 percent in people with prediabetes and type 2 diabetes, improved insulin sensitivity (the ability of cells to use insulin) by up to 34 percent, and lowered postmeal spikes in blood sugar by an average of 20 percent. Research conducted in Greece, Sweden, Japan, and the Middle East has confirmed many of Dr. Johnston's findings.

How it works: The acetic acid in vinegar — the compound that gives vinegar its tart flavor and pungent odor — blunts the activity of disaccharidase enzymes that help break down the type of carbohydrates found in starchy foods such as potatoes, rice, bread, and pasta. As a result, those foods are digested and absorbed more slowly, lowering blood glucose and insulin levels.

Suggested daily intake: Two tablespoons right before or early in the meal. (More is not more effective.)

If you're using vinegar in a salad dressing, the ideal ratio for blood sugar control is two tablespoons of vinegar to one tablespoon of oil. Eat the salad early in the meal so that it disrupts the carb-digesting enzymes before they get a chance to work. Or dip premeal whole-grain bread in a vinaigrette dressing.

Soy Foods

A recent ten-year study published in _Journal of the American Society of Nephrology,_* found that the mortality rate for people with diabetes and kidney disease was more than 31 percent. Statistically, that makes kidney disease the number-one risk factor for death in people with diabetes.

Fortunately, researchers have found that there is a simple way to counter kidney disease in diabetes — eat more soy foods.

Standout scientific research: Dozens of scientific studies show that soy is a nutritional

* M. Afkarian et al., "Kidney Disease and Increased Mortality Risk in Type 2 Diabetes," _Journal of the American Society of Nephrology_ 24, no. 2 (February 2013): 302–308.

ally for diabetes patients with kidney disease. But the best and most recent of these studies, published in *Diabetes Care,* shows that eating lots of soy can help reverse signs of kidney disease, reduce risk factors for heart disease, and reduce blood sugar too.

The study involved forty-one diabetes patients with kidney disease, divided into two groups. One group ate a diet with protein from 70 percent animal and 30 percent vegetable sources. The other group ate a diet with protein from 35 percent animal sources, 35 percent textured soy protein, and 30 percent vegetable proteins. After four years, those eating the soy-rich diet had lower levels of several biomarkers for kidney disease. (In another, smaller experiment, the same researchers found that soy improved biomarkers for kidney disease in just seven weeks.) In fact, the health of the participants' kidneys actually improved, a finding that surprised the researchers, since diabetic nephropathy (diabetes-caused kidney disease) is considered to be a progressive, irreversible disease.

Those eating soy also had lower fasting blood sugar, lower LDL "bad" cholesterol, lower total cholesterol, lower triglycerides, and lower C-reactive protein, a biomarker for chronic inflammation.

How it works: Substituting soy for animal protein may ease stress on the delicate filters of the kidneys. Soy itself also stops the overproduction of cells in the kidney that clog the filters, boosts the production of nitric oxide, which improves blood flow in the kidneys, and normalizes the movement of minerals within the kidneys, thus improving filtration.

Suggested daily intake: The diabetes patients in the study ate 16 g of soy protein daily. Examples: Four ounces of tofu provide 13 g of soy protein; one soy burger, 13 g; one-quarter cup of soy nuts, 11 g; one-half cup of shelled edamame (edible soybeans in the pod), 11 g; one cup of soy milk, 6 g.

What's Wrong with Diabetes Drugs?

Doctors typically try to control high blood sugar with a glucose-lowering medication such as metformin, a drug most experts consider safe. But other diabetes drugs may not be safe.

Example #1: Recent studies show that sitagliptin and exenatide double the risk for hospitalization for pancreatitis (inflamed pancreas) and triple the risk for pancreatic cancer.

Example #2: Pioglitazone can triple the risk for eye problems and vision loss, double the risk for bone fractures in women, and double the risk for bladder cancer.

Bill Gottlieb, CHC, a health coach certified by the American Association of Drugless Practitioners. He is author of several health books that have sold more than two million copies and former editor in chief of Rodale Books and *Prevention Magazine* Health Books. Based in northern California, he is author of *Defeat High Blood Sugar — Naturally! Super-Supplements and Super-Foods Selected by America's Best Alternative Doctors.* BillGottliebHealth.com.

GOT DIABETES? STOP BLOOD SUGAR FROM SPIKING WITH RED GINSENG

Adult-onset (type 2) diabetes is so common that it ultimately impacts a whopping one in four people age sixty-five and older. In this type of diabetes, blood sugar can go way up — or spike — after a meal. You'll know your blood sugar is spiking because instead of feeling energized and fit after nourishing yourself, you'll just crash. More than just wanting to take a nap — you won't be able to do anything but. That's right. You'll have to take a rest after eating a meal because you will feel sleepy, exhausted. Your eyes may even blur. If this happens often enough, hardening of the arteries can occur, which, as you know, can lead to a heart attack. But you can prevent this from happening naturally. Red ginseng extract may be just the thing to keep blood sugar on an even keel.

Why is it called "red" ginseng? Tonics, extracts, and teas of Asian white ginseng (also called Chinese or Korean white panax ginseng) are natural powerhouses of health and vitality made from the raw dried root of the plant. They increase energy and stamina, reduce cholesterol and blood pressure, and fight cancer and aging. But steaming the root before drying it starts a fermentation process that supports wellness even more. Once fermented, the ginseng is called red ginseng, and this is the kind that is especially good for people with diabetes and others who have problems with glucose control. Korean researchers have recently confirmed that red ginseng significantly reduces blood glucose levels and increases insulin levels after meals. That makes it especially helpful in preventing dangerous spikes in blood sugar that can happen after diabetics or borderline diabetics have a meal.

The researchers recruited forty-two healthy men and women between the ages of twenty and seventy-five for their study. Nineteen of these participants had type 2 diabetes, and the remaining twenty-three had prediabetes. Half of the group received capsules of fermented red ginseng extract, and half received capsules of a placebo. They were instructed to take one capsule three times a day for four weeks. The total daily dose of red ginseng for the treatment group was 2.7 grams (0.1 ounces).

The researchers found that red ginseng was able to regulate glucose and insulin after meals, thus preventing blood sugar spikes.

Compared with the placebo group, insulin increased and glucose decreased after meals. And no serious side effects were reported in the Korean study, although one person in the treatment group had to drop out because hypoglycemia (low blood sugar) developed.

Natural but Potent Diabetes Care

"Red ginseng extract may be a good addition to a natural, broader approach to controlling, limiting, or getting rid of type 2 diabetes," says Andrew Rubman, ND, a naturopathic physician and founder of the Southbury Clinic for Traditional Medicines in Southbury, Connecticut. In his opinion, however, alpha-lipoic acid, a powerful antioxidant that helps the body use glucose more efficiently, may be a better choice. Plus, it relieves pain, inflammation, burning, tingling, and numbness in people who have peripheral neuropathy (nerve damage) caused by diabetes. But because it can reduce blood glucose levels (leading to hypoglycemia), it should not be used without the supervision of a health-care professional who can monitor your blood sugar levels.

Another readily available herbal supplement recommended by Dr. Rubman for type 2 diabetes is gymnema extract, used in Ayurvedic medicine for centuries.

As for red ginseng, most people can use it daily with no side effects, according to Dr. Rubman. He cautions that people who are taking several medications, especially antacids or statins, or who have liver or gastrointestinal diseases should hold off on taking ginseng extracts, since they can put an added burden on the liver. He also says that anyone who wants to try red ginseng for diabetes should do so under the supervision of a naturopathic doctor or clinically trained nutritionist — or at least let your doctor know that you are taking the extract so that he or she can monitor and interpret your physical exams and blood tests. Minor side effects include decreased energy, irregularity, and/or intestinal gas.

Red ginseng is widely available online, in Asian food stores, and at large health-food and nutrition shops.

Andrew L. Rubman, ND, founder and medical director, Southbury Clinic for Traditional Medicines, Southbury, Connecticut. South buryClinic.com.

SAY GOODBYE TO YOUR DIABETES MEDICATION WITH BERBERINE

Some of my patients who have type 2 diabetes are able to keep the disease under control with diet, exercise, and supplements. Lucky them! But for other diabetes patients, that's not enough, and they must take pharmaceutical medications.

I'm happy to report that there is another natural treatment option for diabetes patients who currently take pharmaceutical medications. Research has found that a plant extract called berberine can control diabetes as well as, or better than, common medications such as metformin and rosiglitazone. And it does this with no side effects — and without damaging the liver, as some medications do. Here's how berberine can help people with diabetes.

A naturally occurring chemical compound, berberine is found in the roots and stems of several plants, including *Hydrastis canadensis* (goldenseal), *Coptis chinensis* (coptis or goldthread) and *Berberis aquifolium* (Oregon grape). Long used as a remedy in Chinese and Ayurvedic medicines, berberine is known for its antimicrobial properties and as a treatment for bacterial and fungal infections. Several decades ago, berberine was used to treat diarrhea in patients in China. That was when doctors noticed that the blood sugar levels of diabetes patients were lower after taking the herbal extract — and berberine began to be investigated for this purpose.

Over the past twenty years, there has been much research on berberine and its effectiveness in treating diabetes. In 2008, Chinese researchers published a study in *Metabolism* in which adults with newly diagnosed type 2 diabetes were given 500 mg of either berberine or the drug metformin three times a day for three months. Researchers found that berberine did as good a job as metformin at regulating glucose metabolism, as indicated by hemoglobin A1C (a measure of blood glucose over several weeks), fasting blood glucose, blood sugar after eating, and level of insulin after eating. Berberine even reduced the amount of insulin needed to turn glucose into energy by 45 percent! In addition, those taking berberine had noticeably lower triglyceride and total cholesterol levels than those taking metformin.

In another 2008 study published in *Journal of Clinical Endocrinology and Metabolism,* researchers found that type 2 diabetes patients who were given berberine had significant reductions in fasting and postmeal blood glucose, hemoglobin A1C, triglycerides, total cholesterol, and LDL "bad" cholesterol — and also lost an average of five pounds to boot during the three-month study period.

In a 2010 study in *Metabolism,* Chinese researchers compared people with type 2 diabetes who took either 1,000 mg daily of berberine or daily doses of metformin or rosiglitazone. After two months, berberine had lowered subjects' fasting blood glucose levels by an average of about 30 percent, an improvement over the rosiglitazone group and almost as much as people in the metformin group. Berberine also reduced subjects' hemoglobin A1C by 18 percent — equal to rosiglitazone and, again, almost as good as metformin. In addition, berberine lowered serum insulin levels by 28.2 percent (indicating increased insulin sensitivity), lowered triglycerides by 17.5 percent, and actually improved liver enzyme levels. Pharmaceutical medications, on the other hand, have the potential to harm the liver.

These were remarkable findings. Here was a botanical that was holding up to scientific scrutiny and performing as well as, or better than, some drugs that patients had been taking for diabetes for years.

How Berberine Works in the Body

Berberine helps to lower blood glucose in several ways. One of its primary mechanisms involves stimulating the activity of the genes responsible for manufacturing and activating insulin receptors, which are critical for controlling blood glucose.

Berberine also has an effect on blood sugar regulation through activation of incretins, gastrointestinal hormones that affect the amount of insulin released by the body after eating.

How Berberine Can Help

I recommend berberine to my patients with newly diagnosed type 2 diabetes to reduce their blood sugar and prevent them from needing pharmaceutical drugs. When a diet, exercise, and supplement program (including supplements such as chromium) is already helping a diabetes patient, I don't recommend that he/she switch to berberine.

Some patients are able to take berberine — and make dietary changes — and stop taking diabetes drugs altogether. People with severe diabetes can use berberine in conjunction with medication — and this combination treatment allows for fewer side effects and better blood sugar control. I don't recommend berberine for prediabetes unless diet and exercise are not effective. Berberine is sold in health-food stores and online in tablet and capsule form. The dosage I typically recommend for all diabetes patients is 500 mg twice daily.

For patients with diabetes who want to use berberine, I recommend talking to your doctor about taking this supplement. It's also important for every patient with diabetes to participate in a comprehensive diet and exercise program.

Note that berberine helps patients with type 2 diabetes, not type 1 diabetes (in which the body does not produce enough insulin).

Mark A. Stengler, NMD, a naturopathic medical doctor and leading authority on the practice of alternative and integrated medicine. Dr. Stengler is author of the *Health Revelations* newsletter, *The Natural Physician's Healing Therapies,* and *Bottom Line's Prescription for Natural Cures.* He is also the founder and medical director of the Stengler Center for Integrative Medicine in Encinitas, California, and former adjunct associate clinical professor at the National College of Natural Medicine in Portland, Oregon. MarkStengler.com.

PYCNOGENOL:
NATURAL ANTI-INFLAMMATORY
FEW KNOW ABOUT

Growing abundantly in the South of France is the French maritime pine tree, source for Pycnogenol, a special patented, clinically studied pine bark extract. New clinical research finds it effective at lowering risk factors for heart disease and controlling blood sugar in people with type 2 diabetes.

Pine Bark Extract Is Potent Medicine

Pycnogenol, or pine bark, is a medicine with numerous benefits, notes Mark Blumenthal, founder and executive director of the non-profit American Botanical Council. It's theorized that pine bark's high level of inflammation-fighting antioxidant bioflavonoids, known as procyanidins (these are the same potent compounds found in fresh fruits and vegetables), should get credit for these results. In addition, Blumenthal says there are a number of benefits to Pycnogenol, including:

• **Better diabetes control.** At the University of Arizona, researchers found that people with noninsulin-dependent type 2 diabetes who took Pycnogenol for three months experienced a 17 percent drop in blood glucose levels. The study also suggested that

Pycnogenol may protect kidney function in people with diabetes.

- **Improved circulation, blood pressure, and cardiovascular health.** Pycnogenol helps strengthen blood vessel walls, improve cholesterol levels, and reduce the constriction of arteries, platelet stickiness, and clotting that can lead to heart attack or stroke. In the University of Arizona trial, participants — who had mild high blood pressure as well as type 2 diabetes — were able to reduce their antihypertensive medication by 50 percent.

- **Less leg and ankle swelling on long flights.** In 2005, a study published in *Clinical and Applied Thrombosis/ Hemostasis* demonstrated that Pycnogenol reduced edema (leg and ankle swelling) and the risk of deep vein thrombosis (DVT) on long-distance flights of seven to twelve hours. DVT — the formation of a blood clot, usually in the leg — is a dangerous condition, since if the clot breaks loose and travels to the lung, it can cause a potentially fatal pulmonary embolism.

- **Reduced joint pain.** In a study at Italy's Chieti-Pescara University, people with osteoarthritis of the knee took 100 mg of Pycnogenol daily for three months. Participants who took the pine bark extract experienced about a 50 percent decrease in osteoarthritis symptoms. They were able to lower their dosage of nonsteroidal anti-inflammatory drugs (NSAIDs), such as aspirin, by 58 percent.

- **Fewer menopausal symptoms.** Taiwanese researchers found that perimenopausal women who took Pycnogenol for several months experienced improvements in symptoms such as headaches, fatigue, and vaginal dryness. With natural anti-inflammatory properties, this extract may also be helpful in controlling menstrual pain.
- **Other benefits.** More than two hundred scientific studies have been conducted on French maritime pine extract — most of them on Pycnogenol — and research suggests that it may aid in the treatment of other disorders such as asthma, erectile dysfunction, and other conditions.

Demonstrated Safety and Effectiveness

Pycnogenol is a well-researched botanical medicine with demonstrated safety and efficacy in study after study at the prescribed doses, says Blumenthal. Consult a physician trained in botanical medicine to determine what dosage best meets your specific medical needs. To prevent any minor stomach discomfort, it's best to take Pycnogenol with or after meals and, as we always recommend, with doctor oversight.

Mark Blumenthal, founder and executive director of the American Botanical Council and editor of *Herbal Gram,* Austin, Texas. HerbalGram.org.

"SNACK" ON THIS FOR
HIGH BLOOD SUGAR CONTROL

Remember when your mom would snap "No snacks!" before mealtime because it would "ruin" your appetite? It stands to reason that if you eat a rich snack before a meal, you either won't eat your meal, replacing nutritious meal calories with empty snack calories, or you will gobble down both the snack and the meal.

But what if the idea of snack were redefined? What if a snack right before meals could help you regulate your blood sugar and prevent cardiovascular disease? You'd stock up on that snack, wouldn't you? Well, such a snack actually exists, but it's not something you eat — it's something you do. It's a quick, easy, short burst of exercise right before meals, dubbed an "exercise snack."

If you're shaking your head, thinking what kind of gimmick is this, clearly, it's a gimmick to get you to exercise. And it works! Although exercise and diet are proven to prevent type 2 diabetes and related heart disease, less than 10 percent of Americans get the exercise they need, often saying they do not have the time. How to get folks to make the time — and figuring out exactly how much time they need and whether shortcuts can do the trick — have been areas of study for researchers.

So a team from the School of Physical

Education, Sport and Exercise Sciences at the University of Otago in New Zealand co-opted the catchy phrase "exercise snack" to refer to a much less catchy but more technically descriptive term: high-intensity interval training. That's a few brief minutes of intensive exercise, such as fitness walking, running, or resistance training. "Exercise snack" was coined by Harvard cardiologist L. Howard Hartley, MD, in 2007 in a column he wrote for *Newsweek* to define quick bursts of calorie-burning ordinary activity, such as pacing while talking on the phone or taking the stairs instead of the elevator. Studies have shown that exercise snacking in the form of high-intensity interval training is as effective as longer workouts for keeping fit and that it improves glucose control.

The researchers set off to see whether their idea of an exercise snack could help keep blood sugar from spiking — a problem among folks with diabetes and prediabetes whereby blood sugar goes way up after meals. Spiking is directly related to diabetes-associated cardiovascular disease, so prevention is a high priority.

The New Zealand study was small, including seven men and two women who had either prediabetes or newly diagnosed diabetes. The participants all practiced three different exercise regimens, each for five days with a break in between, to examine the impact of each regimen on blood sugar after meals.

One regimen, regarded as a traditional workout regimen, had participants do thirty minutes of moderate-intensity treadmill walking before their evening meals. Another regimen — referred to as an exercise snack — had participants do only six minutes of treadmill walking, alternating one minute at an intensive pace followed by one minute at a slow pace, a half hour before breakfast, lunch, and dinner. The third exercise regimen, also a six-minute exercise snack done half an hour before each meal, involved alternating intensive one-minute walks with one-minute resistance exercises that worked the arms, back, and core.

A Quickie Is Better!

The researchers found that a person doesn't have to huff and puff for thirty minutes a day to keep blood sugar in check — a few minutes of intensive exercise before meals was better in preventing blood sugar from spiking. Exercise snacking (either kind described above) before breakfast reduced postmeal blood sugar by an average 17 percent. Although exercise snacking before lunch didn't have much of an effect on blood sugar levels, exercise snacking before dinner reduced it by an average 13 percent. In comparison, the thirty-minute daily workout had no effect on postmeal blood sugar.

"First and most important, exercise snacks are more time-efficient," says lead researcher and doctoral candidate Monique Francois. "Running an hour or two every day can help reduce blood sugar spikes after meals, but doing this is not feasible for most people. Short, intense exercise done right before a meal gives the same benefit."

How to "Exercise Snack"

You don't have to invest in a treadmill or buy any exercise gear to exercise snack, says Francois. If you want to do it as part of a regimen for blood sugar control, simply take a quick, brisk walk before mealtime. For blood sugar control or simply overall fitness, Francois echoes the advice that Dr. Hartley gave in his *Newsweek* article back in 2007: rather than driving all the way to a destination, bike, jog, or walk at a moderate to fast pace either part or all the way — and take the stairs instead of an elevator or escalator when you can. Francois cautions, though, that people with health conditions such as diabetes should discuss exercise routines with their doctors before they start them to get guidance about doing them safely and effectively. This is one case in which, instead of doing strenuous, time-consuming exercise — which many people are likely to skip precisely because it seems so onerous — giving it all you've got for a few quick minutes brings better health results. So snack away!

Monique Francois, doctoral candidate, exercise metabolism, nutrition, and type 2 diabetes, University of British Columbia, Canada. Ms. Francois was formerly a teaching fellow and research assistant at the School of Physical Education, Sport and Exercise Sciences, University of Otago, Dunedin, New Zealand, where this study was done as part of her master's degree. Her study was published in *Diabetologia*.

SUPPLEMENTS THAT HELP
MANAGE DIABETES

Lifestyle change has always been the cornerstone treatment for people with type 2 diabetes. Beyond that, natural approaches are rarely discussed. Mark Stengler, NMD, author of several books on alternative health, recommends a number of plant-based remedies for those with diabetes, some of which date back hundreds, even thousands, of years.

According to Dr. Stengler, type 2 diabetes absolutely can be prevented and, in certain cases, even reversed with diet, exercise, and appropriate dietary supplements. The following is some of his own "best practice" advice for prevention, maintenance, and symptom management of this lifestyle-related disease.

To prevent diabetes:

- **Curb sugar cravings with *Gymnema sylvestre*.** A staple of Ayurvedic medicine, this herb helps curb cravings for sugary foods that throw your blood glucose levels off balance. Scientists speculate that it works by positively influencing insulin-producing cells in the pancreas.

    Dr. Stengler believes *Gymnema sylvestre* works best when used in combination with other glucose-balancing herbs, such as bitter melon and fenugreek. Ask your doctor for advice on the best combination and dosage for you.

- **Chromium can normalize sugar levels.** Your body requires adequate levels of chromium to properly control blood glucose levels.

This essential trace mineral aids in the uptake of blood sugar into the body's cells, where it can be used to generate energy more efficiently. It's also helpful in reducing sweet cravings.

Dr. Stengler advises up to 1,000 mcg of chromium a day (under your physician's supervision). He adds that this is a good mineral to take with gymnema.

- **Regulate blood sugar with fiber and fiber supplements.** Soluble fiber helps prevent or control prediabetes and diabetes by slowing the rate at which intestines release glucose into the bloodstream, thus modulating fluctuations in blood sugar levels. Rich sources of soluble fiber include plant foods, such as legumes, oat bran, rye, barley, broccoli, carrots, artichokes, peas, prunes, berries, and bananas. In a small study in Taiwan, scientists found that supplementation with glucomannan (a soluble dietary fiber made from konjac flour) lowered elevated levels of blood lipids, cholesterol, and glucose in people with diabetes.

Most Americans eat too much junk food and too little fiber. For his patients who fall into that category, Dr. Stengler typically prescribes one glucomannan capsule thirty minutes before lunch and dinner and another before bedtime with a large glass of water.

To manage symptoms and minimize complications:

- **Boost antioxidant levels with alpha-lipoic acid.** This powerful antioxidant kills free radicals that damage cells and cause pain, inflammation, burning, tingling, and numbness in people who have peripheral neuropathy (nerve damage) caused by diabetes. Studies also suggest that alpha-lipoic acid (ALA) enables the body to utilize glucose more efficiently.

    Dr. Stengler says to take alpha-lipoic acid daily under a physician's supervision.
- **Decrease blood glucose levels with chamomile tea.** Drinking chamomile tea, a rich source of antioxidants, may help prevent diabetes complications, such as blindness, nerve damage, and kidney problems, according to recent research by UK and Japanese scientists.

    Drink chamomile tea along with antioxidant-rich black, white, and green teas, says Dr. Stengler.
- **Take omega-3 fatty acids to reduce inflammation.** These healthy fats improve the body's ability to respond to insulin,

reduce inflammation, lower blood lipids, and prevent excessive blood clotting. Good dietary sources of omega-3 fatty acids include cold-water fish, such as salmon or cod (eat two or three times a week), olive or canola oil, flaxseed, and English walnuts.

Unless you know you are getting sufficient omega-3 fatty acids in your diet, it's good to take a daily fish oil supplement that contains about 1,000 mg of the omega-3 fatty acid eicosapentaenoic acid (EPA) and about 500 mg of the omega-3 fatty acid docosahexaenoic acid (DHA).

Caution: Because many dietary supplements lower blood sugar, and fish oil supplements may alter the way anticoagulant therapy functions, it is critical to work closely with your doctor before and while taking any of the above supplements. He/she will prescribe the right doses for you and may also suggest that you alter other medications accordingly.

Don't Neglect the ABCs of Diabetes Self-Care

When addressing a difficult disease such as diabetes, all the nutrients and vitamins in the world will do no good if you do not also follow the basics of diabetes self-care: maintain a healthy weight, get twenty to thirty minutes of exercise most days of the week, follow a diet that emphasizes lean proteins and healthy fats and limits simple carbohydrates, monitor blood glucose levels, and take diabetes, blood pressure, and cholesterol medicine as prescribed by your physician. Dr. Stengler adds that even as simple a measure as taking a ten-minute walk after each meal can keep blood sugar under control. Start today.

Mark A. Stengler, NMD, a naturopathic medical doctor and leading authority on the practice of alternative and integrated medicine. Dr. Stengler is author of the *Health Revelations* newsletter, *The Natural Physician's Healing Therapies,* and *Bottom Line's Prescription for Natural Cures.* He is also the founder and medical director of the Stengler Center for Integrative Medicine in Encinitas, California, and former adjunct associate clinical professor at the National College of Natural Medicine in Portland, Oregon. MarkStengler.com.

SUPERCHARGE YOUR
DIABETES MEDICATIONS

Alpha-lipoic acid is an endogenous (made in the body) antioxidant that helps transform blood sugar (glucose) into energy. It is found in foods such as red meat and liver, though it is difficult to get enough from food to work effectively with your medication for type 2 diabetes.

When taken in the larger doses that are found in supplements, alpha-lipoic acid lowers blood sugar and may reduce pain, itching, and other symptoms caused by diabetes-related nerve damage (neuropathy). For diabetic neuropathy, I typically recommend 400 to 500 mg of alpha-lipoic acid, twice daily. For general antioxidant benefit, 100 to 300 mg daily is usually sufficient.

If you're taking a diabetes medication that lowers blood sugar, such as metformin or glyburide, the addition of alpha-lipoic acid may allow you to use a smaller drug dose. If your glucose levels are stabilized through diet and regular exercise (without medication), you may want to take alpha-lipoic acid indefinitely.

Caution: Taking too much alpha-lipoic acid with a diabetes drug could lead to excessively low blood sugar, which can cause anxiety, sweating, shakiness, and/or confusion. Alpha-lipoic acid also may interact with chemotherapy drugs and thyroid medication such as levothyroxine. Talk to your doctor before taking alpha-lipoic acid with any prescription medication.

Thomas Kruzel, ND, a naturopathic physician at the Rockwood Natural Medicine Clinic in Scottsdale, Arizona. He is author of *The Homeopathic Emergency Guide.* RockwoodNaturalMedicine.com.

Move Over Blueberries . . . Olive Leaf Extract May Be the New Star

Olive leaf (*Olea europaea*) remedies are popular in countries ranging from Greece and Italy to Australia and New Zealand and in Africa. Leaves from olive trees contain flavonoid polyphenols such as oleuropein and hydroxytyrosol, which have antioxidant, antiviral, anti-inflammatory, and antimicrobial effects. In fact, researchers have found that extract made from olive leaf has a greater antioxidant capacity than other more highly touted sources, including pomegranate, blueberry, cranberry, and even green tea. Multiple studies have demonstrated olive leaf's potential in:

- **Preventing or managing infection.** In lab and animal studies, scientists have discovered that olive leaf is effective against a wide range of bacteria, viruses, fungi, and parasites — and without the worrisome side effects of antibiotics.
- **Lowering blood pressure.** In a South African study, olive leaf extract thwarted the development of severe hypertension in salt-sensitive, insulin-resistant rats.
- **Preventing heart disease.** Laboratory studies in Italy showed that olive leaf extract inhibits low-density lipoprotein (LDL)

oxidation. An Australian study showed that liquid olive leaf extract (tested in vitro) has antiplatelet effects that may help prevent clots.

- **Controlling blood sugar.** Animal studies suggest that olive leaf improves sugar uptake, which may prove helpful in preventing or treating diabetes and metabolic syndrome.

Three Ways to Try It

Olive leaf is readily available online and in health-food stores as an extract and in capsule form, as well as tea, though some find the taste bitter and unappealing.

Advice from Dr. Yanez: At the first sign of a cold or the flu, take three capsules three or four times a day, or, if you prefer the extract, drink it straight (follow the package directions for one serving) or diluted in water or juice three times a day, or drink two cups daily of olive leaf tea.

Olive leaf is generally considered safe, but as always when trying an herbal remedy, check with your doctor first. This is especially important if you have a chronic condition — olive leaf may interact with certain diabetes and blood pressure drugs, and some people are allergic to olive tree pollen and should be on the alert for hives or other signs of allergy to the extract.

JoAnn Yanez, ND, Yanez Consulting, Sioux Falls, South Dakota. She is an expert in health policy and integrative medicine and former vice president of the New York Association of Naturopathic Physicians.

MACA: THE SUPERFOOD THAT HELPS WITH EVERYTHING

Super foods are foods and herbs considered to be especially healthful due to their hefty nutritional content. The list includes familiar favorites, such as blueberries, broccoli, and beans. Now a more exotic superfood you may never have heard of is generating excitement in the world of natural health — a Peruvian root vegetable called maca (*Lepidium meyenii* or *peruvianum*), pronounced MACK-ah.

The root of the maca is shaped like a large radish. It is a cousin to other cruciferous plants, such as cauliflower and Brussels sprouts. Peruvians traditionally boil or roast the maca root or grind it into flour for baking. However, despite maca's popular description as a superfood, you won't see it in food form in this country. Instead, the root is dried and ground into a fine powder. It then is distributed primarily in capsules, although you can also buy the powder to blend into beverages or sprinkle on foods.

In addition to its healthful fiber, complex carbohydrates, and protein, maca provides numerous minerals, including calcium, magnesium, phosphorous, potassium, sulfur, iron, zinc, iodine, and copper; vitamins B-1, B-2, C, and E; nearly twenty amino acids, including linoleic acid, palmitic acid, and oleic acid; as well as various plant sterols, which are natural cholesterol-lowering agents. All of these nutrients have been shown to promote health in a multitude of ways.

Here is what this superfood can do for you.

Fight Stress and Disease

Any kind of stress — from work, personal problems, illness, injury, toxins, hormonal imbalances, or any other source — can negatively affect how our bodies function. Maca is what holistic doctors call an adaptogen, a plant or herb that boosts the body's ability to resist, deal with, and recover from emotional and physical stress.

Practitioners of traditional medicine from China and India have known about and made use of adaptogens for centuries, though the term itself was not coined until the middle of the twentieth century. Well-known adaptogens include the herbs ashwagandha, ginseng, rhodiola, and licorice root, all of which I have prescribed to my patients with much success over the years.

How it works: To be classified as an adaptogen, a natural substance must meet specific criteria. It must be nontoxic, normalize levels of chemicals raised during periods of stress, and produce physical, chemical, and/or biological responses that increase the body's resistance to stress.

Although all adaptogenic plants contain antioxidants, researchers do not believe that antioxidants alone account for adaptogens' normalizing powers. Rather, it is thought that a variety of phytochemicals helps balance the dozens of endocrine, digestive, and neural hormones that operate throughout the body — including insulin (which regulates blood sugar levels) and dopamine (which enhances and stabilizes mood). Many adaptogens also stimulate immune system components, leading to better immune function.

More of Maca's Superpowers

Animal studies suggest that maca may reduce the risk for the following:

- **Arthritis** — by promoting cartilage growth.
- **Blood toxicity** — by improving liver function.
- **Diabetes** — by allowing for better control over blood sugar levels and body weight.
- **Digestive health** — by combating ulcers.
- **Fatigue** — by increasing energy and endurance.
- **Heart disease** — by lowering levels of LDL "bad" cholesterol and triglycerides (a type of blood fat).
- **Memory and mood** — by enhancing certain brain chemicals.

- **Osteoporosis** — by increasing bone density.
- **Prostate problems** — by reducing prostate enlargement.

The Safest Way to Start

Maca generally appears to be safe, given its long history of use by Peruvians, but there are a few guidelines to bear in mind.

Breast cancer patients taking tamoxifen or other estrogen blockers and women who have had breast cancer must not use maca, because it raises estrogen levels. Women in a family with a strong history of breast cancer should discuss maca use with their doctors first. People who take thyroid medication should be monitored by their doctors because maca may increase thyroid activity.

Since its long-term effects have not been scientifically studied, I recommend taking a break from maca now and then in order to give the body's cell receptors a break from any hormone stimulation. People who want to try maca to see if it is a superfood for them should take supplements for three months, then stop using maca for one or two weeks. They may then continue this regimen as needed for symptom relief.

How Much to Take

Maca is available in supplement and powder form. The average dose of maca supplements is 1,000 to 2,000 mg daily — which you can take with or without food at any time of day.

Or you can get your maca by adding powder to your favorite foods and drinks. It has a slightly nutty flavor, so you may enjoy mixing it with almond milk. Other ways to incorporate maca into your diet:

- **Sprinkle on cereal** (hot or cold).
- **Mix into your favorite smoothie or protein shake.**
- **Add to yogurt or applesauce,** perhaps with a little cinnamon.
- **Stir into tea** — especially chai blends, as the flavors complement each other.
- **Use in baking** — substitute maca powder for one-quarter of the flour in any recipe (no more, or it might affect texture or consistency).

Be aware: Maca powder has a high fiber content and may initially cause gassiness. I suggest beginning with one teaspoon a day, then gradually increasing your intake by one teaspoon every five days until you find your comfort zone. The optimum dosage is three to six teaspoons daily.

Mark A. Stengler, NMD, a naturopathic medical doctor and leading authority on the practice of alternative and integrated medicine. Dr. Stengler is author of the *Health Revelations* newsletter, *The Natural Physician's Healing Therapies,* and *Bottom Line's Prescription for Natural Cures.* He is also the founder and medical director of the Stengler Center for Integrative Medicine in Encinitas, California, and former adjunct associate clinical professor at the National College of Natural Medicine in Portland, Oregon. MarkStengler.com.

6
MANAGE YOUR DIABETES

If you are already dealing with a diabetes diagnosis, day-to-day life will obviously be different from your average Joe's or Jane's. And while you would do well to practice the advice on diabetes prevention, it's important to up your game if you are living with the real thing. Your life doesn't have to revolve around medications and measurements, but awareness of all the factors is key.

You may not just be reading about insulin; you may be taking it yourself. What is the safest way to do so? Do you or your caretaker know how to measure your glucose or how it might vary at certain times of the day? Even seemingly irrelevant circumstances such as weather can suddenly come into play, but armed with the following articles (and in some cases, a warm coat), you can brave any storm.

STAY-WELL SECRETS FOR PEOPLE WITH DIABETES OR PREDIABETES

Many people downplay the seriousness of diabetes. That's a mistake. Because elevated glucose can damage blood vessels, nerves, the kidneys, and eyes, people with diabetes are much more likely to die from heart disease and/or kidney disease than people without diabetes — and they are at increased risk for infections, including gum disease, as well as blindness and amputation. (Nerve damage and poor circulation can allow dangerous infections to go undetected.)

And diabetes can be sneaky — increased thirst, urination, and/or hunger are the most common symptoms, but many people have no symptoms and are unaware that they are sick.

Despite these sobering facts, doctors rarely have time to give their patients all the information they need to cope with the complexities of diabetes. Fortunately, diabetes educators — health care professionals, such as registered nurses, registered dietitians, and medical social workers — can give patients practical advice on the best ways to control their condition.*

Good news: Most health insurers, including Medicare, cover the cost of diabetes

---

* See the Resources section for more information on how to find an educator near you.

patients' visits with a diabetes educator.

Savvy Eating Habits

Most doctors advise people with diabetes or prediabetes to cut back on refined carbohydrates, such as cakes and cookies, and eat more fruits, vegetables, and whole grains. This maximizes nutrition and promotes a healthy body weight (being overweight greatly increases diabetes risk). Other steps to take include the following:

• **Drink one extra glass of water each day.** The extra fluid will help prevent dehydration, which can raise glucose levels.
• **Never skip meals — especially breakfast.** Don't assume that bypassing a meal and fasting for more than five to six hours will help lower glucose levels. It actually triggers the liver to release glucose into the bloodstream.

  Better strategy: Eat three small meals daily and have snacks in between. Start with breakfast, such as a cup of low-fat yogurt and whole-wheat toast with peanut butter or a small bowl of whole-grain cereal and a handful of nuts.

  Good snack options: A small apple or three graham crackers. Each of these snacks contains about 15 g of carbohydrates.
• **Practice the "plate method."** Divide a nine-inch plate in half. Fill half with veg-

etables, then split the other half into quarters — one for protein, such as salmon, lean meat, beans, or tofu, and the other for starches, such as one-third cup of pasta or one-half cup of peas or corn. Then have a small piece of fruit. This is an easy way to practice portion control — and get the nutrients you need.

- **Ask yourself if you are satisfied after you take each bite.** If the answer is yes, stop eating. This simple strategy helped one of my clients lose fifty pounds.
- **Be wary of "sugar-free" foods.** These products, including sugar-free cookies and diabetic candy, are often high in carbohydrates, which are the body's primary source of glucose. You may be better off eating the regular product, which is more satisfying. Compare the carbohydrate contents on product labels.

Get Creative with Exercise

If you have diabetes or prediabetes, you've probably been told to get more exercise. Walking is especially helpful. For those with diabetes, walking for at least two hours a week has been shown to reduce the risk for death by 30 percent over an eight-year period. For those with prediabetes, walking for thirty minutes five days a week reduces by about 60 percent the risk that your condition will progress to diabetes. But if you'd like some other options, consider the following:*

- **Armchair workouts.** These exercises, which are performed while seated and are intended for people with physical limitations to standing, increase stamina, muscle tone, flexibility, and coordination.
- **Strength training.** This type of exercise builds muscle, which burns more calories than fat even when you are not exercising.‡ Use hand weights, exercise machines, or the weight of your own body — for example, leg squats or bicep curls with no weights. Aim for two to three sessions of strength training weekly, on alternate days.
- **Stretching,** even while watching TV or talking on the phone. By building a stretching routine into your daily activities, you won't need to set aside a separate time to do it. If your body is flexible, it's easier to perform other kinds of physical activity. Stretching also promotes better circulation. Before stretching, do a brief warm-up, such as walking for five minutes and doing several arm windmills. Aim to do stretching

* Consult your doctor before starting a new exercise program.
‡ Be sure to check with your doctor before starting a strength-training program — this type of exercise can raise blood pressure.

exercises at least three times weekly, including before your other workouts.

Control Your Blood Glucose

If you are diagnosed with diabetes, blood glucose control is the immediate goal. Self-monitoring can be performed using newer devices that test blood glucose levels.

Good choices: LifeScan's OneTouch Ultra, Bayer's Contour, or Abbott Laboratories' FreeStyle.

The hemoglobin A1C test, which is ordered by your doctor and is typically done two to four times a year, determines how well glucose levels have been controlled over the previous two to three months.

If you have prediabetes: Don't settle for a fasting glucose test, which measures blood glucose after you have fasted overnight. It misses two-thirds of all cases of diabetes. The oral glucose tolerance test (OGTT), which involves testing glucose immediately before drinking a premixed glass of glucose and repeating the test two hours later, is more reliable. If you can't get an OGTT, ask for an A1C test and fasting glucose test.

If you have diabetes or prediabetes, you should have your blood pressure and cholesterol checked at every doctor visit and schedule regular eye exams and dental appointments. In addition, don't overlook the following:

- **Proper kidney testing.** Doctors most commonly recommend annual microalbumin and creatinine urine tests to check for kidney disease. You also may want to ask for a glomerular filtration rate test, which measures kidney function.
- **Meticulous foot care.** High glucose levels can reduce sensation in your feet, making it hard to know when you have a cut, blister, or injury. In addition to seeing a podiatrist at least once a year and inspecting your own feet daily, be wary of everyday activities that can be dangerous for people with diabetes.

  Stepping into hot bath water, for example, can cause a blister or skin damage that can become infected. To protect yourself, check the water temperature on your wrist or elbow before you step in. The temperature should be warm to the touch — not hot.

Stay Up to Date on Medications

Once diabetes medication has been prescribed, people with diabetes should review their drug regimen with their doctors at every visit. Insulin is the most commonly used diabetes drug, but you may want to also ask your doctor about these relatively new medications:

- **DPP-4 inhibitors.** These drugs include sitagliptin, which lowers glucose levels by increasing the amount of insulin secreted by the pancreas. DPP-4 inhibitors are used alone or with another type of diabetes medication.

• **Pramlintide.** Administered with an injectable pen, pramlintide helps control blood glucose and reduces appetite, which may help with weight loss. It is used in addition to insulin.

If you have prediabetes or diabetes: Always consult a pharmacist or doctor before taking any over-the-counter products. Cold medicines with a high sugar content may raise your blood glucose, for example, and wart removal products may cause skin ulcers. Pay close attention to drug label warnings.

Theresa Garnero, advanced practice registered nurse (APRN), certified diabetes educator (CDE), and clinical nurse manager of the Center for Diabetes Services at the California Pacific Medical Center in San Francisco. She is author of *Your First Year with Diabetes: What to Do, Month by Month.*

FOUR BIG MISTAKES MOST PEOPLE WITH DIABETES MAKE . . . AND THE RIGHT WAYS TO STAY HEALTHY

If you have diabetes, you may think that you are taking all the right steps with your diet, medication, and exercise habits.

But the truth is, virtually all people with this common disease make mistakes in managing their condition — and unknowingly increase their risk for diabetes complications, such as heart attack, stroke, kidney failure, and blindness.

Small changes can give big results: Fortunately, you can correct these missteps if you understand some of the subtle aspects of diabetes that can easily derail one's care. To learn more, we spoke to Richard K. Bernstein, MD, an outspoken diabetes specialist who gives his patients no-holds-barred advice on controlling their disease.

Guerrilla tactics that really work: Dr. Bernstein, who was diagnosed himself with type 1 diabetes at age twelve, is vigorous and healthy at almost eighty. He swears by the sometimes unconventional but highly effective approach that he has developed and adopted for himself and the thousands of patients with type 1 and type 2 diabetes he has treated.

Here's where Dr. Bernstein thinks people with diabetes — and many mainstream medical authorities — have got it all wrong.

351

***Mistake #1:* Not recognizing hidden causes of elevated blood sugar.** Acute stress — such as a fight with your boss or anxiety about a key presentation — can raise it. If your glucose reading is higher than expected when you're stressed, an injection of rapid-acting insulin will bring it down if you have type 1 diabetes. If you have type 2, your own insulin secretions will likely lower blood sugar within twenty-four hours.

Infection raises blood sugar levels — and high blood sugar increases infection risk. Suspect infection if your glucose level is up and insulin isn't working as well as usual. Get prompt treatment so that your blood sugar will go down and the infection will heal. Beware of dental infections and gum disease.

What I do: I brush twice daily, floss after meals, and get tartar and plaque scrapings from a periodontist every three months.

***Mistake #2:* Using the wrong glucose meter.** Whether you inject insulin for type 1 diabetes, take oral drugs for type 2, or control your disease with diet and exercise alone, you must accurately track your blood sugar with home testing.

My advice: Test a meter you are considering buying in the store — take ten readings in succession using the manufacturer's "normal" control solution. A pharmacy with glucose meters on display will usually let you test them — ask the pharmacist. Readings should be within 6 mg/dL of the midpoint of that normal range.

Important: Make sure that you can return the device if you find it to be inaccurate later. If your insurance company won't cover a meter you like, file an appeal.

My favorite glucose meter: Of the many glucose meters for home use that I have tried, the FreeStyle Freedom Lite by Abbott, available at most drugstores or online for about twenty dollars, has been the most accurate.

Mistake #3: **Pricking your finger the wrong way.** If you use a glucose meter, your doctor will probably tell you to wipe the site with alcohol before pricking it. I disagree.

First, it isn't necessary to wipe your finger with alcohol — this dries out the skin and can lead to calluses, which makes it difficult to get a blood sample. Neither my patients nor I have ever developed an infection from not using alcohol.

However, you should wash your hands before drawing blood. This is especially true if you've been handling food or glucose tablets or applied hand cream — all of which can cause false high readings.

Helpful: Rinse your finger with warm water to get the blood flowing, and prick the back of your finger between the joints — this area may produce more blood and cause less pain.

***Mistake #4:* Overdoing vitamin C.** In excess, vitamin C raises blood sugar and inactivates the glucose-processing enzyme in the test strip, resulting in deceptively low glucose readings. You'll probably get all the vitamin C you need from vegetables (you shouldn't rely on fruit — it has too much natural sugar). If you must take supplements, 250 mg daily in a sustained-release form is tops. These formulations are less likely to cause blood sugar spikes.

How to Use Insulin the Right Way
Insulin injections are crucial for type 1 diabetes and often needed for type 2 diabetes. To use effectively:

- **Change with the seasons.** Most people need less insulin in summer than winter (or during a warm spell in colder months). Capillaries dilate when warm, and more blood containing insulin is delivered to peripheral tissues. Adjust your dose accordingly.
- **Prevent blood sugar spikes** by correctly gauging how much insulin you need to cover each meal and when to inject it. With regular (a type of short-acting insulin), that's usually thirty to forty-five minutes before the meal.

To determine your best timing: Inject an insulin dose, and check blood sugar after twenty-five minutes, then at five-minute intervals. When it has dropped by 5 mg/dL, it's time to eat. This may not work for people who have diabetic gastroparesis, which causes unpredictable stomach emptying.

Richard K. Bernstein, MD, a diabetes specialist in private practice in Mamaroneck, New York. Dr. Bernstein is also author of several books on diabetes, including *Dr. Bernstein's Diabetes Solution: A Complete Guide to Achieving Normal Blood Sugars,* DiabetesBook.com. His free monthly teleseminars are available at AskDrBernstein .net.

The All-Day, All-Night Guide to Controlling Your Diabetes

From the time you wake up until you go to bed, it is essential to keep your blood sugar as stable as possible if you have diabetes.

Reasons: Over time, uncontrolled elevated blood sugar harms the blood vessels, kidneys, eyes, and nerves, increasing the risk for heart attack, stroke, kidney failure, blindness, and tissue damage that can require limb amputation.

Diabetes Is Also Linked to Dementia

Despite these dangers, scarcely half of the twenty-three million Americans who have been diagnosed with diabetes have their disease under control. If you're struggling, you can significantly improve your blood sugar control by eating the right foods and doing the right things at the right times of day.

Throughout the Day

It is key to eat foods that digest slowly, so blood sugar remains relatively stable, and avoid foods that are digested quickly, triggering rapid blood sugar spikes. This also helps control weight — an important factor because excess weight contributes to diabetes complications. Follow these guidelines:

- **Have 40 to 50 g of carbohydrates at each meal.** Stick with mostly complex carbs (whole grains, vegetables, nuts), and limit refined carbs (cakes, white pasta). Check labels!
- **Avoid foods with more than 10 g of sugar per serving.**
- **Have some lean protein every day** — chicken, fish, lean beef, low-fat dairy, eggs, tofu. Most people get enough protein, so you do not need protein with each meal unless your doctor recommends this.
- **Limit starches** (corn, peas, potatoes, sweet potatoes) to one serving per meal.
- **Limit fruit to two servings per day.** A serving equals one small handheld fruit (peach, plum), half an apple or half a banana, twelve grapes, one cup of strawberries, or one-half cup of blueberries, raspberries, or diced fruit (such as melon). Avoid pineapples and dried fruits, which are high in sugar.
- **At wake-up time:** Test your blood sugar before breakfast. If it is high, you may have eaten too many carbohydrates too close to bedtime the night before. Or your levels may have fallen too low during the night, so your liver released more glucose, causing a blood sugar "rebound." Talk to your doctor — you may need to adjust your medication dosage and/or timing.
- **At breakfast:** The morning meal helps get

357

your metabolism running efficiently, so don't skip it.

Ideal: One or two slices of wholegrain bread with a soft spread that contains cholesterol-lowering plant sterols, such as Smart Balance or Promise Activ, plus a two-egg vegetable omelet. It is fine to use whole eggs, but if you have high cholesterol, make your omelet with egg whites instead and limit egg yolks to two per week.

Another good choice: One cup of unsweetened or lightly sweetened whole-grain cereal that contains no more than 25 g of carbohydrates per cup, such as Cheerios or Product 19, plus one-half cup of blueberries and one cup of low-fat milk. Don't be fooled into thinking that high-fiber necessarily equals healthful — you still must check labels to see if the food is too high in carbs.

Your doctor may advise you to take a dose of diabetes medication right before breakfast.

Also: If you have diabetic nerve damage, take 100 mcg of vitamin B-12 daily. If you take blood pressure medication, morning is the best time, because blood pressure typically is higher during the day than at night. If you plan to drive, test your blood sugar before leaving home.

• **In midmorning:** A midmorning snack is generally not necessary unless your doctor advises you to have one (for instance, due to the type of insulin you are on). However, if you start to feel weak or dizzy, have a snack that provides no more than 10 g of carbohydrates — for instance, a small tangerine, half a banana, or two graham cracker squares.

- **At lunch:** Good choices include a sandwich, such as turkey, lettuce, and tomato on whole-wheat bread, or sushi with rice (preferably brown).

  Common mistakes: Eating too much (especially at restaurants), choosing a fruit plate (too much sugar and no protein), overdoing it on chips or condiments (which can be high in fat or sugar).

- **In midafternoon:** Again, have a snack only if you feel weak or your doctor recommends it, and limit yourself to no more than 10 g of carbs.

  Good choices: About fifteen pistachios, ten almonds, or one-third of an ounce of whole grain crackers.

- **At dinner:** Check your blood sugar before dinner. If you are on oral diabetes medication, take it just before your meal.

  Dinner should include four ounces of lean protein, several generous servings of vegetables, and one serving of a starch. Have a green salad, but skip the high-carb, high-fat dressings. Instead, drizzle greens with lemon juice, balsamic vinegar, safflower oil, and/or olive oil.

Limit: One alcoholic drink daily, consumed with a meal. Opt for five ounces of wine, twelve ounces of a low-carb beer, such as Miller Lite, or one ounce of distilled liquor (Scotch, vodka). Avoid mixed drinks, which are often high in carbs.

Dessert options: A scoop of low-carb, no-sugar-added ice cream, berries, two Lorna Doone cookies, or three Social Tea Biscuits.

- **In the evening:** This is the best time to exercise to maximize muscle cells' absorption of glucose. Strength training and stretching are good, but aerobic exercise is most important because it increases insulin sensitivity (cells' ability to respond to insulin) for up to fourteen hours. Each week, aim for two and a half hours of moderate-intensity aerobic exercise, such as walking, or one and a half hours of strenuous activity. For blood sugar control, thirty-minute workouts are generally most effective. As part of your exercise regimen, consider tai chi. In one study, diabetes patients who did this martial art significantly lowered their blood sugar levels.

  Caution: Ask your doctor before starting an exercise program. Test blood sugar before each workout. If it is below 100 mg/dL, have a snack before exercising. Do not work out when your blood sugar is higher than 250 mg/dL — when blood sugar is this high, exercise may elevate it even further. If you have retinopathy (damaged blood vessels in the retina), to protect vision, do not lift weights above eye level.

- **At bedtime:** If you are on long-acting insulin, a bedtime injection controls night-time glucose levels. If you take cholesterol-lowering medication, do so now — it is most effective at night. Test your blood sugar at bedtime. If it is somewhat elevated (but not above 250 mg/dL), lower it with ten minutes of moderate exercise.

Insomnia doesn't raise blood sugar, but the stress it creates can.

To promote sleep: Turn off the cell phone, TV, and computer at least thirty minutes before bedtime so your mind can quiet down. Take a warm bath, checking your feet for wounds or signs of infection, because diabetes often damages nerves in the feet.

Have you been told that you snore? Diabetes patients are prone to sleep apnea (repeated halts in breathing during sleep), which contributes to poor blood sugar control. Do you frequently get up at night to urinate? It could be a sign that your medication needs adjusting. If you have either symptom, tell your doctor.

The late Stanley Mirsky, MD, coauthor of the *Diabetes Survival Guide.* Dr. Mirsky was a practicing internist and diabetologist, a past president of the American Diabetes Association of New York State, and a board member of the Joslin Diabetes Center. He was named Endocrinologist of the Year for 2005 at the Mount Sinai School of Medicine.

MINOR MISSTEPS CAN MAKE
YOUR DIABETES WORSE

Despite what you may have heard, type 2 diabetes doesn't have to be a lifelong condition. It can be controlled and even reversed in the early stages or stopped from progressing in the later stages — with none of the dire consequences of out-of-control blood sugar.

The problem is, even people who are following all the doctor's orders may still be sabotaging their efforts with seemingly minor missteps that can have big consequences. Among the most common mistakes that harm people with diabetes are oversights in the way they eat and exercise. For example:

Skimping on protein. The majority of people with type 2 diabetes are overweight or obese. These individuals know that they need to lose weight but sometimes fail despite their best efforts.

Here's what often happens: We have had it drummed into our heads that the best way to lose weight is to go on a low-fat diet. However, these diets tend to be low in protein — and you need more protein, not less, if you have type 2 diabetes and are cutting calories to lose weight.

What's so special about protein? You need protein to maintain muscle mass. The average adult starts losing lean muscle mass every year after about age forty. If you have diabetes, you'll probably lose more muscle mass than someone without it. And the loss will be even greater if your diabetes is not well controlled.

Muscle is important because it burns more calories than other tissues in your body. Also, people with a higher and more active muscle mass find it easier to maintain healthy blood glucose levels, since active muscle doesn't require insulin to clear high glucose from the blood.

My advice: Protein should provide 20 to 30 percent of total daily calories. For example, if you're on an 1,800-calorie diet, that's about 90 to 135 g of protein a day. If you're on a 1,200-to 1,500-calorie diet, that's about 60 to 113 g of protein a day.

Examples: Good protein sources include fish, skinless poultry, nonfat or low-fat dairy, legumes, and nuts and seeds. A three-ounce chicken breast has about 30 g of protein; a three-ounce piece of haddock, 17 g; one-half cup of low-fat cottage cheese, 14 g; and one-quarter cup of whole almonds, 7 g of protein.

Note: If you have kidney problems, you may need to limit your protein intake. Check with your doctor.

Not doing resistance training. It's widely known that aerobic exercise is good for weight loss and blood sugar control. What usually gets short shrift (especially among older people) is resistance training, such as lifting weights and using stretch bands.

When you build muscle, you use more glucose, which helps reduce glucose levels in the blood. If you take insulin for your diabetes (see below), toned muscles will also make your body more sensitive to it.

An added benefit: People who do resistance training can often reduce their doses of insulin or other medications within a few months.

My advice: Do a combination of resistance, aerobic, and flexibility exercises. Start with twenty minutes total, four days a week, splitting the time equally among the three types of exercise. Try to work up to sixty minutes total, six days a week. An exercise physiologist or personal trainer certified in resistance training can help choose the best workout for you.

If You Take Diabetes Meds
Sometimes, diet and exercise aren't enough to tame out-of-control blood sugar. Avoid the following traps:

• **Drug-induced weight gain.** Ironically, the drugs that are used to treat diabetes also can cause weight gain as a side effect. If you start taking insulin, you can expect to gain about ten pounds within six months. With oral drugs, such as glipizide, you'll probably gain from four to seven pounds.
  My advice: Ask your doctor if you can

switch to one of the newer, "weight-friendly" medications.

Examples: A form of insulin called insulin detemir causes less weight gain than insulin glargine or insulin isophane. Newer oral drugs called DPP-4 inhibitors, such as sitagliptin, saxagliptin, and alogliptin, don't have weight gain as a side effect.

Important: The newer drugs are more expensive and may not be covered by insurance. But if they don't cause you to gain weight, you might get by with a lower dose — and reduced cost.

• **Erratic testing.** You should test your blood sugar levels at least four to six times a day, particularly when you're making lifestyle changes that could affect the frequency and doses of medication. Your doctor has probably advised you to test before and after exercise and before meals.

My advice: Be sure to also test after meals. This will help determine the effects of different types and amounts of foods.

Osama Hamdy, MD, PhD, medical director of the Joslin Diabetes Center's Obesity Clinical Program and an assistant professor of medicine at Harvard Medical School, both in Boston. He is also coauthor of *The Diabetes Breakthrough.*

No Two Diabetes Patients Are the Same

Chances are you know one or more people who have type 2 diabetes, or perhaps you have been diagnosed with the condition yourself.

The number of Americans with diabetes is truly staggering — a new case is diagnosed every seventeen seconds. And of course, the consequences of uncontrolled diabetes are dire, including increased risk for heart attack and other cardiovascular problems, blindness, leg amputation, kidney failure, and, ultimately, premature death.

To help meet this enormous challenge, medical research has been stepped up.

Now: American researchers have joined forces with their European counterparts to devise new strategies to diagnose and manage diabetes more effectively than ever before.

Easier Diagnosis

In the United States, twenty-nine million people have diabetes. This includes roughly twenty-one million who have been diagnosed and an estimated eight million who are undiagnosed. To break it down even further, more than 25 percent of the U.S. population aged over sixty-five years has diabetes!*

* Centers for Disease Control and Prevention. National Diabetes Fact Sheet: General Information

Experts hope that a change in the diagnostic process will lead to more widespread testing and fewer undiagnosed cases.

Until recently, diabetes was typically diagnosed using one of two standard tests — a blood test that requires an overnight fast to measure blood glucose levels and an oral glucose tolerance test, which involves drinking a high-sugar mixture and then having blood drawn thirty minutes, one hour, and two hours later to show how long it takes blood glucose levels to return to normal.

The problem: Both of these tests are inconvenient for the patient, and they measure blood glucose levels only at the time of the test. Many people never get tested because they don't like the idea of having to fast overnight or wait hours to complete a test.

New approach: More widespread use of the A1C test. For decades, the A1C test, which provides a person's average blood glucose levels over a period of two to three months, has been used to monitor how well people with diabetes were controlling their disease. However, it wasn't deemed a reliable tool for

---

and National Estimates on Diabetes in the United States, 2011. Atlanta, Georgia, U.S. Department of Health and Human Services, Centers for Disease Control and Prevention, 2011, http://care.diabetes journals.org/content/35/12/2650.full.

diagnosis.

Now, after major improvements that have standardized the measurements from laboratory to laboratory, the A1C test is considered a practical and convenient diagnostic option.

The A1C requires no fasting or special preparation, so it's the perfect "no excuses" test. A1C tests analyzed by accredited labs (such as LabCorp and Quest Diagnostics) meet the latest standardization criteria.

Updated Treatment Guidelines

Recently, the American Diabetes Association and the European Association for the Study of Diabetes collaborated on recommendations for best treatment practices for type 2 diabetes. The most significant change in the recent guidelines is the concept of individualized treatment.

The problem: In the past, diabetes care was based on a one-size-fits-all strategy — with few exceptions, everyone with the condition got basically the same treatment.

New approach: The recently released guidelines acknowledge that there are multiple treatment options for each patient and that the best treatment for one patient may be different from what another patient requires.

This is important because diabetes affects an enormously wide range of people. For example, diabetes can strike a thin seventy-seven-year-old woman or a three-hundred-pound teenage boy, and their treatment needs and goals will be as different as their characteristics.

After reviewing a patient's medical history and individual lifestyle, the doctor and patient consider treatment options together and decide on the best fit. Factors that are more explicitly spelled out in the new guidelines include:

- **Other medical conditions and medications.** If diabetes treatments interact badly with a patient's current medications, it may cause one of the medications to become ineffective, amplify the effects of the drugs, or cause allergic reactions or serious, even life-threatening side effects. This is especially true for people being treated for kidney disease or heart problems, as many diabetes medications may exacerbate those health issues.
- **Lifestyle and daily schedule.** Diabetes management is easier for people who have predictable schedules. For example, a full-time worker who regularly wakes up at seven a.m., eats breakfast, takes a lunch hour, and is home for dinner will have simpler treatment needs than a college student who sleeps past noon, eats cold pizza for breakfast, then pulls an all-nighter.

If a physician gives standard insulin recommendations to someone who has an unusual eating and sleeping schedule, it is easy to have blood sugar drop too low, a dangerous condition called hypoglycemia. That's why it is important that patients share as many details of their lives as possible, even if the information seems irrelevant.

Best Treatment Strategies

Until recently, diabetes has been treated with a stepwise approach — starting with conservative treatment, adding medication later only when needed. This sounds good, except that new treatments are incorporated only after previous treatments fail and blood glucose rises.

The problem: Depending on scheduled doctor visits, blood sugar may remain elevated for months or even years before anyone catches the change.

New approach: Research suggests that if physicians intervene more intensively at the beginning, they have the potential to stop the progression of diabetes. With this in mind, treatment aims to decrease the rate at which the body loses insulin-producing ability and prevent diabetes complications by not allowing blood sugar to exceed safe levels.

Under this new scenario, doctors hit diabetes full force with the patient's individualized treatment plan (including lifestyle changes and medication), instead of with graduated, step-up treatments.

What the new guidelines mean for anyone diagnosed with diabetes: If your current diabetes treatment plan does not address the points described in this article, see your doctor. Your treatment may need to be more customized.

Ildiko Lingvay, MD, MPH, an assistant professor in the departments of internal medicine and clinical science and a practicing endocrinologist at the University of Texas Southwestern Medical Center in Dallas. Dr. Lingvay is an internationally recognized researcher who has authored several dozen articles related to type 2 diabetes, obesity, and metabolic syndrome.

IF YOU HAVE DIABETES . . . HOW TO FAST SAFELY FOR A MEDICAL TEST

Recently, an employee at Bottom Line Publications was scheduled for a colonoscopy, the screening test for colon cancer. The medical test turned into medical mayhem.

The day before the test, the woman followed her doctor's orders to start ingesting a "clear liquid" diet, which includes soft drinks, Jell-O, and other clear beverages. But when she drank the "prep" — the bowel-cleaning solution that is consumed the evening before a colonoscopy (and sometimes also the morning of) — she vomited. Over and over. As a result, her colon wasn't sufficiently emptied to conduct the test, which had to be postponed.

What went wrong?

The woman has diabetes, and her glucose (blood sugar) levels had become unstable, triggering nausea and vomiting. Yet not one medical professional — not a doctor, not a nurse, not a medical technician — had warned her that people with diabetes need to take special precautions with food and diabetes medicine whenever they have any medical test that involves an extended period of little or no eating. Unfortunately, this lack of diabetes-customized instruction about medical tests is very common.

Do It Early

If you're undergoing a test that requires only overnight fasting, which includes many types of CT scans, MRIs, and X-rays, make sure that the test is scheduled for early in the morning — no later than nine a.m. That way, you will be able to eat after the test by ten or eleven a.m., which will help to stabilize your blood sugar as much as possible.

Don't expect your blood sugar levels to be perfect after the test. The important thing is to keep them from getting too high or too low.

The Right Clear Liquids

Conventional dietitians and doctors specify clear liquids and foods that reflect the conventional American diet, such as regular soda, sports drinks, Popsicles, Kool-Aid, and Jell-O (no red or purple). But the pH of these products is highly acidic. And that could contribute to diabetic ketoacidosis, a potentially life-threatening condition where the body burns fat instead of glucose for fuel, producing ketones, substances toxic to the liver and brain.

When my clients with diabetes are on a clear-liquid diet before a test, I recommend that they consume liquids with essential nutrients and a more balanced pH, such as apple juice, white grape juice, and clear, fat-free broth (vegetable, chicken or beef). A typical dinner could include up to three-quarters cup of juice (to limit sugar) and any amount of broth. A bedtime snack could include one-half cup of juice and any amount of broth. Plenty of good pure water between meals is also important to stay well-hydrated.

Check Blood Sugar Often

Many people with diabetes check their blood sugar a few times a day, typically right before a meal and again one to two hours afterward. But if you're on a clear-liquid diet or fasting before a medical test, you should check your glucose level every two to three hours. If it's too low, correct it with a fast-acting carbohydrate, such as four ounces of 100 percent fruit juice or a glucose gel (a squeezable, over-the-counter product).

Important: Take fruit juice or a glucose gel with you to the test — if the test is delayed for any reason, you can ingest the carb and keep your blood sugar on track.

Stop Taking Metformin

Your doctor likely will recommend that you stop taking the diabetes medication metformin twenty-four hours before the test. Metformin also can contribute to acidosis and typically is stopped twenty-four hours before and up to seventy-two hours after any test that requires a contrast agent (an injected dye often used in an X-ray, CT scan, or MRI that helps create the image). Talk to your doctor about when to stop taking your medication and when to resume or about the possible need for an alternative diabetes drug during this period.

An unexpected threat: Metformin is a component of many multi-ingredient diabetes drugs, so you may not realize you're taking it and therefore may need to discontinue it. Drugs that include metformin are Actoplus Met and Actoplus Met XR, Glucovance, Janumet and Janumet XR, Jentadueto, Kazano, Kombiglyze XR, and PrandiMet. New drugs are being developed constantly, so check with your pharmacist to see if yours contains metformin.

Also important: Many X-rays, CT scans, and MRIs utilize an injected dye or a contrast agent that can damage the kidneys in people with diabetes (contrast-induced nephropathy). Before restarting metformin, have a kidney function test (such as blood urea nitrogen, which requires a blood sample, and creatinine clearance, which requires a urine sample and a blood sample) that confirms that your kidneys are working normally. These tests are recommended twenty-four to forty-eight hours after your procedure is completed and usually are covered by insurance.

Decrease Insulin

Insulin is the hormone used by the body to regulate blood sugar — and many people with advanced diabetes give themselves shots of short- and/or long-acting insulin to keep glucose levels steady. But if you're consuming only clear liquids or fasting before a medical test, you likely will need to take less insulin.

Excellent guidelines for insulin use before a medical procedure have been created by the University of Michigan Comprehensive Diabetes Center. In general, it recommends:

• Take one-half of your usual dose of long-acting insulin the evening before the procedure.
• Take one-half of your usual dose of long-acting insulin the morning of the test and no short-acting insulin the morning of the test.

You can find the complete guidelines in downloadable PDF form at the University of Michigan website (link in Resources section at the back of the book). Print them out, and discuss them with your doctor.

Reduce Anxiety

Anxiety triggers the release of the stress hormone cortisol, which in turn sparks the production of glucose. To keep blood sugar balanced before a test, use these two methods to keep anxiety in check:

- **Get all your questions answered.** Fear of the unknown is the greatest stress. Before your procedure, create a list of questions to ask your doctor or nurse practitioner. Examples: What is going to happen during the procedure? What is it going to feel like? What are the potential side effects from the test, and how can I best avoid them? When will I be informed of the test results? How will the test results affect future decision-making about my health?
- **Breathe deeply.** Deep breathing is the easiest and simplest way to reduce anxiety. My recommendation, based on the approach of Andrew Weil, MD:
  Repeat this breathing exercise three times, and do it three times a day every day: Inhale for a count of four, hold for a count of seven, and exhale for a count of eight. (Don't worry if you can't do the entire count — shorter counts also work.) Do this exercise when you get up in the morning, at midday, and at bedtime. You can do it more often, but most people find three times simple and easy to integrate into their routines.

  Also, you can use this breathing technique in any situation that you find anxiety-producing, such as before and during the test itself. Breathe deeply three times every ten or fifteen minutes, and be sure to keep the 4:7:8 ratio — inhale for four, hold for seven, exhale for eight.

Paula Vetter, RN, MSN, a diabetes educator, holistic family nurse practitioner, personal wellness coach and former critical care nursing instructor at the Cleveland Clinic.

JEWELRY THAT CAN SAVE YOUR LIFE

Medical ID jewelry has evolved. Those simple and basic necklaces and ID bracelets that people used to wear to alert others to medical problems, such as a heart condition or a seizure disorder, have gone high-tech, offering an array of data-sharing options so emergency responders can gain instant access to your comprehensive medical information. The new generation of medical emergency bracelets and tags uses portable computer memory devices (typically a USB drive) or an internet component to store and share your medical information. Here's a sampling of what's available:

- **The CARE medical history bracelet** is basically a USB drive you wear strapped to your wrist. It holds software and forms. It alerts emergency personnel that you have a medical condition and, once plugged into a computer (it works on both PC and Mac), downloads a detailed medical history. The waterproof bracelet comes in five colors.
- Similar in appearance to a traditional dog tag, the **American Medical ID** is a USB drive that carries a summary of medical information. It is easy to use and update. The tag can be engraved with four lines summarizing your critical medical information, such as food or drug allergies or a seizure disorder.

- **ICEdot invisible bracelet,** a web-based service supported by the American Ambulance Association, assigns each wearer a personal identification number (PIN) that first responders use to trigger a text message detailing critical medical information, emergency contacts, or whatever other data you choose to provide.

  How it works: Your ten-dollar-per-year membership buys a sticker pack displaying the PIN (to be displayed in convenient places, for instance on your driver's license) that allows emergency responders to access your information.
- **Road ID Interactive** is an ID band, tag, or pouch you can wear on your wrist, ankle, or shoe. It is engraved with two lines of personal information (name, address) and a toll-free phone number, web address, and PIN that responders can use to get more details.
- **MedicAlert** is the classic line of jewelry, now in an updated variety of attractive styles (for instance, made with Swarovski beads or sterling silver), including bracelets, necklaces, sports bands, shoe tags, and even a watch. These pieces can be engraved with medical information and also provide phone access to a twenty-four-hour emergency service that provides more detailed information. The service notifies anyone you designate that you've had an emergency

381

and provides information on where you're being treated.

How to Choose

Only about 20 percent of patients come in to a hospital emergency department with any sort of information at all. Yet these products can provide comprehensive information very quickly.

This is especially helpful for patients with chronic conditions, but even healthy folks would be well advised to take a few minutes to consider and make notes on their medical history in order to have important information at the ready in the event of an emergency. At minimum, write down your information on an index card, have it laminated (you can do this at many office-supply stores), and store it in your wallet, as EMTs know to look there.

Information that emergency physicians would like to get from every patient in order to deliver the best possible emergency care includes:

• Name, date of birth, address(es)
• Your phone numbers.
• Contact for next of kin or significant other(s)
• Identifying features — moles, tattoos, scars, etc. — that can positively distinguish you from others
• Contact information for your primary care

physician and relevant specialists, including name, phone number, location
- A list of all known allergies
- An up-to-date list of medications and any supplements you take
- Information on previous surgery or planned elective surgery (such as an upcoming gallbladder surgery or a scheduled biopsy)
- Current immunization information, including flu and other vaccines, along with the date of your most recent tetanus shot and others as appropriate
- List of other medical problems such as diabetes, cancer, etc.
- List of any medical devices that you have or use, such as pacemaker, prosthesis, cochlear implant, etc.

Whether it is recorded on a flash drive, a bracelet, an index card, or elsewhere, putting this information together and keeping it with you can make all the difference — at the very least, by expediting treatment in the event of an emergency and quite possibly even saving your life.

The late Richard O'Brien, MD, former spokesperson, American College of Emergency Physicians, and associate professor, the Commonwealth Medical College of Pennsylvania, Scranton.

Don't Be One of the Millions of Americans Overtreated for Diabetes

Bringing blood sugar down with diabetes drugs might be too simple an approach and, worse, ineffective and even harmful for some of us, especially those of us who are sixty-five or older. What's more, the reason why so many Americans have diabetes might not be because their blood sugar levels are dangerously high but because the system that defines what constitutes diabetes is rigged. And even doctors might not realize it!

Here's how to really protect your health and protect yourself from overtreatment when a doctor tells you that your blood sugar is high.

Follow the Money

Diabetes management has become big business, amassing billions of dollars in annual sales. In 2014, sales of diabetes drugs alone reached $23 billion. For this, we can thank, in part, the changing definition of what exactly diabetes is. Since 1997, the American Diabetes Association and other professional endocrinology groups have twice lowered blood sugar thresholds for type 2 diabetes and prediabetes. Each time they did this, millions more Americans were suddenly considered, by definition, diabetic or prediabetic.

But the doctors making these blood sugar

threshold changes have strong incentives to do so that have nothing to do with your well-being, according to a recent exposé published by the medical news outlet *MedPage Today* and the *Milwaukee Journal Sentinel.* Many of these doctors receive speaking and consulting fees from diabetes-drug manufacturers. In one analysis, the authors of the exposé found that thirteen of nineteen members of a committee responsible for diabetes guidelines accumulated a combined sum of more than $2 million in speaking and consulting fees from companies that make diabetes drugs. Whether doctors responsible for diabetes guidelines are intentionally and systematically basing their decisions on their bank account balances isn't known, but the findings do reveal an obvious and material conflict of interest.

Effectiveness of Therapies Questioned

The authors of the exposé also pointed out that although they reduce blood sugar, none of the thirty diabetes drugs approved since 2004 has been definitively proven to reduce the risk of heart attack and stroke, blindness, or any other diabetes-related complication. "In order to approve a new diabetes drug, the FDA requires evidence that the drug effectively reduces hemoglobin A1C levels — a measure of blood glucose — and that it doesn't result in an unacceptable increase in heart disease risk. The evidence that the drug reduces the risk of complications of diabetes, such as heart attacks and stroke, is not required," explains endocrinologist Kasia Lipska, MD, assistant professor of medicine at Yale School of Medicine. She is the leader of a recent, related study that showed that mature adults are being treated too aggressively for diabetes, sometimes with dangerous consequences. The study population of nearly thirteen hundred adults, selected from the National Health and Nutrition Examination Survey database, represents a cross section of senior Americans with diabetes.

Similar to a recent study showing that tight blood pressure control may not be beneficial in older adults, prior studies suggest that tight blood sugar control in people sixty-five and older who have serious health problems actually may do more harm than good. Tight blood sugar control is defined by the American Diabetes Association as a hemoglobin A1C level of less than 7 percent.

Dangerous Side Effects

When it comes to drug treatment for diabetes, most doctors will turn to the older drug metformin first, says Dr. Lipska. It has been used in the United States since 1994 and has had a good safety record here and in Europe, where it has been used much longer. It is considered safe and effective. In addition, it does not cause low blood sugar reactions or weight gain. However, after metformin, there is no clear winner among the diabetes drugs, and the choice of drug depends on a number of trade-offs and risks, particularly for older adults, she says. Insulin and sulfonylurea drugs such as glipizide, glyburide, and glimepiride have been associated with dangerously low blood sugar (hypoglycemia), and other drugs, such as pioglitazone, with risk of fluid retention and fractures. Some drugs, such as saxagliptin, may be associated with heart failure, while, for very new drugs, such as canagliflozin, the risks are not yet known.

Although the American Diabetes Association and other professional groups have been lowering the threshold for what constitutes diabetes (and, thereby, driving the market for diabetes drugs, at least according to the *MedPage* exposé), the American Diabetes Association and the American Geriatrics Society discourage tight blood sugar control in older adults. They acknowledge that older adults whose blood sugar is too aggressively controlled are more vulnerable to the dangerous side effects mentioned above, says Dr. Lipska. She adds that one treatment standard does not fit all in older adults, because their health and treatment preferences vary greatly. Tight control may be safe and appropriate for one person and not another.

Avoid Treatment

Diabetes in older people should be generally managed through lifestyle modification first, including exercise, according to Dr. Lipska. Nevertheless, medications are often required to bring down blood sugar levels, she says. "For many older people with serious health problems or a history of hypoglycemia, tight blood sugar control may not be worth the risks involved. But for some relatively healthy people, tight blood sugar control may make sense. Treatment should be individualized, which requires a careful case-by-case approach," she says. Unfortunately, this is not always the case in practice. Her study found absolutely no difference in how people were treated based on their health. In other words, patients in poor health and at risk for hypoglycemia tended to be treated as aggressively as far healthier patients. What's more, 55 percent of older adults with diabetes who achieved tight blood sugar control were taking insulin or sulfonylureas — drugs that can lead to hypoglycemia — regardless of whether they were healthy, had complex health issues, and/or were in poor health.

To avoid overtreatment for diabetes, Dr. Lipska recommends that you make the necessary lifestyle changes and work together with doctors and other healthcare providers on a personalized approach to your specific health needs and safety. You need to be engaged and part of the plan. The plan should involve much more than simply prescribing a diabetes drug if your blood sugar is above the recommended threshold.

Kasia Joanna Lipska, MD, MHS, assistant professor of medicine (endocrinology), department of internal medicine, Yale School of Medicine, New Haven, Connecticut. Her study was published in *JAMA Internal Medicine*.

TEST YOUR GLUCOSE METER FOR ACCURACY

Glucose meters that check blood sugar should be tested for accuracy every time users open a new pack of test strips, get a new meter, or suspect a malfunction. A recent survey found that only 23 percent of patients with diabetes who use glucose meters said they followed these manufacturer recommendations.

Here's how to test a glucose meter: Use one drop of the control-solution liquid on the test strip (just like you would check your own blood sugar) to test the accuracy of both the meter and packages of test strips.

Katherine O'Neal, PharmD, assistant professor, University of Oklahoma College of Pharmacy, Tulsa.

TIMING IS EVERYTHING . . .
ESPECIALLY WITH YOUR MEDICATIONS

The time of day that you take your medication can make a big difference in how well you do.

Few doctors talk to their patients about the best time of day to take medication or undergo surgery, but it can make a big difference.

If you have high blood pressure, it's usually best to take slow-release medication at bedtime. For osteoarthritis, your pain reliever needs to work hardest in the afternoon. Why does the timing matter?

Virtually every bodily function — including blood pressure, heart rate, and body temperature — is influenced by our circadian (twenty-four-hour) clocks. External factors, such as seasonal rhythms, also play a role in certain medical conditions.

Physiological reactions that are more detrimental at night than in the morning are believed to play a role in both type 2 diabetes and metabolic syndrome — a constellation of conditions that includes insulin resistance (in which the body's cells don't use insulin properly), abdominal obesity, high blood pressure, and elevated LDL "bad" cholesterol.

The body produces and uses insulin most effectively in the daytime hours, and its metabolism is most active during the day. The liver, pancreas, and muscles are better able to utilize blood sugar (glucose) and burn calories when metabolism is high. Because metabolism slows at night, someone who eats a lot of snack foods, for example, at night will be unable to efficiently remove the resulting glucose and fats from the blood. Over time, this can cause a chronic rise in insulin and cholesterol and may lead to metabolic syndrome.

For best results: People with metabolic syndrome or diabetes (or those who are at increased risk for either condition due to obesity or high blood pressure) should synchronize their meals with their metabolic rhythms. Consume most of your calories early in the day. Eat a relatively light supper — for example, a piece of fish, a green salad, and vegetables — preferably at least a few hours before going to bed. Diabetes drugs, such as insulin, should be taken in anticipation of daytime calories and carbohydrates.

William J. M. Hrushesky, MD, principal investigator at the Chronobiology and Oncology Research Laboratory at the Dorn Research Institute VA Medical Center in Columbia, South Carolina. He is also an adjunct professor of epidemiology and biostatistics at the University of South Carolina School of Medicine in Columbia and author of *Circadian Cancer Therapy*.

MEASURE SUGAR BEFORE MEALS

Diabetics should measure blood sugar before meals to best establish their long-term blood sugar levels. Premeal sugar level is more closely aligned with long-term levels than standard blood sugar measurements taken two hours after a meal. Postmeal levels are still important to measure the effects of the meal on blood sugar.

Important: Those with diabetes should maintain a low-sugar and low-carbohydrate diet.

The late Stanley Mirsky, MD, coauthor of the *Diabetes Survival Guide.* Dr. Mirsky was a practicing internist and diabetologist, a past president of the American Diabetes Association of New York State, and a board member of the Joslin Diabetes Center. He was named Endocrinologist of the Year for 2005 at the Mount Sinai School of Medicine.

CHAMOMILE TEA PROTECTS
AGAINST DIABETES DAMAGE

Chamomile is one of the most popular herbal teas. Moms give it to their children to soothe tummy aches and may have a cup themselves to relieve stress or gastrointestinal discomfort. People turn to chamomile tea to calm themselves at bedtime or to reduce cold and flu symptoms, and now evidence has emerged that it may also be helpful in preventing complications of type 2 diabetes.

Chamomile Quenches Free Radicals

According to Stanley Mirsky, MD, former associate clinical professor of medicine at the Mount Sinai School of Medicine in New York and coauthor of the *Diabetes Survival Guide,* chamomile is thought to be beneficial for people with diabetes because it is so rich in antioxidants, which quench free radicals in the body that contribute to disease by allowing inflammation to flourish. In Japan and the United Kingdom, multiple researchers fed diabetic rats a chamomile extract prepared from the dried flowers of *Matricaria chamomilla* for twenty-one days. When compared with a similar group of rats who also had diabetes and were fed the same diet but without the chamomile, the chamomile-treated animals had a significant drop in blood sugar. There was also a decline in two enzymes that are associated with dangerous diabetic complications such as loss of vision, nerve damage, and kidney damage.

Results of the study were published in the *Journal of Agricultural and Food Chemistry*. The researchers expressed hope that these preliminary findings might one day lead to a chamomile-based treatment for diabetes that would be cheaper and have less side effects than pharmaceutical treatments.

Even as this research continues, it may be helpful to add chamomile tea to your diet. For those who like it (and have no contraindications, as it is known to interact with certain medications), it may be a good substitute for sugary sodas or fruit juices, which can wreak havoc on blood sugar levels. Check with your doctor first.

The late Stanley Mirsky, MD, coauthor of the *Diabetes Survival Guide.* Dr. Mirsky was a practicing internist and diabetologist, a past president of the American Diabetes Association of New York State, and a board member of the Joslin Diabetes Center. He was named Endocrinologist of the Year for 2005 at the Mount Sinai School of Medicine.

CONTROL DIABETES WITH QIGONG

Wouldn't it be great if you could just wave your arms to get better control over your blood sugar? A research scientist at Bastyr University in Washington has adapted the ancient Chinese practice of movement called qigong (pronounced chee-GOONG) to help people with type 2 diabetes achieve better blood sugar control, feel better, and even reduce their reliance on drugs.

Study author Guan-Cheng Sun, PhD, assistant research scientist at Bastyr University, qigong teacher, and executive director and founder of the Institute of Qigong & Internal Alternative Medicine in Seattle, says there are many types of qigong. What makes his version unique is the way it explicitly incorporates a specific energy component.

Dr. Sun named his new system Yi Ren Qigong (Yi means "change" and Ren means "human") and says it works by teaching patients with diabetes to calm the chi, or "life energy," of the liver (to slow production of glucose) and to enhance the chi of the pancreas (exhausted by overproducing insulin). The goal of this practice is to "improve the harmony between these organs and increase energy overall," he says, noting that his patients have achieved significant results — reduced blood glucose levels, lower stress, and less insulin resistance. Some were even able to cut back the dosages of their medications.

How Do They Know It Worked?

Dr. Sun's research team studied thirty-two patients, all on medication for their diabetes. They were divided into three groups. One group practiced qigong on their own at home twice a week for thirty minutes and also attended a one-hour weekly session led by an instructor. The second group engaged in a prescribed program of gentle exercise that included movements similar to the qigong practice but without the energy component for an equivalent period of time. And the third group continued their regular medication and medical care but did not engage in structured exercise.

The results: After twelve weeks, the qigong patients had lowered their fasting blood glucose and their levels of self-reported stress and improved their insulin resistance. The gentle exercise group also brought down blood glucose levels, though somewhat less, and lowered stress. It was worse yet for the third group — blood glucose levels climbed, and so did insulin resistance, while there was no reported change in their stress levels. The study was published in *Diabetes Care*.

While Yi Ren Qigong is not available anywhere beyond Bastyr, Dr. Sun is developing a training program for instructors who can then teach in their own communities.

Guan-Cheng Sun, PhD, assistant research scientist at Bastyr University, Kenmore, Washington, qigong teacher, and executive director and founder of the Institute of Qigong & Integrative Medicine, Seattle.

THE MARTIAL ART THAT
DEFENDS AGAINST DIABETES

"People with diabetes often assume that for exercise to be beneficial, you have to be huffing and puffing, sweating, and red-faced afterward," says Beverly Roberts, PhD, RN, a professor at University of Florida College of Nursing. "However, we found that a gentle activity such as tai chi can be just as beneficial in improving the health of people with diabetes."

Dr. Roberts is talking about a recent study that she and her colleagues conducted showing that regular practice of tai chi — an ancient martial art from China consisting of deep breathing and gentle, flowing movements — can help you lower blood sugar, manage diabetes more effectively, improve mood, and boost energy levels.

Tai Chi for Glucose Control

A team of researchers from Korea and the United States studied sixty-two people with type 2 diabetes. Thirty-one practiced tai chi twice a week, and thirty-one didn't.

After six months, those practicing tai chi had a greater drop in fasting blood sugar (a test that measures blood sugar after you haven't eaten for eight hours); a bigger decrease in A1C (a measurement of long-term blood sugar levels); more participation in diabetic self-care activities, such as daily measuring of glucose levels; happier social interactions; better mood; and more energy.

"For those with type 2 diabetes, tai chi could be an alternative exercise to increase glucose control, diabetic self-care activities, and quality of life," conclude the researchers in the *Journal of Alternative and Complementary Medicine.*

"Tai chi has similar effects as other exercises on diabetic control," says Dr. Roberts. "The difference is that tai chi is a low-impact exercise, which means that it's less stressful on the bones, joints, and muscles than more strenuous exercise.

"Tai chi provides a great alternative for people who want the benefits of exercise on diabetic control but may be physically unable to complete strenuous activities because of age, health condition, or injury."

Helps in Several Ways

"These and other studies show that tai chi can have a significant effect on the management and treatment of diabetes," says Paul Lam, MD, of the University of South Wales School of Public Health, the author of five scientific studies on tai chi and diabetes.

"Tai chi can help with diabetes in several ways," he continues. "It can help you control blood sugar, reduce stress, and minimize the complications of diabetes, such as high blood pressure, high cholesterol, and the balance and mobility problems that accompany peripheral neuropathy."

Dr. Lam developed the tai chi program that was used in several studies on tai chi and diabetes — Tai Chi for Diabetes. It is available on DVD and includes a complete tai chi routine, along with a warm-up, stretches, and qigong exercises (also from China) that increase the flow of chi (life force) in the parts of the body affected by diabetes.

Dr. Lam is also the coauthor of the book *Tai Chi for Diabetes: Living Well with Diabetes,* which supplements the DVD.

Both the DVD and the book are available at www.amazon.com. You can also learn more about the Tai Chi for Diabetes program at Dr. Lam's website www.taichifordiabetes.com, where you can order his DVD and book.

Also helpful: If you decide to take a tai chi class, look for an instructor who has practiced for at least three to four years and who inspires you to the regular practice of tai chi, says Daniel Caulfield, a teacher of tai chi at Flow Martial and Meditative Arts in Keene, New Hampshire. "The greatest benefit from tai chi comes from both taking a class with a qualified instructor and practicing at home at least twenty minutes a day."

Beverly Roberts, PhD, RN, professor, University of Florida College of Nursing.

Paul Lam, MD, family physician, tai chi master, clinical teacher and lecturer, University of South Wales, Australia.

Daniel Caulfield, tai chi instructor at Flow Martial and Meditative Arts, in Keene, New Hampshire. FlowMMA.org.

WATCH OUT FOR EXTREME WEATHER

Extreme heat is more dangerous for individuals with diabetes.

Recent finding: People who have type 1 or type 2 diabetes often have difficulty adjusting to rises in temperature. Also, due to nerve damage associated with diabetes, their sweat glands may not produce enough perspiration to cool them down. This may explain why people with diabetes have higher rates of hospitalization, dehydration, and death in warmer months. Winter also can be a problem for diabetics because poor circulation increases the likelihood of skin damage in the cold weather.

Jerrold S. Petrofsky, PhD, professor of physical therapy, School of Allied Health Professions, Loma Linda University, Loma Linda, California, and coauthor of a study published in the *Journal of Applied Research.*

7

COMPLICATIONS: WHAT DIABETES CAN CAUSE

If all of the previous information on diabetes prevention and management hasn't inspired you to take better care of yourself, then what you read here may scare you into it.

At a certain age, you begin to naturally have more to worry about when it comes to hearing, eyesight, and chronic pain. When you add in diabetes, the serious complications can lead to pain, amputation, and even death. But there is plenty that you can do to protect yourself, from simple solutions to big-picture ideas. It's also important to make sure that the community around you is made aware of how to handle themselves should an emergency arise. This includes your doctor, any family or close friends, and certainly a caregiver if you have one.

THE DIABETES COMPLICATION THAT KILLS MORE PEOPLE THAN MOST CANCERS

A foot or leg amputation is one of the most dreaded complications of diabetes. In the

United States, more than sixty-five thousand such amputations occur each year.

But the tragedy does not stop there. According to recent research, about half of all people who have a foot amputation die within five years of the surgery — a worse mortality rate than most cancers. That's partly because people with diabetes who have amputations often have poorer glycemic control and more complications such as kidney disease. Amputation also can lead to increased pressure on the remaining limb and the possibility of new ulcers and infections.

Latest development: To combat the increasingly widespread problem of foot infections and amputations, new guidelines for the diagnosis and treatment of diabetic foot infections have been created by the Infectious Diseases Society of America (IDSA).

How Foot Infections Start

Diabetes can lead to foot infections in two main ways — peripheral neuropathy (nerve damage that can cause loss of sensation in the feet), and ischemia (inadequate blood flow).

To understand why these conditions can be so dangerous, think back to the last time you had a pebble inside your shoe. How long did it take before the irritation became unbearable? Individuals with peripheral neuropathy and ischemia usually don't feel any pain in their feet. Without pain, the pebble will stay in the shoe and eventually cause a sore on the sole of the foot.

Similarly, people with diabetes will not feel the rub of an ill-fitting shoe or the pressure of standing on one foot too long, so they are at risk of developing pressure sores or blisters.

These small wounds can lead to big trouble. About 25 percent of people with diabetes will develop a foot ulcer — ranging from mild to severe — at some point in their lives. Any ulcer, blister, cut, or irritation has the potential to become infected. If the infection becomes too severe to treat effectively with antibiotics, amputation of a foot or leg may be the only way to prevent the infection from spreading throughout the body and save the person's life.

A Fast-Moving Danger

Sores on the foot can progress rapidly. While some foot sores remain unchanged for months, it is possible for an irritation to lead to an open wound (ulcer), infection, and amputation in as little as a few days. That is why experts recommend that people with diabetes seek medical care promptly for any open sore on the feet or any new area of redness or irritation that could possibly lead to an open wound.

Important: Fully half of diabetic foot ulcers are infected and require immediate medical treatment and sometimes hospitalization.

Don't try to diagnose yourself — diagnosis requires a trained medical expert. An ulcer that appears very small on the surface could have actually spread underneath the skin, so you very well could be seeing just a small portion of the infection.

What Your Doctor Will Do

The first step is to identify the bacteria causing the infection. To do this, physicians collect specimens from deep inside the wound. Once the bacteria have been identified, the proper antibiotics can be prescribed.

Physicians also need to know the magnitude of the infection — for example, whether there is bone infection, abscesses, or other internal problems. Therefore, all diabetes patients who have new foot infections should have X-rays. If more detailed imaging is needed, an MRI or a bone scan may be ordered.

The doctor will then classify the wound and infection as mild, moderate, or severe and create a treatment plan.

How to Get the Best Treatment

Each person's wound is unique, so there are no cookie-cutter treatment plans. However, most treatment plans should include the following:

• **A diabetes foot-care team.** For moderate or severe infections, a team of experts should coordinate treatment. This will be done for you — by the hospital or your primary care physician. The number of specialists on the team depends on the patient's specific needs but may include experts in podiatry and vascular surgery. In rural or smaller communities, this may be done via online communication with experts from larger hospitals (telemedicine).

- **Antibiotic treatment.** Milder infections usually involve a single bacterium. Antibiotics will typically be needed for about one week. With more severe infections, multiple bacteria are likely involved, so you will require multiple antibiotics, and treatment will need to continue for a longer period — sometimes four weeks or more if bone is affected.

  If the infection is severe or even moderate but complicated by, say, poor blood circulation, hospitalization may be required for a few days to a few weeks, depending on the course of the recovery.

- **Wound care.** Many patients who have foot infections receive antibiotic therapy only, which is often insufficient. Proper wound care is also necessary. In addition to frequent wound cleansing and dressing changes, this may include surgical removal of dead tissue (debridement) and the use of specially designed shoes or shoe inserts — provided by a podiatrist — to redistribute pressure off the wound (off-loading).

- **Surgery.** Surgery doesn't always mean amputation. It is sometimes used not only to remove dead or damaged tissue or bone but also to improve blood flow to the foot.

If an infection fails to improve: The first question physicians know to ask is: "Is the patient complying with wound care instructions?" Too many patients lose a leg because they don't take their antibiotics as prescribed or care for the injury as prescribed.

Never forget: Following your doctors' specific orders could literally mean the difference between having one leg or two.

James M. Horton, MD, chair of the Standards and Practice Guidelines Committee of the Infectious Diseases Society of America, www.idsociety.org. Dr. Horton is also chief of the department of infectious disease and attending faculty physician in the department of internal medicine, both at Carolinas Medical Center in Charlotte, North Carolina.

Foot Care Is Critical If You Have Diabetes

To protect yourself from foot injuries:

- **Never walk barefoot,** even around the house.
- **Don't wear sandals** — the straps can irritate the side of the foot.
- **Wear thick socks with soft leather shoes.** Leather is a good choice because it breathes, molds to the feet, and does not retain moisture. Laced-up shoes with cushioned soles provide the most support.

  In addition, pharmacies carry special diabetic socks that protect and cushion your feet without cutting off circulation at the ankle. These socks usually have no seams that could chafe. They also wick moisture away from feet, which reduces risk for infection and foot ulcers.
- **See a podiatrist.** This physician can advise you on the proper care of common foot problems, such as blisters, corns, and ingrown toenails. A podiatrist can also help you find appropriate footwear — even if you have foot deformities.

  Ask your primary care physician or endocrinologist for a recommendation, or consult the American Podiatric Medical Association.

Also: Inspect your feet every day. Otherwise, you may miss a developing infection. Look for areas of redness, blisters, or open sores, particularly in the areas most prone to injury — the bottoms and bony inner and outer edges of the feet.

If you see any sign of a sore, seek prompt medical care. You should also see a doctor if you experience an infected or ingrown toenail, callus formation, bunions or other deformity, fissured (cracked) skin on your feet, or you notice any change in sensation.

James M. Horton, MD, chair of the Standards and Practice Guidelines Committee of the Infectious Diseases Society of America, www.idsociety.org. Dr. Horton is also chief of the department of infectious disease and attending faculty physician in the department of internal medicine, both at Carolinas Medical Center in Charlotte, North Carolina.

IF YOU HAVE DIABETES, A JOINT REPLACEMENT, OR ARTHRITIS

When most people think of bone problems, broken bones and osteoporosis (reduced bone density and strength) come to mind. But our bones also can be the site of infections that can sometimes go unrecognized for months or even years.

This is especially the case if the only symptoms of bone infection (a condition known as osteomyelitis) are ones that are commonly mistaken for common health problems, such as ordinary back pain or fatigue.

Are You at Risk?

Older adults (age seventy and older), people with diabetes or arthritis, and anyone with a weakened immune system (due to chronic disease, such as cancer, for example) are among those at greatest risk for osteomyelitis.

Anyone who has an artificial joint (such as a total hip replacement or total knee replacement) or metal implants attached to a bone also is at increased risk for osteomyelitis and should discuss the use of antibiotics before any type of surgery, including routine dental and oral surgery. Bacteria in the mouth can enter the bloodstream and cause a bone infection.

Types of Bone Infections

Before the advent of joint-replacement surgery, most bone infections were caused by injuries that expose the bone to bacteria in the environment (such as those caused by a car accident) or a broken bone or an infection elsewhere in the body, such as pneumonia or a urinary tract infection, that spreads to the bone through the bloodstream.

Now: About half the cases of osteomyelitis are complications of surgery in which large metal implants are used to stabilize or replace bones and joints (such as in the hip or knee).

Osteomyelitis is divided into three main categories, depending on the origin of the infection:

- **Blood-borne osteomyelitis** occurs when bacteria that originate elsewhere in the body migrate to and infect bone. People with osteoarthritis or rheumatoid arthritis are prone to blood-borne infections in their affected joints due to injury to cells in the lining of the joints that normally prevent bacteria from entering the bloodstream.
- **Contiguous-focus osteomyelitis** occurs when organisms — usually bacteria, but sometimes fungi — infect bone tissue. These cases usually occur in people with diabetes, who often develop pressure sores on the soles of their feet or buttocks due to poor circulation and impaired immunity.

- **Post-traumatic osteomyelitis** occurs after trauma or surgery to a bone and/or surrounding tissue opens the area to bacteria and other microbes. The use of prosthetic joints, surgical screws, pins, or plates also makes it easier for bacteria to enter and infect the bone.

Important: Any of the three types of bone infections described above can lead to chronic osteomyelitis, an initially low-grade infection that can persist for months or even years with few or no symptoms. Eventually, it gets severe enough to literally destroy bone. Left untreated, the affected bone may have to be amputated.

Difficult to Diagnose

When osteomyelitis first develops (acute osteomyelitis), the symptoms — such as pain, swelling, and tenderness — are usually the same as those caused by other infections.

If the initial infection is subtle (low-grade) or doesn't resolve completely with treatment, it can result in chronic osteomyelitis. In this case, you may have no symptoms or symptoms that are nonspecific. For example, someone who has had surgery might blame discomfort on delayed recovery, not realizing that what they have is a bone infection.

Surprising finding: When we studied the histories of more than two thousand osteomyelitis patients, we found that most of those with chronic infections had relatively little pain from the infection itself. About 28 percent of those who required surgery for infection had normal white blood cell counts — suggesting that, over time, the body adjusts to lingering infections.

If a doctor suspects that you may have osteomyelitis because of chronic pain, swelling, possibly fever, fatigue, or other symptoms, he/she will usually order special laboratory tests that detect the formation of antibodies. If the results indicate the presence of infection, he may then order an X-ray or magnetic resonance imaging (MRI) scan. These and other imaging tests can readily detect damaged bone tissue and reveal the presence of infection.

Best Treatment Options

About 60 to 70 percent of people with acute osteomyelitis can be cured with antibiotics (or antifungal agents, if a fungal infection is present) if treatment begins early enough to prevent the infection from becoming chronic. In these cases, patients exhibit symptoms, test positive for infection, and readily respond to drug treatments. Most patients can be cured with a four- to six-week course of antibiotics. Fungal infections are more resistant to treatment — antifungal drugs may be needed for several months.

For chronic osteomyelitis, surgical debridement (the removal of damaged tissue and bone using such instruments as a scalpel or scissors) is usually necessary.

Reasons: Damaged bone can lose its blood supply and remain in the body as "dead bone" — without living cells or circulation. Such bone is invulnerable to the effects of antibiotics.

After debridement, the surgeon may insert a slow-release antibiotic depot, a small pouch that releases the antibiotic for up to a month. This approach can increase drug concentrations up to one hundred times more than oral antibiotic therapy.

Even with these treatments, in people with chronic osteomyelitis who are otherwise healthy, up to 6 percent may require a second or even a third operation to cure the infection. In people with diabetes or other disorders, the percentage may be as high as 25 percent.

To improve your chances of a full recovery from chronic osteomyelitis: Eat well, maintain healthy blood sugar levels, stay active after treatment (to promote blood circulation, prevent blood clots, and help maintain an appetite), and don't use tobacco products.

George Cierny, MD, and Doreen Di-Pasquale, MD, physician-partners at RE-Orthopaedics in San Diego. Dr. Cierny was an international lecturer in orthopedic surgery who published more than one hundred scientific papers and book chapters in the field of musculoskeletal pathology and infection. Dr. DiPasquale, an orthopedic surgeon, was residency program director at George Washington University in Washington, DC, and National Naval Medical Center in Bethesda, Maryland.

NATURAL CURES FOR PAINFUL NEUROPATHY

Peripheral neuropathy may be one of the most common conditions you've never heard of — and it is indeed common. Estimates are that it affects as many as two-thirds of people with diabetes, 10 to 20 percent of people with cancer, and 8 percent of all people over age fifty-five. One reason may be that neuropathy is not an isolated medical condition. Rather, it results from other medical problems including vitamin deficiencies, autoimmune disorders, and heavy metal exposure, in addition to diabetes and cancer. Symptoms generally come on gradually over a period of weeks or even months, starting in the toes and sometimes the fingers. They include burning and tingling sensations, numbness, and occasional sharp, sudden pains similar to electrical shocks. Intensity of symptoms varies widely, from mild annoyance to numbness severe enough to impair function to debilitating pain.

Medical Treatments

Mainstream medical doctors often treat peripheral neuropathy with pharmaceutical drugs, but they all have serious side effects, including dizziness, sleepiness, dry mouth, blurred vision, weight gain, nausea, headache, and in serious cases, allergic reaction and confusion, among others.

Given the problems with pharmaceuticals, it's good to be aware about natural approaches to the problem. The first step is to find the root cause and correct it as much as possible. For example, people with diabetes must control blood sugar levels to help slow further peripheral neuropathy development. People who suspect vitamin deficiencies should see a holistic physician for blood level tests and to help them establish a healthy diet and vitamin protocol. They must also avoid or greatly reduce alcohol consumption. Those having chemotherapy should alert the supervising doctor immediately if numbness or tingling starts in their feet or hands. The doctor may be able to alter the drugs somewhat to keep the neuropathy from escalating. However, when chemo-related peripheral neuropathy begins weeks or even months after completion of chemotherapy — as is often the case — the next step is to seek treatment to alleviate the discomfort and possibly help reduce or even heal it. This advice holds true for other causes of peripheral neuropathy as well, although you should check with your doctor to be sure it is appropriate for you.

Natural Approaches

The natural substance with the longest record for helping both diabetic peripheral neuropathy and chemotherapy-induced peripheral neuropathy is alpha-lipoic acid, a powerful antioxidant that scavenges many harmful free radicals. (Note: Alpha-lipoic acid can reduce blood sugar levels, so your doctor should monitor your medication and blood sugar for the duration.) It's not a quick solution however — you should wait eight to twelve weeks before assessing results. The other natural substance I recommend is acetyl-L-carnitine, which has a regenerative effect on the nerves. Again, stay on acetyl-L-carnitine therapy for eight to twelve weeks to assess its efficacy. To further reduce nerve irritation, I often prescribe a vitamin B complex including B-12, as well as vitamins E and C, selenium, and Pycnogenol, a plant-derived substance that has antioxidant, anti-inflammatory, and other powerful properties. Injections or sublingual doses of vitamins B-12 and B-1, which you can get from your doctor, are also helpful.

Acupuncture

Acupuncture is an increasingly popular treatment for peripheral neuropathy, in particular that caused by chemotherapy. Yi Hung Chan, LAc, DPM, is a staff member at the Bendheim Integrative Medicine Center of the Memorial Sloan-Kettering Cancer Center in New York City. Dr. Chan treats many neuropathy patients, some of whom are still in chemo and others who develop peripheral neuropathy after chemo completion. To attain the greatest relief, he recommends starting acupuncture treatment at the first sign of symptoms — early intervention helps to avoid full-blown neuropathy and may reverse symptoms. In his clinical practice, Dr. Chan has found that about 80 percent of patients show substantial improvement after eight to twelve sessions of treatment.

Patients start acupuncture with one to two appointments per week. Those still in chemotherapy continue acupuncture sessions for about six weeks after completion of cancer treatment and taper off from there. When peripheral neuropathy begins after chemo, Dr. Chan recommends one to two sessions per week for six or so months with occasional follow-up sessions after that. Although Dr. Chan's experience is mostly with chemo-related peripheral neuropathy, he notes that in a small study of seven individuals with diabetes, done at Harvard in 2007, acupuncture eased their neuropathy pain as well.

Healthy Habits

All people with peripheral neuropathy should maintain a healthy lifestyle and keep their weight normal to lessen pressure on the feet. A regular practice of meditation, yoga, or any other calming technique helps provide relaxation when neuropathy flares. Other ways to increase comfort are to keep the feet warm, wear soft-leather shoes with good support, and sleep with light blankets to avoid pressure on sensitive feet. Though some people are unable to obtain full relief from peripheral neuropathy, there is fortunately much you can do to make it bearable.

Mark A. Stengler, NMD, a naturopathic medical doctor and leading authority on the practice of alternative and integrated medicine. Dr. Stengler is author of the *Health Revelations* newsletter, *The Natural Physician's Healing Therapies,* and *Bottom Line's Prescription for Natural Cures.* He is also the founder and medical director of the Stengler Center for Integrative Medicine in Encinitas, California, and former adjunct associate clinical professor at the National College of Natural Medicine in Portland, Oregon. MarkStengler.com.

VITAMIN B-12 — BETTER THAN A DRUG FOR DIABETIC NEUROPATHY

Twenty-five percent of people with diabetes develop diabetic neuropathy — glucose-caused damage to nerves throughout the body, particularly in the hands, arms, feet, and legs (peripheral neuropathy).

You experience tingling and prickling. Numbness. And pain — from annoying, to burning, to stabbing, to excruciating. Drugs hardly help.

"Many studies have been conducted on drugs for diabetic neuropathy, and no drug is really effective," says Anne L. Peters, MD, professor of medicine and director of the University of Southern California Westside Center for Diabetes and author of *Conquering Diabetes*.

But a new study says a vitamin can help.

Less Pain and Burning

Researchers in Iran studied one hundred people with diabetic neuropathy, dividing them into two groups. One group received nortriptyline, an antidepressant medication that has been used to treat neuropathy. The other group received vitamin B-12, a nutrient known to nourish and protect nerves.

After several weeks of treatment, the B-12 group had:

- 78 percent greater reduction in pain
- 71 percent greater reduction in tingling and prickling
- 65 percent greater reduction in burning

"Vitamin B-12 is more effective than nortriptyline for the treatment of painful diabetic neuropathy," conclude the researchers in the *International Journal of Food Science and Nutrition.*

Latest development: A few months after the Iranian doctors conducted their study, research in the United States involving seventy-six people with diabetes showed that the widely prescribed diabetes drug metformin may cause vitamin B-12 deficiency — and that 77 percent of those with the deficiency also suffered from peripheral neuropathy!

Anyone already diagnosed with peripheral neuropathy who uses metformin should be tested for low blood levels of B-12, says Mariejane Braza, MD, of the University of Texas Health Science Center and the study leader. If B-12 levels are low, she recommends supplementing with the vitamin, to reduce the risk of nerve damage.

Heal the Nerves

"If you take metformin, definitely take at least 500 mcg a day of vitamin B-12, in either a multivitamin or B-complex supplement," advises Jacob Teitelbaum, MD, author of *Pain-Free 1-2-3!* "It's the single, most effective nutrient for helping prevent and reverse diabetic neuropathy.

"On a good day, the best that medications can do for neuropathy is mask the pain," he continues. "But vitamin B-12 gradually heals the nerves."

Best: If you already have neuropathy, Dr. Teitelbaum recommends finding a holistic physician and asking for fifteen intramuscular injections of 3,000 to 5,000 mcg of methylcobalamin, the best form of B-12 to treat peripheral neuropathy. "Receive those shots daily to weekly — at whatever speed is convenient to quickly optimize levels of B-12," says Dr. Teitelbaum.

Resource: To find a holistic physician, Dr. Teitelbaum recommends visiting the website of the American Board of Integrative Holistic Medicine, www.abihm.org.

If you can't find a holistic physician near you, he suggests taking a daily sublingual (dissolving under the tongue) dose of 5,000 mcg for four weeks. (Daily, because you only absorb a small portion of the sublingual vitamin B-12, compared with intramuscular injections.)

At the same time that you take B-12, also take a high-dose B-complex supplement (B-50). "The body is happiest when it gets all the B-vitamins together," says Dr. Teitel-baum.

He points out that it can take three to twelve months for nerves to heal, but that the neuropathy should progressively improve during that time.

Also helpful: Other nutrients that Dr. Teitelbaum recommends to help ease periph-eral neuropathy include:

- **Alpha-lipoic acid** (300 mg, twice a day)
- **Acetyl-l-carnitine** (500 mg, three times a day)

Anne L. Peters, MD, professor of medicine and director of the University of Southern California Westside Center for Diabetes and author of *Conquering Diabetes.*

Mariejane Braza, MD, researcher, Univer-sity of Texas Health Science Center, and internist, Valley Baptist Medical Center, Harlingen, Texas.

Jacob Teitelbaum, MD, author of *Pain-Free 1-2-3!* and *From Fatigued to Fantastic!* EndFatigue.com.

HELP FOR DIABETIC FOOT ULCERS

Diabetic foot ulcers can be healed by acne medication.

Recent finding: In a study of twenty-two men with diabetes, more than 84 percent of ulcers treated with topical tretinoin, a popular acne medication, and antibacterial cadexomer iodine gel shrunk by at least half. In the group treated with a placebo solution and cadexomer iodine gel, 45.4 percent of ulcers shrunk by half.

Theory: Tretinoin stimulates blood vessel growth, which helps deliver oxygen to the wound site. Left untreated, diabetic ulcers may increase risk for amputation.

Wynnis Tom, MD, assistant clinical professor of medicine, University of California, San Diego.

BETTER FOOT CARE WITH CHARCOT

Charcot foot (a condition in which bones in the foot weaken and break) is common in people with diabetes and/ or peripheral neuropathy. They may have a loss of feeling in the feet due to nerve damage and are sometimes unaware that they have Charcot foot until it causes severe deformities.

If you have diabetes and/or peripheral neuropathy: See a podiatrist or orthopedic surgeon to be monitored for Charcot foot, which can be treated with surgery and/ or specialized footwear. Warning signs include sudden swelling or pain of the foot and/or leg.

Valerie L. Schade, DPM, FACFAS, podiatric surgeon, Tacoma, Washington.

TOENAIL FUNGUS TROUBLE . . .
AND A UNIQUE CURE

When is the last time you took a good look at your toenails? If it has been a while, you may be in for an unpleasant surprise — in fungal form. Toenail fungus infection, also called onychomycosis, is a common condition that turns nails a yellow or brown color. In some cases, the nail thickens or splits and may fall off. Sufferers may experience pain around the nail and notice a foul smell. The infection is typically caused by any one of several types of fungi that feed on keratin, the protein surface of the nail. Occasionally, different yeasts and molds may cause the infection.

By age seventy, almost half of Americans have had at least one affected toe. While the infection can occur in fingernails, it most often affects toenails, because feet are confined to the dark, warm environment of shoes, where fungi can thrive. The nails of the big toe and little toe are particularly susceptible, because friction from the sides of shoes can cause trauma to the nail surface, making it easier for fungi to penetrate. Nail fungus is not the same as athlete's foot — because athlete's foot affects the skin rather than the nail itself — but the two conditions may coexist and can be caused by the same type of fungus.

I find that athletes and others who commonly use gym locker rooms and showers are more likely to develop toenail fungus due to the damp floors and shared environment. Women who wear toenail polish are at increased risk because moisture can get trapped beneath the polish. Tight-fitting shoes and hosiery that rub the toenails also contribute to the problem. People with diabetes and other circulation problems that prevent infection-fighting white blood cells from adequately reaching the toes are particularly susceptible to the fungus, as are people with compromised immune systems, such as those with cancer or HIV.

Toenail fungus doesn't usually clear up on its own. In fact, it tends to get more severe over time, affecting a larger portion of the nail and spreading to adjacent toes and to the other foot. Therefore, I recommend starting treatment as early as possible.

Conventional Treatments

Medical doctors generally turn to topical and oral antifungal treatments. For mild cases that involve a small area of the nail, a medicated nail polish containing an antifungal agent, such as ciclopirox, is often prescribed. For toenail fungus that covers a large portion of a nail or affects several nails, the typical medical approach is to prescribe oral antifungal medications, such as itraconazole or terbinafine. These are quite powerful medications and may need to be taken for up to twelve weeks until the infection clears up. In 10 to 20 percent of cases, the fungus returns within several months.

The most worrisome side effect of oral antifungals is liver damage. To monitor the effect of these medications, liver enzyme tests should be performed before beginning treatment and every four to six weeks during treatment. An elevation in liver enzymes means that the drugs are irritating the liver and need to be discontinued. Several patients who were being treated by other doctors have come to see me after elevated liver enzymes forced them to stop this pharmaceutical treatment. As a last resort, the nail can be surgically removed, at which point the infection will clear up, and the nail will slowly grow back.

An Unusual Cure

The typical natural treatment for toenail fungus is to apply tea tree oil or oregano oil. Using a cotton swab, apply nightly to the affected area, continuing treatment for eight to twelve weeks. These oils work well to clear up mild toenail fungus, but they are often not strong enough for moderate to severe cases. There is an unusual yet effective therapy for severe toenail fungus developed by Mark Cooper, ND, an innovative naturopathic doctor. Years ago, Dr. Cooper treated an HIV-positive patient who commented on an article he had read stating that bleach killed HIV on surfaces (not in the body). Knowing that hospital bedsheets and floor surfaces are washed with bleach to kill all types of fungi, viruses, and bacteria, Dr. Cooper theorized that bleach might also kill toenail fungus and clear up persistent cases of infection.

Dr. Cooper, who practices at Alpine Naturopathic Clinic in Colorado Springs, has treated hundreds of his patients with this topical bleach treatment. My patients have responded very well to it too.

How it works: Mix one cup of household bleach with ten cups of warm water. Soak the toes of the affected foot for three minutes, then thoroughly rinse off the bleach solution with water and dry the feet completely. Do this twice weekly, with three days between treatments. Most cases resolve in two to three months. Severe cases may take longer.

Boosting the strength of the bleach-and-water mixture beyond the one-to-ten ratio will not increase the effectiveness of the treatment, and it could irritate the skin. Nor is it wise to increase the frequency or duration of treatments. Dr. Cooper told me about a seventy-four-year-old man who misunderstood the directions — instead of soaking his toes for three minutes, he tried to soak them for thirty minutes. The burning pain was so intense that he had to stop the soaking after twenty minutes. Obviously, this treatment needs to be used with caution and should not be used when there is an open wound near the infection site.

Interesting: Bleach is composed of sodium hypochlorite (NaOCl). Household bleach usually contains 3 to 6 percent NaOCl, while industrial-strength bleach contains 10 to 12 percent. Near the end of the nineteenth century, after Louis Pasteur discovered its powerful effectiveness against disease-causing bacteria, bleach became popular as a disinfectant. It is still used today for household cleaning, removing laundry stains, treating waste water, sterilizing medical equipment, and disinfecting hospital linens and surfaces.

Fungus-Fighting Foods and Supplements

Dr. Cooper explains that the topical bleach treatment is even more effective when combined with an antifungal diet. Avoid simple sugars (white breads, pastas, cookies, and soda) and alcohol — they suppress immune function and contribute to fungal growth. Eat raw or cooked onions, shallots, and leeks, plus garlic (as a food or an extract) as often as possible for their antifungal action.

I also have found that severe cases of toenail fungus, especially in people with diabetes, clear up more quickly when natural antifungal supplements are taken orally. The most potent is oregano oil. It contains plant compounds, such as carvacrol and thymol, that have strong antifungal properties. I recommend taking three doses daily for four to eight weeks. Each dose equals one 500-mg capsule or five to fifteen drops of the liquid form mixed with two to four ounces of water. Some people may experience heartburn from oregano oil, so if you are prone to heartburn, you may need to reduce the dosage. Oregano oil should not be ingested by people with active stomach ulcers (since it can irritate the stomach lining) or by pregnant or nursing women (as a general precaution). It should be given to children only under the guidance of a doctor.

How will you know when the fungal infection is gone? When the discolored nail returns to its normal hue or when the damaged nail grows out and a new nail grows in normally.

Fungus Prevention Strategies

- **Wash your feet every day using calendula soap.** Made from the marigold plant, it is gentle yet antiseptic. Find it in health-food stores.
- **Always dry feet thoroughly with a clean towel.** Do not share towels with other people.
- **Keep toenails clipped short** to reduce the protein surface on which fungi feed.
- **Avoid going barefoot in public places.** Wear plastic sandals in community showers

and locker rooms and at poolside.
- **Choose socks made of breathable fabrics,** such as cotton. Change socks immediately after exercising and whenever feet perspire.
- **Be sure your shoes are not too tight.** If shoes get damp, change them promptly.

Mark A. Stengler, NMD, a naturopathic medical doctor and leading authority on the practice of alternative and integrated medicine. Dr. Stengler is author of the *Health Revelations* newsletter, *The Natural Physician's Healing Therapies,* and *Bottom Line's Prescription for Natural Cures.* He is also the founder and medical director of the Stengler Center for Integrative Medicine in Encinitas, California, and former adjunct associate clinical professor at the National College of Natural Medicine in Portland, Oregon. MarkStengler.com.

FREE YOURSELF FROM CHRONIC PAIN

Talk about piling on — many people who are chronically ill, for instance with diabetes or cancer or who have suffered a traumatic injury, ultimately end up with a condition called neuropathy, where their nervous systems turn against them, randomly sending out pain signals that can range from tingling that is merely uncomfortable to stabbing sensations so painful that they are debilitating. Opioids and antidepressants can help, but these drugs have side effects that can make them less-than-great choices. Acupuncture can be helpful too, but generally speaking, treatment is not all that effective.

So here's information from a recent study that's good news, even though the study was very small, did not include a control group, and the treatment worked for only about one-third of the patients who tried it. New research evaluated the use of a therapy called transcutaneous electrical nerve stimulation (TENS) in people with neuropathy as the result of a spinal cord injury. This form of treatment involves placing electrodes (attached to a battery pack) on the skin along both sides of the spine at the level of and just above the spinal cord injury to deliver electrical current. The same technique has been used to treat other forms of chronic pain and muscle spasms.

Shocking but Effective

Twenty-four patients were given TENS units and taught to self-administer the treatment three times a day for thirty to forty minutes at a time. They did this for two weeks at high frequency and then for another two weeks at low frequency.

Results: About one-third of the patients reported pain was reduced at least somewhat — 29 percent were helped by high-frequency stimulation and 38 percent by low-frequency stimulation. But what I thought was most notable about this study was that six patients — one-quarter of those who tried this therapy — asked if they could keep their TENS units so they could continue the treatments themselves at home. Clearly, they experienced some benefit.

To those who've never tried it, TENS may sound more like torture than treatment — after all, you'd think that stimulating nerves that have already gone haywire would simply cause more pain. According to Cecilia Norrbrink, RPT, PhD, from the department of clinical sciences at the Karolinska Institute in Stockholm, Sweden, where the study was done, TENS is not painful, and it does work well for some people. She says scientists believe that it works by using the body's own pain-inhibiting systems.

Her very simplified explanation: High-frequency TENS activates large nerve fibers, which are the ones carrying nonpainful signals such as touch. Stimulating these nerve fibers releases transmitter signals in the spinal cord that can inhibit the pain signals coming from small nerve fibers. Low-frequency TENS, on the other hand, seems to activate neurons in the brain stem (where inhibitory pathways start) by releasing pain-blocking endorphins.

Another option: There's a form of Japanese acupuncture that incorporates electrical stimulation through the needles, according to contributing medical editor Andrew L. Rubman, ND. It is called electroacupuncture, and it might be a good option to explore with your acupuncturist or naturopathic doctor.

Can You Do This at Home?

Side effects from the treatment are minimal — some patients experience muscle spasms, and others find the electrodes irritating to their skin. But those are minor complaints compared with the pain relief the treatments sometimes deliver. If you're interested in exploring TENS treatment for neuropathic pain, discuss it with your doctor — there's a long list of medical cautions that are considered contraindications for its use. If you are among the lucky ones, this might provide welcome relief.

Cecilia Norrbrink, RPT, PhD, department of clinical sciences, Danderyd Hospital, Karolinska Institute, Stockholm, Sweden.

SAY WHAT? A SURPRISING LINK TO HEARING LOSS FOR WOMEN

You might expect to lose your hearing a little bit as you age, but you may be shocked by a recent study that points to a risk factor that may make hearing loss even worse. Women with this specific condition need to listen up!

Needing to turn up the volume on the TV or radio yet again, straining to catch a dinner companion's words in a crowded restaurant, having trouble identifying background noises — it's normal to notice an increase in such experiences as we get older.

But: This recent study has highlighted an important and often overlooked risk factor that can make age-related hearing loss among women much worse than usual — diabetes that is not well controlled.

Study Details

Researchers reviewed the medical charts of 990 women and men who, between 2000 and 2008, had had audiograms to test their ability to hear sounds at various frequencies; participants were also scored on speech recognition. Study participants were classified by age, sex, and whether they had diabetes (and, if so, how well controlled their blood glucose levels were).

Results: Among women ages sixty to seventy-five, those whose diabetes was well controlled were able to hear about equally as well as women who did not have diabetes, but those with poorly controlled diabetes had significantly worse hearing.

For men in this specific study, there was no significant difference in hearing ability between those with and without diabetes, no matter how well controlled the disease was, though this finding could have been influenced by the fact that men generally had worse hearing than women regardless of health status. But smaller studies have shown that diabetes can have an impact on hearing, no matter what your sex (see article that follows).

Now Hear This

Are you still not convinced this is a dangerous disease? Diabetes also increases the risk for heart disease, vision loss, kidney dysfunction, nerve problems, and other serious ailments, so this recent study gives women with diabetes yet one more important motivation for keeping blood glucose levels well under control with diet, exercise, and/or medication.

If you have not been diagnosed with diabetes: If your hearing seems to be worsening, ask your doctor to check for diabetes, particularly if you have other possible warning signs, such as frequent urination, unusual thirst, slow wound healing, blurred vision, and/or numbness in the hands and feet.

Derek J. Handzo, DO, an otolaryngology resident, and Kathleen Yaremchuk, MD, chair of the department of otolaryngology–head and neck surgery at Henry Ford Hospital in Detroit. They are coauthors of a study on diabetes and hearing loss presented at a recent Triological Society Combined Sections Meeting.

CONTROL YOUR BLOOD SUGAR . . .
PROTECT YOUR HEARING

If you're like most people, you probably assume that hearing loss is an inevitable part of growing older and that you can't do anything about it other than get a hearing aid. But that's not always true.

Most of the nearly forty million Americans who don't hear as well as they used to have sensorineural hearing loss (SNHL) — damage to delicate, hairlike nerve endings (hair cells) in the inner ear. These tiny hair cells translate sound vibrations into electrical impulses that are sent to the brain.

While SNHL does often result from aging or loud noise (repeated exposure or a single exposure to a very loud noise, such as an explosion), it also can be due to unexpected causes such as certain health problems or even prescription or over-the-counter (OTC) drugs.

Latest development: Recent scientific research is revealing that there may be more opportunities to prevent or slow SNHL than once thought. The following are some of the surprising causes of SNHL and what you can do to prevent it.

Viagra and Other Drugs
There are hundreds of ototoxic drugs that can damage hearing. For example, in a study

published in 2011 in *Laryngoscope,* researchers in the UK identified forty-seven cases in which men who took sildenafil or other drugs for erectile dysfunction experienced SNHL — and 67 percent of them developed it within twenty-four hours of starting the medication. Other ototoxic drugs include:

- **Nonsteroidal anti-inflammatory drugs (NSAIDs),** such as aspirin, ibuprofen, and naproxen.
- **Loop diuretics,** such as furosemide used for high blood pressure, congestive heart failure, and kidney disease.
- **Antidepressants,** such as fluoxetine, clomipramine, and amitriptyline.
- **Antianxiety medications,** such as alprazolam.
- **Certain antibiotics,** including erythromycin, gentamicin, neomycin, and tetracycline.
- **Chemotherapy drugs,** such as cisplatin and carboplatin.
- **Quinine-based antimalarial drugs.**

Important: The hearing loss caused by these drugs may be temporary or permanent depending on factors such as dosage and the length of time the medication was taken.

Self-defense: If your doctor prescribes a new medication, ask whether it could cause hearing loss. You can also research drug side effects online at the Physicians' Desk Reference website, www.pdrhealth.com.

If the medication can affect hearing, ask your doctor if there are alternatives that are suitable for your particular condition. If not, an audiologist should conduct hearing tests before you begin taking the medication to obtain a baseline. These tests should be repeated several times during the course of treatment with the drug.

For the greatest protection: Normally, an audiologist checks hearing in the 250- to 8,000-hertz (Hz) range, but to monitor drug-related hearing loss, it is best to examine the high-frequency range (between 9,000 and 20,000 Hz), where damage is likely to occur first.

If your hearing is affected, the prescribing physician should reconsider how best to treat the condition for which you were prescribed medication.

If you're already taking a drug that you suspect may be causing hearing loss, see an ear, nose, and throat (ENT) specialist for advice. Also notify an ENT specialist if you develop a sense of fullness in one or both ears (which could signal hearing loss) or tinnitus (ringing, buzzing, or other unwanted sounds with or without hearing loss).

Blood Sugar Problems and Hearing Loss

Most physicians realize that diabetes slowly destroys blood vessels throughout the body, increasing risk for heart disease, stroke, Alzheimer's disease, chronic kidney disease, blindness, and even amputation of circulation-starved limbs. Now, hearing loss has been identified as an underrecognized complication of diabetes.

Recent research: In a study of forty-six people with type 2 diabetes and forty-seven with rheumatoid arthritis, those with diabetes had three times more cases of hearing loss than the study participants with arthritis.

Possible mechanism: Diabetes reduces circulation and causes nerve degeneration — two factors that can affect the viability of hair cells involved in hearing.

Another danger: Studies have linked obesity and high triglyceride levels — both of which often accompany diabetes — to SNHL.

To preserve your hearing: Take steps to prevent high blood sugar. Weight loss, regular exercise, and a diet that limits processed foods and emphasizes unprocessed foods (such as vegetables, fruits, whole grains, legumes, fish, lean meat, and poultry) are the best approaches to take.

Riding in a Convertible and Loud Noises

Most people know that loud noises such as jackhammers and explosions can damage hearing. But other causes are being discovered. For example, researchers at the St. Louis University School of Medicine tested noise levels while riding in a convertible at fifty-five miles per hour or faster with the top down and windows open. Levels were found to be above 85 decibels (dB) — the point at which hearing damage begins.

Self-defense: Avoid regularly exposing your ears to any sounds above 85 dB. To protect yourself:

• **Use earplugs** when you operate noisy equipment of any kind, such as a lawn mower, power saw, chain saw, snowmobile — or even your vacuum cleaner.

Also helpful: If you are in an environment where you can't hear another person talking to you who is three feet away or closer, wear earplugs — or leave.

• **Lower the volume of your iPod** or other music player if you notice any signs of hearing damage, such as your ears feeling muffled or full or ringing in your ears.

Antioxidants = Better Hearing

In many cases, you may be able to prevent hearing loss that could require a hearing aid by consuming an abundance of certain anti-oxidants.* For example:

- **Coenzyme Q10 (CoQ10).** In people with SNHL, those who took the powerful anti-oxidant CoQ10 daily experienced improved hearing, according to recent research by Italian scientists.
- **Fish oil.** Several studies link diets high in omega-3 fatty acids from fish to preventing or delaying age-related SNHL.

    Important: I recommend using molecu-larly distilled fish oil (check the label) — it is less likely to contain toxins such as mercury than other fish oil products.

Also helpful: Diets rich in vitamin C, vitamin E, the B-vitamin riboflavin, magne-sium, and the antioxidant lycopene were linked to better hearing, according to a recent study from researchers at Vanderbilt Univer-sity in Nashville. Other nutrients that may help prevent hearing loss include resveratrol, lecithin, alpha-lipoic acid, acetyl-L-carnitine, and N-acetylcysteine.

Talk to an integrative physician for advice on the specific nutrients and dosages that would be best for you. To find an integrative

* Consult your doctor before starting this or any other supplement regimen.

physician, consult the Academy of Integrative Health and Medicine, www.aihm.org.

Michael Seidman, MD, director of the Otolaryngology Research Laboratory and the division of otologic/neurotologic surgery and chair of the Center for Integrative Medicine at the Henry Ford Health System in Detroit. Dr. Seidman is coauthor, with Marie Moneysmith, of *Save Your Hearing Now: The Revolutionary Program That Can Prevent and May Even Reverse Hearing Loss.* His formulations for preventing and treating hearing loss are available at BodyLanguageVitamins.com.

ALZHEIMER'S: IS IT "TYPE 3" DIABETES?

For years, scientists from around the world have investigated various causes of Alzheimer's disease. Cardiovascular disease factors, such as hypertension, stroke and heart failure; other neurological diseases, such as Parkinson's disease; accumulated toxins and heavy metals, such as aluminum, lead, and mercury; nutrient deficiencies, including vitamins B and E; infections, such as the herpes virus and the stomach bacterium H. pylori; and head injuries have each been considered at one time or another to be a possible contributor to the development of this mind-robbing disease.

However, as researchers continue to piece together the results of literally thousands of studies, one particular theory is now emerging as perhaps the most plausible and convincing of them all in explaining why some people — and not others — develop Alzheimer's disease.

A Pattern Emerges

Five million Americans are now living with Alzheimer's, and the number of cases is skyrocketing. Interestingly, so are the rates of obesity, diabetes, and metabolic syndrome (a constellation of risk factors including elevated blood sugar, high blood pressure, abnormal cholesterol levels, and abdominal fat).

What's the potential link? Doctors have long suspected that diabetes increases risk for Alzheimer's. The exact mechanism is not known, but many experts believe that people with diabetes are more likely to develop Alzheimer's because their bodies don't properly use blood sugar (glucose) and the blood sugar–regulating hormone insulin.

Now research shows increased dementia risk in people with high blood sugar — even if they do not have diabetes. A problem with insulin appears to be the cause. How does insulin dysfunction affect the brain? Neurons are starved of energy, and there's an increase in brain cell death, DNA damage, inflammation, and the formation of plaques in the brain — a main characteristic of Alzheimer's disease.

An Alzheimer's-Fighting Regimen

Even though experimental treatments with antidiabetes drugs that improve insulin function have been shown to reduce symptoms of early Alzheimer's disease, it is my belief, as an integrative physician, that targeted non-drug therapies are preferable in preventing the brain degeneration that leads to Alzheimer's and fuels its progression. These approaches won't necessarily reverse Alzheimer's, but they may help protect your brain if you are not currently fighting this disease or help slow the progression of early-stage Alzheimer's.

My advice includes:

- **Follow a low-glycemic (low-sugar) diet.** This is essential for maintaining healthy glucose and insulin function as well as supporting brain and overall health. An effective way to maintain a low-sugar diet is to use the glycemic index (GI), a scale that ranks foods according to how quickly they raise blood sugar levels.

  Here's what happens: High-GI foods (such as white rice, white potatoes, and refined sugars) are rapidly digested and absorbed. As a result, these foods cause dangerous spikes in blood sugar levels.

  Low-GI foods (such as green vegetables, fiber-rich foods including whole grains, and plant proteins including legumes, nuts, and seeds) are digested slowly, so they gradually raise blood sugar and insulin levels. This is critical for maintaining glucose and insulin function and controlling inflammation.

  Helpful: www.glycemicindex.com gives glucose ratings of common foods and recipes.

- **Consider trying brain-supporting nutrients and herbs.*** These supplements,

---

* Consult your doctor before trying these supplements, especially if you take any medications or have a chronic health condition, such as liver or kidney

which help promote insulin function, can be used alone or taken together for better results (dosages may be lower if supplements are combined due to the ingredients' synergistic effects).

▶ **Alpha-lipoic acid** is an antioxidant shown to support insulin sensitivity and protect neurons from inflammation-related damage.

Typical dosage: 500 to 1,000 mg per day.

▶ **Chromium** improves glucose regulation.

Typical dosage: 350 to 700 mcg per day.

▶ **Alginates** from seaweed help reduce glucose spikes and crashes.

Typical dosage: 250 to 1,000 mg before meals.

▶ **L-Taurine,** an amino acid, helps maintain healthy glucose and lipid (blood fat) levels.

Typical dosage: 1,000 to 2,000 mg per day.

---

disease. If he/she is not well versed in the use of these therapies, consider seeing an integrative physician. To find one near you, consult the Institute for Functional Medicine, www.functionalmedicine.org.

Kick up Your Heels!

Regular exercise, such as walking, swimming, and tennis, is known to improve insulin function and support cognitive health by increasing circulation to the brain. Dancing, however, may be the ultimate brain-protective exercise. Why might dancing be better than other brain-body coordination exercises, such as tennis? Because dancing is mainly noncompetitive, there isn't the added stress of contending with an opponent, which increases risk for temporary cognitive impairment.

Best: Aerobic dances with a social component, such as Latin, swing, or ballroom, performed at least three times weekly for ninety minutes each session. (Dancing for less time also provides some brain benefits.) If you don't like dancing, brisk walking for thirty minutes a day, five days a week, is also shown to help protect the brain against dementia.

Free courses: In addition to getting regular physical activity, it's helpful to learn challenging new material to exercise the brain. For free online lectures provided by professors at top universities such as Stanford and Johns Hopkins, go to openculture.com/freeonlinecourses. Subjects include art, history, geography, international relations, and biology, among many others.

Isaac Eliaz, MD, LAc, an integrative physician and medical director of the Amitabha Medical Clinic & Healing Center in Sebastopol, California, an integrative health center specializing in chronic conditions. Dr. Eliaz is a licensed acupuncturist and homeopath and an expert in mind/body medicine. He has coauthored dozens of peer-reviewed scientific papers on natural healing. DrEliaz.org.

BLOOD SUGAR PROBLEMS? TAKE ACTION NOW TO PROTECT YOUR BRAIN

Knowledge is power — so even though the news from a recent study on dementia is not exactly welcome, the information is indeed beneficial if it inspires people to take steps that can help keep their brains healthy. The findings are particularly important for people with diabetes, and also, surprisingly, for those with prediabetes, a condition that now affects half of Americans ages sixty-five and older.

In the study, 1,017 seniors did oral glucose tolerance tests (in which blood sugar is measured after fasting and again after consuming a sweet drink) to determine whether they had normal blood sugar levels, impaired glucose tolerance (a prediabetic condition), or diabetes. Participants were then followed for fifteen years to see who developed Alzheimer's disease, vascular dementia (caused by blood vessel damage), or some other form of dementia.

Findings: Compared with participants who had normal blood sugar levels, those with prediabetes were 35 percent more likely to develop some type of dementia and 60 percent more likely to develop Alzheimer's. People with diabetes fared even worse, having a 74 percent higher risk for dementia of any kind, an 82 percent higher risk for vascular dementia, and more than double the risk for Alzheimer's.

The connection: Diabetes and prediabetes can damage blood vessels, causing inflammation and lack of blood flow to the brain, which in turn lead to brain cell death, and/or excess glucose carried through the blood vessels to the brain may allow accumulation of proteins that damage nerve cells.

Self-defense: More research is needed, but for now, maintaining good blood sugar control seems like a sensible way to reduce dementia risk. Ask your doctor about getting screened for prediabetes and diabetes, particularly if you are over age forty-five, are overweight, have high blood pressure, have a family history of diabetes, and/or have a history of diabetes during pregnancy.

If you have prediabetes: According to the American Diabetes Association, you can reduce your odds of developing diabetes by more than half by doing moderate exercise (such as brisk walking) for thirty minutes five days per week and losing 7 percent of your body weight (about fourteen pounds if you currently weigh 200 or about ten pounds if you weigh 150).

If you have diabetes: Be conscientious about controlling blood sugar through diet, exercise, and/or medication, and talk to your doctor about seeing a neurologist if you notice signs of cognitive problems, such as memory loss.

Yutaka Kiyohara, MD, a professor in the department of environmental medicine in the Graduate School of Medical Sciences at Kyushu University in Fukuoka, Japan, and coauthor of a study on diabetes and dementia risk published in *Neurology*.

A Cup of Decaf
May Prevent Memory Loss

When you need a boost, chances are you reach for a cup of caffeinated coffee.

And if you find that it's helping you to remember things more vividly and think more clearly while you're working on an important task, you probably chalk that up to the caffeine.

Well, the caffeine might help in the short term. But recent research conducted at Mount Sinai School of Medicine in New York City shows that coffee itself also may provide a long-term memory benefit — even when it's decaf!

In fact, the study showed that drinking a certain amount of decaf over the long term might reduce the odds of developing the neurological impairment that's associated with the early stages of Alzheimer's disease.

This is certainly promising news for those of us who are overly sensitive to caffeine but love the taste of coffee. And it's even more promising for people with type 2 diabetes, because they're often told by doctors to avoid caffeine to keep their blood sugar under control, and they're also at higher risk for Alzheimer's disease.

Coffee's Secret Weapon
To learn more, we contacted Giulio M. Pasinetti, MD, PhD, professor of neurology and

psychiatry at Mount Sinai School of Medicine and the lead researcher in the study. Before the study, Dr. Pasinetti and his team had become interested in how chlorogenic acids — types of antioxidants found in coffee, as well as in grapes, cocoa, and other foods — affect the brain. They were interested in seeing whether the positive health effects of chlorogenic acids could come from coffee without caffeine. And they wanted to analyze how decaf could affect people with type 2 diabetes, since, as mentioned earlier, people with that condition are usually advised by doctors to avoid caffeine.

Researchers used mice in the study, because they could completely control what they ate. They gave the mice a high-fat diet that triggered the onset of type 2 diabetes. At the same time, they fed half of the mice a daily extract of decaffeinated coffee made from unroasted coffee beans.

What the Decaf Did
What they found? The decaf-drinking mice's brains used 25 percent more oxygen — meaning that these mice were less likely to experience neurological impairment. Researchers suspect that the chlorogenic acids in decaf are the reason for this result.

Will It Translate to Humans?

Of course, just because decaf helps mouse brains doesn't necessarily mean that it helps human brains, but Dr. Pasinetti is hopeful, because a great deal of previous medical research using mice has, in fact, been followed by similar results in humans. (That's a big reason mice are so often used in research.)

How much might humans consume to get a similar benefit? Dr. Pasinetti recommends asking your doctor about taking a daily supplement that contains 400 mg extract of decaf green (aka "unroasted") coffee. (Dr. Pasinetti used an extract called Svetol, which can be found at www.swansonvitamins.com. A month's supply costs ten dollars.) Or drink the equivalent (two cups of decaf per day), but Dr. Pasinetti says that roasting coffee beans sucks out some of the beneficial chlorogenic acids, so the benefit would not be as much as from the extract.

Another question is whether the results would be the same with regular (caffeinated) coffee. "Since we suspect that the benefits come from the chlorogenic acids in the coffee itself — and not the caffeine — caffeinated coffee is likely to prevent neurological impairment too," says Dr. Pasinetti. "Other foods rich in chlorogenic acids, such as grapes and cocoa, are also likely to have similar benefits, but more research needs to examine that."

Giulio M. Pasinetti, MD, PhD, professor of neurology and psychiatry, Mount Sinai School of Medicine, New York City, and lead researcher of a study reported in *Nutritional Neuroscience.*

STATINS CAN HELP
DIABETES COMPLICATIONS

In addition to lowering risk for heart attack and stroke, statins lowered risk for diabetes complications, according to a recent finding. People with diabetes taking statins were 34 percent less likely to be diagnosed with diabetes-related nerve damage (neuropathy), 40 percent less likely to develop diabetes-related damage to the retina, and 12 percent less likely to develop gangrene than diabetics not taking statins.

Børge G. Nordestgaard, MD, DMSc, chief physician at Copenhagen University Hospital, Herlev, Denmark, and leader of a study of sixty thousand people, published in *The Lancet Diabetes & Endocrinology.*

Remedies for Edema: Swollen Feet, Swollen Ankles, Swollen Hands, and the Rest of You

If you are someone who puffs up with water retention in the warm weather, the prospect of cooler days might be a relief (although damp, heavy weather can make you swell up too). Or you may be someone whose calves, ankles, and feet are often a little "cushiony" with water retention despite the weather. They may be so cushiony that they dimple when you press into them. That kind of swelling can be painful too — and it can be a sign of a serious health problem, even a medical emergency. But for most people who deal with limb swelling — men and women alike — it is simply a recurring nuisance that a doctor may or may not be able to diagnose. Here are some surefire remedies to soothe the swelling and also advice for when limb swelling might be life-threatening.

Why We Swell

Swelling caused by fluid buildup is called edema (pronounced ih-DEE-mah). When it affects only your arms, legs, hands, and feet, it is called peripheral edema. We retain water because blood vessels in our arms, legs, hands, and feet expand or dilate. This dilation can be caused by hot or humid weather or a number of other causes. The dilation makes it easier for fluid to leak out of blood vessels into surrounding tissue, causing the tissue to swell. Sitting or standing in one position for a long time without moving makes the swelling worse because gravity just pulls all that fluid down to pool in your hands, legs, and feet.

Relief for Swollen Limbs

Besides weather-related effects on blood vessels, the reason why some people swell can't always be figured out, but common disease-related causes of swelling are kidney and cardiovascular disease. Whether a doctor can or cannot pinpoint the cause of peripheral edema, he or she too often prescribes a diuretic and suggests that you cut back on salt.

Although cutting back on salt may be great advice, taking a diuretic may not be unless the swelling is related to high blood pressure or high blood pressure medication. But there are safe, natural ways to relieve swelling, including the following:

• **Leg elevation.** Keep your legs elevated while sitting for prolonged periods. Yes, put a comfy, compact ottoman under your desk, or put your legs up and rest your feet on that extra chair. Also, prop your feet up on a few pillows while lying on the sofa or in bed. Don't just bear with swelling, because if it happens often, it can cause your skin and tissue to stretch and change. It can also lead to more serious and lasting edema.

- **Walking breaks.** If you really can't plop your feet up on a chair in a place where you regularly spend time — such as in an office or another noncasual setting — then make a point of getting up from the chair and taking five-minute walking breaks every hour or so. This increases circulation and gets your lymphatic system to pump out excess fluid.
- **Compression stockings.** If you need to stand for a long time during the day, wear support hose or compression knee-highs or stockings. These help blood circulation between your feet and your heart, with one benefit being more spring in your step. In fact, athletes often use compression stockings to enhance their performance.

  Compression stockings come in many styles and colors, price ranges (from about ten to one hundred dollars), sizes, and pressures. So when buying compression stockings online, you will need to find sellers that provide guidance on sizing and compression needs. One source is Bright Life Direct, which carries all the major brands and has easy-to-follow guidance and FAQs to figure out what size and kind of compression stocking is right for you — and right for your budget.
- **Massage your hands.** Swollen hands? To

enhance circulation and lymphatic drainage, apply lotion to your hands and massage one hand and then the other, starting with the fingertips and moving down the hand to the wrist. Also exercise the hands by holding them at chest level and clenching and unclenching them. To do this effectively, gently make a fist and then open your fist and spread your fingers. Massage and exercise your hands several times a day when edema is acting up.

When Edema Is Dangerous

There are other factors that can cause edema, and they can be life-threatening. Besides cardiovascular and kidney disease, other causes, which were spelled out by the American Academy of Family Physicians in a recent article by and for doctors, include liver disease, sleep apnea, allergies, use of certain medications (such as nonsteroidal anti-inflammatory drugs, antihypertensives, corticosteroids, antidepressants, diabetes medications, hormone replacement therapy), and chemotherapy. Edema also can be caused by surgical removal or malfunction of the lymph nodes, which, as part of the lymphatic system, filter fluid and cleanse the body of bacteria, viruses, and other debris.

What's the danger of unchecked edema? Besides the fact that you might have a serious underlying condition needing treatment, all that swelling and stretching of the skin can cause a flaky, eczema-like appearance and even skin ulcers. Ulcers, in turn, can lead to serious skin infections, such as cellulitis, where the infection bores through the skin and into underlying tissue. And you probably also know that chronic swollen legs and feet can put you at risk for blood clots that can lodge in a leg or travel up to the lungs, heart, brain, or another part of your body. This is called thromboembolism (or stroke when it hits your brain) — and, just like a stroke, it can kill you.

If you are having symptoms such as shortness of breath, rapid heartbeat, or pain and heat in a limb, be sure to get to a doctor or even an emergency room right away. You could be experiencing thromboembolism. The symptoms may be accompanied by chest pain, fever, or intense anxiety (a feeling of doom). Once treated for a thromboembolic attack, you may be put on a medication to prevent blood clots and be instructed to wear compression stockings.

For all these reasons, if you have chronic edema — even if you can get relief from the self-treatments described above — it's a good idea to get it checked out by a doctor. In addition to the suggestions listed above, additional steps a doctor might take if you have severe chronic edema include:

- **Checking for clots.** Even if you are not having a thromboembolic emergency, your doctor may order an ultrasound of the swollen limb to see whether clots have formed. If so, he or she will likely put you on a blood-thinning drug to prevent a thromboembolic event.
- **Prescribing pneumatic compression.** If swelling is severe and related to surgical removal or malfunction of lymph nodes, you might be instructed in the use of a pneumatic compression device, an inflatable garment resembling a boot, sock, or sleeve that does the work of a compression stocking but with greater intensity.
- **Recommending physiotherapy.** You also may be referred to a physiotherapist for massage and movement therapy and specialized compression techniques that involve use of bandage wrappings.

So do not endure swollen limbs simply because it's something that you've put up with for years. Keeping the swelling in check and getting a handle on the underlying cause, when possible, can save you from major health woes down the line.

Study titled "Edema: Diagnosis and Management," published in *American Family Physician*.

A Cancer and Diabetes Risk Your Doctor May Not Know About

If you don't have any of the well-known risk factors for cancer, including smoking, a family history of cancer, or long-term exposure to a carcinogen such as asbestos, you may think that your risk for the disease is average or even less than average.

What you may not realize: Although most of the cancer predispositions (genetic, lifestyle, and environmental factors that increase risk for the disease) are commonly known, there are several medical conditions that also can increase your risk, such as diabetes.

Unfortunately, many primary care physicians do not link diabetes to cancer. As a result, they fail to prescribe the tests and treatments that could keep cancer at bay or reduce the condition's cancer-causing potential.

The high blood sugar levels that occur with type 2 diabetes predispose you to heart attack, stroke, nerve pain, blindness, kidney failure, a need for amputation — and cancer.

New research: For every 1 percent increase in HbA1C — a measurement of blood sugar levels over the previous three months — there is an 18 percent increase in the risk for cancer, according to a study published in *Current Diabetes Reports.*

Other current studies have linked type 2 diabetes to a 94 percent increased risk for pancreatic cancer, a 38 percent increased risk for colon cancer, a 15 to 20 percent higher risk for postmenopausal breast cancer, and a 20 percent higher risk for blood cancers such as non-Hodgkin's lymphoma and leukemia.

What to do: If you have type 2 diabetes, make sure your primary care physician orders regular screening tests for cancer, such as colonoscopy and mammogram.

Screening for pancreatic cancer is not widely available, but some of the larger cancer centers (such as the H. Lee Moffitt Cancer Center & Research Institute in Tampa, Florida, and the Mayo Clinic in Rochester, Minnesota) offer it to high-risk individuals.

This typically includes people with long-standing diabetes (more than twenty years) and/or a family history of pancreatic cancer. The test involves an ultrasound of both the stomach and small intestine, where telltale signs of pancreatic cancer can be detected.

Also work with your doctor to minimize the cancer-promoting effects of diabetes. For example, control blood sugar levels through a diet that emphasizes slow-digesting foods that don't create spikes in blood sugar levels, such as vegetables and beans. Also, try to get regular exercise — for example, thirty minutes of walking five or six days a week. Studies have shown that regular exercise helps to control blood sugar. And consider medical interventions, such as use of the diabetes drug metformin.

Lynne Eldridge, MD, medical manager of the Lung Cancer site for About.com and a former clinical preceptor at the University of Minnesota Medical School in Minneapolis. Dr. Eldridge practiced family medicine for fifteen years and now devotes herself full time to researching and speaking on cancer prevention. She is author of *Avoiding Cancer One Day at a Time.*

DIABETICS: THE BODY PART THAT'S AGING FASTER THAN THE REST OF YOU

People with type 2 diabetes have a lot of balls to keep in the air, medically speaking.

They need to, of course, keep their blood sugar in check, get regular eye screenings, and monitor their feet, which often can suffer from nerve damage.

Now new research may add another item to that already-long checklist.

It suggests that people with type 2 diabetes should start getting colonoscopies earlier and, perhaps, get them more frequently. Here's why.

Type 2 Diabetics Have "Older" Colons

Researchers from Washington University in St. Louis reviewed colonoscopy records of male and female patients over a six-year span, comparing the incidence of precancerous polyps in three groups — those ages forty to forty-nine with type 2 diabetes, those ages forty to forty-nine without type 2 diabetes, and those ages fifty to fifty-nine without type 2 diabetes.

Their first finding was expected, since age increases the risk for precancerous polyps. Nondiabetics in their fifties had a much higher rate of precancerous polyps (32 percent) than nondiabetics in their forties (14 percent).

But their second finding was alarming. Diabetics in their forties had nearly the same rate of precancerous polyps (30 percent) as nondiabetics in their fifties (again, 32 percent). And this was after individual cancer risk factors — such as sex, race, obesity, smoking, high cholesterol, and alcohol use — were taken into account.

"It's almost as if the colons of diabetics are ten years older," study author Hongha Vu-James, MD, formerly clinical gastroenterology fellow at the university, says. It's believed that the culprit is a high level of insulin in type 2 diabetics, since insulin is thought to promote cell growth in the colon, she says.

Should Screening Guidelines Change?
Current guidelines from the American Cancer Society (ACS) suggest that colorectal cancer screenings should begin at age fifty for people at average risk for colon cancer. ACS advises those at high risk (anyone with inflammatory bowel disease, a personal history of colorectal cancer, or a family history of colorectal cancer) to get screened even earlier (the age varies by risk factor). In addition, the site for the American College of Gastroenterology says, "Recent evidence suggests that African Americans should begin screening earlier at the age of forty-five."

What about people with type 2 diabetes? The American Diabetes Association, while acknowledging that type 2 diabetes is linked with a higher risk for colorectal and other cancers, urges diabetics to reduce lifestyle-related cancer risk factors but doesn't deviate from the "begin screening at age fifty" recommendation for those at average risk.

Dr. Vu-James, however, is hoping that her research — and future studies that replicate it — will change that. Her study suggests that people with type 2 diabetes should consider getting their first colorectal cancer screening earlier than age fifty.

In her view, doctors should be open to discussing the idea of earlier colorectal cancer screenings with diabetic patients based on their overall risk factors, and it might help to bring a copy of this article with you if you want to broach the idea with your physician. Unfortunately, if you have type 2 diabetes and you want to get a colorectal cancer screening before the age of fifty but you're considered to be at average risk, according to the current guidelines, it's unlikely that insurance will cover it, says Dr. Vu-James, and a colonoscopy can cost around $1,200 or more. If more research confirms Dr. Vu-James's findings and screening guidelines change, colonoscopies are more likely to be covered in the future.

If you have type 2 diabetes and are over the age of fifty and you've already started getting colorectal cancer screenings, Dr. Vu-James says that there is no data yet on whether or not more frequent screenings are necessary, but if you're concerned, talk to your doctor.

Also: This increased risk for colorectal cancer does not apply to people of any age with type 1 diabetes, says Dr. Vu-James, because type 1 is caused by a lack of insulin.

Hongha Vu-James, MD, formerly clinical gastroenterology fellow, Washington University, St. Louis, and lead author of a study presented at a Digestive Disease Week conference in San Diego.

DIABETIC WOMEN AT RISK FOR COLORECTAL CANCER

There seems to be no end to the health risks associated with diabetes, a truly insidious disease that can lead to other serious health problems. Having diabetes increases risk for cardiovascular disease, kidney failure, hypertension, stroke, and damage to the nerves and eyes. Recent research has also linked diabetes to a greater risk of certain cancers, including colorectal (colon or rectum) cancer. And now a study from Washington University in St. Louis concludes that diabetic women are at greater risk for developing colorectal adenomas — polyps that can turn into cancer. This is especially true for diabetic women who are also obese, defined in this study as having a body mass index of over 30.

The study compared the colonoscopy records of one hundred women with type 2 diabetes with those of five hundred nondiabetic women to evaluate the rate of adenomas in these women.

The results: Diabetic women had a significantly higher rate of adenomas compared with those who did not have the disease — 37 percent versus 24 percent. Furthermore, women with type 2 diabetes were also more apt to have advanced adenomas — 14 percent versus 6 percent. Apparently, at greatest risk of all are women who are obese and have diabetes. In fact, when compared with nonobese, nondiabetic women, these women faced nearly twice as high a risk of having any kind of adenoma and more than two times greater risk for having advanced adenoma.

We spoke with the study's lead author, Jill E. Elwing, MD, about these results. She explains that insulin is in itself a growth factor and that might be what is behind the link between diabetes and colorectal adenoma — the growth factor could produce a pro-cancerous effect. The immediate takeaway from this study, she says, is that medical professionals and this group of vulnerable women should have greater awareness and pay more attention to regular screening. Women of any age who have type 2 diabetes should discuss a colorectal screening schedule with their doctors. And because being over age fifty is also considered a risk factor for colorectal cancer, diabetic women over that age should be particularly careful to follow their doctor's advice about regular screenings, she says.

Jill E. Elwing, MD, is in private practice in St. Louis, Missouri.

A WALK DOES WONDERS FOR CHRONIC KIDNEY DISEASE

If you have chronic kidney disease (CKD), there is a simple way that you might save yourself from needing dialysis or a kidney transplant. CKD, a condition in which the kidneys struggle to filter waste from the blood, is a silent health threat that you can be completely unaware of until serious damage is done. One in three adults with diabetes and one in five with high blood pressure has CKD, and like so many illnesses, incidence increases after age fifty. If left unchecked, end-stage renal disease — kidney failure — occurs. That's when you'll need to be hooked up to a dialysis machine to filter your blood or will require a kidney transplant to stay alive.

Although there is no cure once CKD sets in, it can often be kept from advancing, and now doctors have confirmed that a certain simple exercise can not only help you avoid dialysis or transplantation but also add years to your life. And that exercise is walking!

A Proven Benefit

We all know that exercise improves cardiovascular fitness, and researchers had already confirmed that it improves fitness in people with CKD. But could walking actually help with the disease itself — and in a significant way? That question had never been tested by research, so a group of Taiwanese researchers decided to find out.

The study started out with 6,363 patients whose average age was seventy. All had moderate to severe CKD, and 53 percent had CKD severe enough to need dialysis or a kidney transplant. The researchers recorded and monitored exercise activity and a range of other health and medical measurements in the group and identified 1,341 people who walked as their favorite form of exercise. These patients were compared with patients who did not walk nor exercise in any other way.

The results: Walkers were 33 percent less likely to die of kidney disease and 21 percent less likely to need dialysis or a kidney transplant than nonwalkers/nonexercisers. And the more a person walked, the more likely he or she was not on dialysis or in need of a kidney transplant and still alive when the study ended. So, for example, someone who walked once or twice a week for an average thirty minutes to an hour had a 17 percent lower risk of death and a 19 percent lower risk of needing dialysis or a kidney transplant compared with someone who didn't walk or exercise. And someone who walked for an average thirty minutes to an hour seven or more times a week had a 59 percent lower risk of death and a 44 percent lower risk of needing dialysis or a kidney transplant.

Now, when researchers see this kind of dramatic result, they should always explore whether there was some reason other than the activity that was studied (in this case, walking) that could explain things. These are called confounding factors — for example, could it be that walkers walked because they were healthier, as opposed to being healthier because they walked? But no confounding factors were found. The average age, average body size, and degree of kidney disease was the same in the two groups, as was the prevalence of diabetes-associated coronary artery disease, cigarette smoking, and use of medications for CKD.

The bottom line for people with CKD — walk! Walk everywhere! Walk often! Even a thirty-minute walk once or twice a week can help. The more you walk, the greater the benefit.

Are You at Risk?
If you have diabetes or high blood pressure, your doctor should give you a simple blood test to see whether CKD is developing. Otherwise, here are telltale signs to keep an eye out for — these may signal that you should be evaluated for CKD:

• Unexplained fatigue
• Trouble concentrating
• Poor appetite

481

- Trouble sleeping
- Nighttime muscle cramps
- Swollen feet and ankles
- Eye puffiness, especially in the morning
- Dry, itchy skin
- Frequent urination, especially at night

Be sure to tell your doctor what medications you're on when you are examined for CKD. Because the kidneys also filter medications out of your body, meds can build up to toxic levels in your system if the kidneys aren't doing their job. If you have CKD, your doctor may take you off some medications and lower the dose of others.

While there's no cure for CKD once it sets in, it need not advance to severe and deadly stages that require dialysis or a kidney transplant. Besides exercising and keeping the underlying cause (whether it be diabetes, high blood pressure, or something else) in check, mild CKD is managed by diet. To do it right:

- **Make walking a priority.**
- **Work with your doctor to manage the underlying cause,** and work with a dietitian to manage your nutrition requirements. A dietitian will plan a regimen that controls the amount of protein, salt, potassium, and phosphorus you consume, all of which can build up to toxic levels in people with CKD. A dietitian will also balance your CKD diet

needs with those related to glucose control or whatever condition may be associated with your CKD.

Che-Yi Chou, MD, PhD, Kidney Institute, division of nephrology, department of internal medicine, both at China Medical University Hospital, Taiwan. Dr. Chou's study appeared in the *Clinical Journal of the American Society of Nephrology*.

483

DANGERS OF A "SLOW STOMACH"

When you eat a meal, you probably don't think about the amount of time it takes your body to digest the food. But for many people, this is the key to uncovering a host of digestive ills — and even some seemingly unrelated concerns such as chronic fatigue.

When Food Moves Too Slowly

In healthy adults, digestion time varies, but it generally takes about four hours for a meal to leave the stomach before passing on to the small intestine and colon.

What happens: When food enters the stomach, signals from hormones and nerve cells trigger stomach acid, digestive enzymes, and wavelike peristaltic contractions of the muscles in the stomach wall. Together, they break down the meal into a soupy mixture called chyme, which peristalsis then pushes into the small intestine.

This process is known as gastric motility. And when gastric motility is impeded — when stomach emptying slows to a crawl, even though nothing is blocking the stomach outlet — it's called gastroparesis.

Surprising fact: An estimated one out of every fifty-five Americans suffers from gastroparesis — but the condition is diagnosed in only one out of every ninety people who have it.

When gastroparesis goes undetected: The

symptoms of gastroparesis are often obvious — for example, nausea, vomiting, feeling full right after starting to eat a meal, bloating, and abdominal pain. But the condition can cause other health problems such as unwanted weight loss and even malnutrition. It also can interfere with the absorption of medications and wear you down physically (one study found that 93 percent of people with gastroparesis were fatigued).

Getting the Right Diagnosis

If you're experiencing the symptoms of gastroparesis, see your primary care physician. He/she may refer you to a gastroenterologist. It's likely the specialist will order the "gold standard" for diagnosing gastroparesis, a test called gastric emptying scintigraphy.

Next step: At the test, you'll eat a meal that contains radioactive isotopes. (Radio-labeled Egg Beaters with jam, toast, and water are typical.) A scan is taken at one, two, and four hours after the meal with a scintigraph or gamma camera. A one-hour scan after drinking liquid is also recommended. If images from any of the scans show that your stomach isn't emptying normally, you are diagnosed with gastroparesis.

Another approach: When I perform an endoscopy on a patient with gastroparesis-like symptoms (a thin, flexible tube with a light and camera on the end is inserted down the esophagus and into the stomach), if I see a significant amount of retained fluids or food despite an overnight fast, I make the diagnosis then and there, saving time and money.

Finding the Cause

Experts haven't discovered the exact mechanisms underlying gastroparesis. In fact, an estimated 40 percent of cases are idiopathic — the cause is unknown. Gastroparesis is a complication for about 30 percent of people with type 1 or type 2 diabetes.

What happens: Diabetes can damage the vagus nerve, which runs from the cranium to the abdomen and plays a key role in digestion.

Medication also can cause gastroparesis.

Examples: Narcotic pain relievers, such as oxycodone, and anticholinergics, a class of drugs that includes certain antihistamines and overactive bladder medications.

Small intestine bacterial overgrowth, in which abnormally large numbers of bacteria grow in the small intestine, also can lead to gastroparesis.

Getting the Best Medical Care

I have found that an integrative approach that combines conventional and alternative medicine is the best way to control gastroparesis.

Conventional treatment typically includes

medications that either speed stomach emptying or help control the symptoms of gastroparesis such as nausea and vomiting. For example:

- **Metoclopramide.** This is currently the only FDA-approved medication for gastroparesis. Metoclopramide works by blocking receptors of the neurotransmitter dopamine, which accelerates gastric motility.

  Problem: The FDA has approved metoclopramide for no more than twelve weeks of use because long-term intake can cause tardive dyskinesia — involuntary, repetitive body movements, such as grimacing. Because of this risk, I rarely prescribe metoclopramide for my patients.

  Another medication option: The drug domperidone has the same dopamine-suppressing action in the digestive tract as metoclopramide, but it does not cross the blood-brain barrier and therefore is much less likely to cause tardive dyskinesia. Risks include breast tenderness and worsening of the heart condition long QT syndrome.

  However, according to clinical guidelines for the management of gastroparesis published in the *American Journal of Gastroenterology,* domperidone "is generally as effective" as metoclopramide with "lower risk of adverse effects."

Domperidone is readily available in most countries, where it is a standard treatment for heartburn, but not in the United States. However, your doctor can obtain it under the FDA's Investigational New Drug program.

- **Antinausea drugs.** Prochlorperazine and ondansetron are commonly prescribed for gastroparesis.
- **Botox.** Injections of botulinum toxin into the pylorus (the opening from the stomach into the small intestine) can help some patients for four to six months, after which the injection must be repeated.

New approaches: Physicians at Johns Hopkins are now using a new and effective procedure called through-the-scope transpyloric stent placement. With this procedure, an endoscope is used to place a stent (tube) that helps transfer stomach contents into the small intestine.

Another new approach, pioneered by John Clarke, MD, of Johns Hopkins, involves placing a stent across the pylorus to drain the stomach.

Alternative Therapies

Certain alternative therapies may also help with stomach motility and/or with nausea and vomiting:*

- **Peppermint oil.** This can help gastroparesis, but it also can worsen heartburn in people with gastroesophageal reflux disease (GERD). If you have gastroparesis but not GERD, an enteric-coated softgel of peppermint oil may help you.
  Recommended dose: 90 mg daily.
- **Iberogast.** Studies have shown that this pharmaceutical-grade, multiherbal tincture can help with gastroparesis.
  Recommended dose: twenty drops, two to three times a day, before meals. (Iberogast does contain alcohol.)
- **Ginger.** Gingerroot may help with nausea and improve gastric motility.
  Recommended dose: 1,200 mg daily.
- **Acupuncture.** This treatment can help control the symptoms of gastroparesis. Acupuncture has been shown to be effective for nausea and vomiting and abdominal pain and bloating.

* Be sure to check with your doctor before trying these therapies, which are available online and at most health-food stores.

489

Diet/Lifestyle Tips

Many dietary and lifestyle habits can improve stomach motility:

- **Eat smaller, more frequent meals.** Eat smaller amounts of food every two, three, or four hours.
- **Reduce dietary fiber and fat.** Both slow stomach emptying.
- **Chew food thoroughly.**
- **Chew sugarless gum.** Do so for about one hour after eating to stimulate peristalsis.
- **Take a leisurely five- or ten-minute (or longer) walk** after every meal.

Gerard Mullin, MD, an associate professor of medicine at the Johns Hopkins University School of Medicine and director of the Celiac Disease Clinic, Integrative GI Nutrition Services and the Capsule Endoscopy Program at Johns Hopkins Hospital, all in Baltimore. He is author of *The Inside Tract,* editor of *Integrative Gastroenterology* and several other textbooks, and the author or coauthor of more than fifty scientific papers.

How to Prevent Glaucoma Vision Loss Before It's Too Late

Imagine that, as you read on your computer screen, the many pixels on the screen begin to stop working, a few at a time, not right in the center, but in clusters all around the screen. It happens slowly, eventually wiping out all but a tiny central spot, which eventually drops out too. The screen is blank then.

That's a pretty close analogy of what happens when glaucoma runs its course. You'll start losing your peripheral vision first, one eye at a time, and you likely won't even realize that it's happening until much of the damage has been done. The damage is irreversible, but the process can be stopped with early detection and treatment.

Are You at Risk?

Glaucoma is the second-leading cause of blindness in the world after cataracts, and it mostly affects people as they age past sixty. The disease is characterized by dying ganglion nerve cells in the retina, the light-sensitive tissue at the back of the eye that catches the images we see. Once these cells die, they are never replaced, which makes early detection of glaucoma critical.

Among the many different types of glaucoma, the most common is open-angle glaucoma, caused by clogging of the eyes' drainage canals in people who have a wide angle between the iris and cornea. Besides older age, risk factors include genetic predisposition, nearsightedness, higher eye pressure, high and low blood pressure, diabetes, and hypothyroidism.

Detection

The lack of symptoms is a major reason why glaucoma is often not detected early. And the idea that glaucoma always has something to do with high eye pressure is a prime reason why diagnosis is often missed by eye specialists during regular eye exams. Although high eye pressure is a hallmark of a condition called angle-closure glaucoma, it is not necessarily present in the more common open-angle glaucoma.

Annual eye exams are recommended for people who are over age sixty and anyone with a first-degree relative (parent, sibling, or child) who has or had glaucoma. People younger than sixty should consider getting eye exams, including glaucoma screening, every two years.

To ensure that your exams are thorough enough to detect glaucoma, make sure that, besides having eye pressure measured, you receive a side vision test, which examines peripheral vision, or a visual field test, which examines both peripheral and central vision. The optic nerve head or optic disc (a part of the eye where ganglion cells enter the optic nerve) should also be examined by the eye specialist to evaluate the health of those ganglion cells.

Treatment

If glaucoma is detected, treatment can prevent further damage by restoring eye-fluid drainage and/or relieving eye pressure. This is accomplished by use of daily eye drops or a combination of eye drops and oral medication. Many different types of eye drops — some known as prostaglandin analogs, some alpha agonists, and some carbonic anhydrase inhibitors — are prescribed, depending on glaucoma symptoms that need to be managed. Laser eye surgery or traditional types of eye surgery that relieve pressure and correct blocked drainage ducts are options for people who don't get adequate relief from eye drops or who experience allergy or severe side effects from medications, but these people may still need to continue using some form of medication after surgery until eye pressure and drainage correct themselves.

Side effects of eye drops can include change in color of the iris and eyelid skin, stinging and burning of the eye, blurred vision, and related problems. But most people who become lax about eye drop use don't do so because of side effects. They do so because they forget to use them, sabotaging their fight against glaucoma symptoms.

In a study in which we electronically monitored people who were using eye drops for glaucoma management, we discovered that, under the best of circumstances, patients were taking their eye drops only 70 percent of the time. Of course, eye drops can't help relieve glaucoma unless they are consistently used.

Helpful: Set up a reminder system. For example, set your cell phone alarm to alert you when to use the drops.

As for alternative treatments for prevention of open-angle glaucoma beyond early detection and management, scientific evidence shows no association between glaucoma and a person's personal habits, such as diet, use of vitamins and supplements, alcohol consumption, and caffeine intake. Altering these behaviors, unfortunately, will not decrease your chances of getting glaucoma or prevent it from getting worse. However, aerobic exercise (twenty minutes four times a week) can increase blood flow and reduce eye pressure, which can keep glaucoma from worsening.

Where to Get Treatment

Optometrists can diagnose glaucoma and treat it with eye drops. Ophthalmologists can diagnose it and treat it with a wider range of therapies — eye drops as well as laser treatments and eye surgery. But whichever type of specialist you consult, make sure that he is up-to-date on how best to detect glaucoma during an eye exam. To find optometrists and ophthalmologists in your area who have specialized training in glaucoma diagnosis and treatment and have been given a seal of approval by glaucoma experts, visit the Glaucoma Research Foundation website.

Harry A. Quigley, MD, A. Edward Maumenee Professor of Ophthalmology and director, Glaucoma Center of Excellence, Wilmer Eye Institute, Johns Hopkins University, Baltimore. Dr. Quigley's book is *Glaucoma: What Every Patient Should Know: A Guide from Dr. Harry Quigley.*

PYCNOGENOL HELPS
DIABETIC RETINOPATHY

Pycnogenol (pronounced pic-NOJ-en-all), an extract from the bark of the French maritime pine, is known to improve circulation, reduce swelling, and ease asthma. Now Italian researchers have found another use for it — it helps patients with diabetes who are in the early stages of diabetic retinopathy, a complication of diabetes in which the retina becomes damaged, resulting in vision impairment, including blurred vision, seeing dark spots, impaired night vision, reduced color perception, and even blindness.

All people with diabetes are at risk for diabetic retinopathy, and it's estimated that as many as 80 percent of people with diabetes for ten years or more will have this complication.

Participants in the Italian study had been diagnosed with diabetes (the researchers did not specify whether the patients had type 1 or 2 diabetes) for four years, and their diabetes was well controlled by diet and oral medication. Study participants had early-stage retinopathy and moderately impaired vision. After two months of treatment, the patients given Pycnogenol had less retinal swelling as measured by ultrasound testing. Most important, their vision was significantly improved. This was especially noticeable because the vision of those in the control group did not improve.

My view: If you have type 1 or 2 diabetes, undergo a comprehensive eye exam at least once a year. If retinopathy is detected, it would be wise to supplement with Pycnogenol (150 mg daily). Because retinopathy among diabetes patients is so prevalent, I recommend this amount to all my patients with diabetes to protect their vision. Pycnogenol has a blood-thinning effect, so people who take blood-thinning medication, such as warfarin, should use it only while being monitored by a doctor.

Mark A. Stengler, NMD, a naturopathic medical doctor and leading authority on the practice of alternative and integrated medicine. Dr. Stengler is author of the *Health Revelations* newsletter, *The Natural Physician's Healing Therapies,* and *Bottom Line's Prescription for Natural Cures.* He is also the founder and medical director of the Stengler Center for Integrative Medicine in Encinitas, California, and former adjunct associate clinical professor at the National College of Natural Medicine in Portland, Oregon. MarkStengler.com.

HOW TO SEE BETTER IN THE DARK

Aging often brings a reduction in the ability to see well in low light.

Reasons: Night vision has two elements. First, the pupils must dilate to let in as much light as possible. Normally, this happens within seconds of entering a darkened environment, but as we age, the muscles that control pupil dilation weaken, slowing down and/or limiting dilation. Second, chemical changes must occur in the light-sensitive photoreceptors (called rods and cones) of the retina at the back of the eyeball. Some of these changes take several minutes, and some take longer, so normally, full night vision is not achieved for about twenty minutes. Even brief exposure to bright light (such as oncoming headlights) reverses these chemical changes, so the processes must start over. With age, these chemical changes occur more slowly, and some of our photoreceptors may be lost.

While we cannot restore the eyes' full youthful function, we can take steps to preserve and even improve our ability to see in low light. Here's how:

• **First, see your eye doctor to investigate possible underlying medical problems.** Various eye disorders can cause or contribute to reduced night vision, including cataracts (clouding of the eye's lens), retinitis pigmentosa (a disease that damages the retina's rods and cones), and macular degeneration (in which objects in the center of the field of vision cannot be seen). Night vision also can be compromised by liver cirrhosis or the digestive disorder celiac disease, which can lead to deficiencies of eye-protecting nutrients, or diabetes, which can damage eye nerves and blood vessels. Diagnosing any underlying disorder is vital, because the sooner it is treated, the better the outcome is likely to be.

• **Adopt an eye-healthy diet.** Eat foods rich in the vision-supporting nutrients below, and ask your doctor whether supplementation is right for you. Especially important:

▶ **Lutein,** a yellow pigment and antioxidant found in corn, dark green leafy vegetables, egg yolks, kiwi fruit, oranges, and yellow squash.
Typical supplement dosage: 6 mg daily.

▶ **Vitamin A,** found in carrots, Chinese cabbage, dark green leafy vegetables, pumpkin, sweet potatoes, and winter squash.
Typical supplement dosage: 10,000 international units (IU) daily.

▶ **Zeaxanthin,** a yellow pigment and antioxidant found in corn, egg yolks, kiwi fruit, orange peppers, and oranges.

Typical supplement dosage: 300 mcg daily.

▶ **Zinc,** found in beans, beef, crab, duck, lamb, oat bran, oysters, ricotta cheese, turkey, and yogurt.

Typical supplement dosage: 20 mg daily.

• **Update prescription lenses.** Many people just keep wearing the same old glasses even though vision tends to change over time, Dr. Grossman says, so new glasses with the correct prescription often can improve night vision.

• **Keep eyeglasses and contacts clean.** Smudges bend rays of light and distort what you see.

• **Wear sunglasses outdoors on sunny days, especially between noon and three p.m.** This is particularly important for people with light-colored eyes, which are more vulnerable to the sun's damaging ultraviolet rays. Excessive sun exposure is a leading cause of eye disorders (such as cataracts) that can impair eyesight, including night vision. Amber or gray lenses are best for sunglasses, Dr. Grossman says, because they absorb light frequencies most evenly.

• **Do not use yellow-tinted lenses at night.** These often are marketed as "night driving" glasses, implying that they sharpen contrast and reduce glare in low light. However, Dr. Grossman cautions that any tint only further impairs night vision.

Safest: If you wear prescription glasses, stick to untinted, clear lenses — but do ask your optometrist about adding an antireflective or antiglare coating.

- **Exercise your night vision.** This won't speed up the eyes' process of adjusting to the dark, but it may encourage a mental focus that helps the brain and eyes work better together, thus improving your ability to perceive objects in a darkened environment.

  What to do: For twenty minutes four times per week, go into a familiar room at night and turn off the lights. As your eyes are adjusting, look directly toward a specific object that you know is there. Focus on it, trying to make out its shape and details and to distinguish it from surrounding shadows. With practice, your visual perception should improve. For an additional challenge, do the exercise outdoors at night, while looking at unfamiliar objects in a dark room, or while using peripheral vision rather than looking directly at an object.

- **When driving at night, avoid looking directly at oncoming headlights.** Shifting your gaze slightly to the right of center minimizes the eye changes that would temporarily impair your night vision, yet still allows you to see traffic.

Also: Use the night setting on rearview mirrors to reduce reflected glare.

• **Clean car windows and lights.** When was the last time you used glass cleaner on the inside of your windshield or on rear and side windows or on headlights and taillights? For the clearest possible view and minimal distortion from smudges, keep all windows and lights squeaky clean.

Marc Grossman, OD, LAc, holistic developmental/ behavioral optometrist, licensed acupuncturist and medical director, Natural Eye Care, New Paltz, New York. He is coauthor of *Greater Vision and Natural Eye Care.* NaturalEyeCare.com.

Beware of Eye Floaters — They Can Be a Telltale Sign of a Vision-Robbing Eye Condition

If you have ever noticed a few tiny dots, blobs, squiggly lines, or cobweb-like images drifting across your field of vision, you are not alone. These visual disturbances, called floaters, are common, and most people simply dismiss them as a normal part of growing older. But that's not always the case.

When it could be serious: In about 15 percent of cases, floaters are a symptom of a harmful condition known as a retinal tear, which can, in turn, lead to a vision-robbing retinal detachment in a matter of hours to days.

How Does It Happen?

The retina, which is an extremely thin, delicate membrane that lines the inside of the back of the eye, converts light into signals that your brain recognizes as images. However, with age, a jelly-like material called the vitreous that fills much of the eyeball commonly shrinks a bit and separates from the retina. If the shrinkage or some other injury exerts enough force, the retina can actually tear.

You might notice a sudden shower of new floaters or flashes of light that look like shooting stars or lightning bolts. What you're seeing when this occurs are actually shadows that are being cast on the retina by the tiny clumps of collagen fibers that comprise the floaters. The flashes of light are caused by the tugging of the vitreous on the retina, which stimulates the photoreceptors that sense light.

Why floaters and/or flashes are a red flag: The retina lacks nerves that signal pain, so these visual disturbances are the only way you will be alerted to a tear. Left untreated, fluid can leak through the retinal tear, and the retina can detach like wallpaper peeling off a wall. A retinal detachment is an emergency — if it's not treated promptly, it can lead to a complete loss of vision in the affected eye.

Are You at Risk?

Changes in the eye that increase risk for a retinal tear or detachment begin primarily in your fifties and sixties and continue to increase as you grow older.

In addition to age, you can also be at increased risk for a retinal tear or detachment due to the following:

• **Nearsightedness.** People of any age with nearsightedness greater than six diopters (requiring eyeglasses or contact lenses with a vision correction of more than minus six) are five to six times more likely to develop a retinal tear or detachment. That's because nearsighted eyeballs are larger than normal.

Therefore, the retina is spread thinner, making it more prone to tearing.

Important: If you're nearsighted, don't assume that corrective eyewear or LASIK surgery decreases your risk for a retinal tear or detachment. Neither does.

- **Cataract surgery.** This surgery alters the vitreous jelly, increasing the risk that the vitreous will pull away from the retina, possibly giving way to a retinal detachment.

  Cataract surgery has been known to double one's detachment risk, but a new Australian study suggests that improvements in technology, such as phacoemulsification, which uses an ultrasonic device to break up and remove the cloudy lens, have cut the risk from one in one hundred to one in four hundred.

- **Diabetes.** Because it impairs circulation to the retina over time, diabetes leads to a higher risk for a severe type of retinal detachment that is not associated with floaters and flashes and can be initially asymptomatic.

  Individuals who have diabetes should be sure to have annual eye exams with dilation of the pupils to check for this and other ocular complications of diabetes. The Optomap test provides a wide view of the retina, but you also need pupil dilation for a thorough screening.

The Danger of a Retinal Tear

Anyone who experiences a sudden burst of floaters or flashes, especially if they are large or appear in any way different from how they have in the past, should contact an ophthalmologist right away for advice.

If an eye exam confirms a retinal tear, it can be treated in an eye doctor's office, using either lasers or freezing equipment to "spot-weld" the area surrounding the tear. (Anesthetic eye drops are used to numb the eye, but the procedure can still be uncomfortable.)

The resulting scar tissue will seal off the tear so the fluid doesn't leak behind the retina and pull it away. The good news is that both laser photocoagulation and freezing are more than 90 percent effective in preventing detachment. There is a small risk for tiny blind spots.

What If a Detachment Occurs?

If you suffer a retinal tear but don't get treatment within a day or two, the fluid can seep through the tear, detaching the retina.

Red flag for detachment: A gradual shading in your vision, like a curtain being drawn on the sides or top or bottom of your eye, means that a retinal detachment may have occurred. If your central vision rapidly changes, this may also signal a retinal detachment or even a stroke.

Retinal detachment is an emergency! When your doctor examines you, he/she will be able to see whether the center of your retina is detached. When the center is involved, vision often cannot be fully restored.

If you have suffered a retinal detachment, your doctor will help you decide among the following treatments:

- **Vitrectomy.** This one- to three-hour surgery is performed in a hospital operating room, usually with sedation anesthesia plus localized numbing of the eye. The vitreous is removed, tears are treated with lasers or freezing, and a bubble (typically gas) is injected to replace the missing gel and hold the retina in place until the spot-welding treatment can take effect. (The bubble will gradually disappear.)

  Important: It is necessary to keep your head in the same position for seven to fourteen days in order to "keep the bubble on the trouble," as doctors say. Therefore, you will need a week or two of bed rest at home. You may have to keep your head facedown or on one side.

- **Scleral buckle.** With this procedure, a clear band of silicone is placed around the outside of the eyeball, where it acts like a belt, holding the retina against the wall of the eyeball.

  Also performed in a hospital operating

room, scleral buckle involves freezing the retina or treating it with a laser to create localized inflammation that forms a seal, securing the retina and keeping fluid out.

Scleral buckle takes from one to two hours and is sometimes combined with vitrectomy to improve the outcome. It is frequently used for younger patients and those who have not had cataract surgery.

- **Pneumatic retinopexy.** Depending on where the retinal detachment is located, a twenty-minute, in-office procedure called a pneumatic retinopexy is an option for patients with smaller tears. With this procedure, a gas bubble is injected, and retinal tears are frozen or treated with a laser.

This is followed by up to two weeks of bed rest. Your head may need to be held in a certain position, such as upright at an angle, depending on the location of your tear.

With pneumatic retinopexy, the reattachment success rate is lower than that of scleral buckle or vitrectomy (70 percent versus 90 percent), but it is less invasive, and no hospital visit is required. In addition, pneumatic retinopexy costs less than a hospital-based procedure, which could range from $5,000 to $10,000.

Even with a successful procedure, 40 percent of patients who suffer retinal detachments see 20/50 or worse afterward even when using glasses. The remainder have better vision.

Adam Wenick, MD, PhD, assistant professor of ophthalmology in the Retina Division at the Wilmer Eye Institute at the Johns Hopkins School of Medicine in Baltimore. He is board-certified by the American Board of Ophthalmology, with special expertise in retinal tears and detachment as well as other diseases of the retina.

8
DIABETES AND YOUR HEART

The heart is such an important organ and affects virtually everything else in your body that it deserves a separate discussion. From heart attacks to high blood pressure, the connection with diabetes is especially important to be aware of.

According to the American Diabetes Association, having both hypertension and type 2 diabetes is particularly lethal and can significantly raise a person's risk of heart attack or stroke as well as increase chances of developing other diabetes-related diseases, such as kidney disease, and retinopathy, which may cause blindness. Additionally, having hypertension increases risk of stroke and Alzheimer's, and those with type 2 diabetes are even more susceptible.

The striking relevancy of heart health today means there is ample support — tests, treatments, tips on eating and drinking, and even simple exercises that can lower stress. Although you also have diabetes to contend with, the overlap in advice leaves you with a wealth of information and inspiration.

NATURAL HELP FOR THE DIABETIC HEART

If you have type 2 diabetes, you've already had a heart attack — whether you've had one or not!

"The guidelines for physicians from the American Heart Association are to treat a person with diabetes as if that individual has already had a heart attack," says cardiologist Seth Baum, MD, medical director of Integrative Heart Care in Boca Raton, Florida, and author of *The Total Guide to a Healthy Heart*.

How Does Diabetes Hurt Your Heart?

As excess sugar careens through the bloodstream, it roughs up the linings of the arteries.

Insulin resistance (the subpar performance of the hormone that moves glucose out of the bloodstream and into muscle and fat cells) raises blood pressure, damaging arteries.

Diabetes also injures tiny blood vessels called capillaries, which hurts your kidneys and nerves — damage that in turn stresses the heart.

The end result — an up to seven-fold increase in the risk of heart disease and stroke, the cardiovascular diseases (CVD) that kill four out of five people with diabetes.

But recent studies show there are several natural ways for people with diabetes to reverse the risk factors that cause heart disease.

Recent Research

It's never too late to exercise — and a little goes a long way. Researchers at the University of British Columbia in Vancouver, Canada, studied thirty-six older people (average age seventy-one) with type 2 diabetes, high blood pressure, and high cholesterol, dividing them into two groups.

One group walked on a treadmill or cycled on a stationary bicycle for forty minutes, three days a week. The other group didn't.

To find out if the exercise was helping with CVD, the researchers measured the elasticity of the arteries — a fundamental indicator of arterial youth and health, with arterial stiffness increasing the risk of dying from CVD.

Results: After three months, the exercisers had a decrease in arterial stiffness of 15 to 20 percent.

"Aerobic exercise should be the first-line treatment to reduce arterial stiffness in older adults with type 2 diabetes, even if the patient has advanced cardiovascular risk factors" such as high blood pressure and high cholesterol, conclude the researchers in *Diabetes Care.*

What to Do

Kenneth Madden, MD, the study leader and associate professor of geriatric medicine at the University of British Columbia, says, "You can improve every risk factor for diabetes and heart disease — and you can do it in a very short period of time."

Dr. Madden recommends that older people with diabetes and cardiovascular disease see a doctor for a checkup before starting an exercise program.

Once you get the okay from your physician, he says to purchase and use a heart monitor during exercise, so you're sure that you're exercising at the level used by the participants in his study — 60 to 75 percent of maximum heart rate.

Example: An estimate of your maximum heart rate is 220, minus your age. If you're sixty, that would be $220 - 60 = 160$. Exercising at between 60 and 75 percent of your maximum heart rate means maintaining a heart rate of between 96 and 120 beats per minute.

Finally, Dr. Madden advises you exercise the amount proven to improve arterial elasticity — a minimum of three sessions of aerobic exercise a week of forty minutes each.

Here are some other natural ways to reduce risk:

- **Maximize magnesium.** Researchers in Mexico studied seventy-nine people with diabetes and high blood pressure, dividing them into two groups. One group received a daily 450-mg magnesium supplement; one didn't.

Results: After four months, those on magnesium had an average drop of twenty points systolic (the higher number in the blood pressure reading) and nine points diastolic (the lower number). Those on the placebo had corresponding drops of five points and one point.

"Magnesium supplementation should be considered as an additional or alternative treatment for high blood pressure in people with diabetes," says Fernando Guerrero-Romero, MD, the study leader.

What to do: "Magnesium acts as a natural vasodilator, relaxing arteries and lowering blood pressure," says Dr. Baum. "People with diabetes should incorporate a magnesium supplement into their regimen."

He suggests a daily supplement of 400 mg, about the level used in the study.

"People with diabetes and high blood pressure should also be encouraged to increase their dietary intake of magnesium, through eating more whole grains, leafy green vegetables, legumes, nuts, and fish," says Dr. Guerrero-Romero.

- **Eat like a Neanderthal.** Researchers in

Sweden tested two diets in thirteen people with type 2 diabetes — the diet recommended by the American Diabetes Association (ADA), a generally healthful diet limiting calories, fat, and refined carbohydrates; and a "Paleolithic" diet, consisting of lean meat, fish, fruits, vegetables, root vegetables, eggs, and nuts — and no dairy products, refined carbohydrates, or highly processed foods whatsoever.

In terms of lowering risk factors for heart disease, the Paleolithic diet clubbed the ADA diet.

Results: After three months, it had done a better job of decreasing:

▶ High LDL "bad" cholesterol
▶ High blood pressure
▶ High triglycerides (a blood fat linked to heart disease)
▶ Too-big waist size (excess stomach fat is linked to heart disease)

The diet was also more effective at increasing HDL "good" cholesterol.

And it was superior in decreasing glycated hemoglobin (A1C), a measure of long-term blood sugar control.

"Foods that were regularly eaten during the Paleolithic, or Old Stone Age, may be optimal for prevention and treatment of type 2 diabetes, cardiovascular disease, and insulin resistance," concludes Tommy Jönsson, MD, in *Cardiovascular Diabetology.*

What to do: "Eating a Paleolithic diet is far easier than most people think," says Robb Wolf, owner of NorCal Strength & Conditioning in Chico, California, and author of *The Paleo Solution.* The basic diet: eat more lean meat, fish, shellfish, fruits, vegetables, eggs, and nuts. Eat less (or eliminate) grains, dairy products, salt, refined fats, and refined sugar.

- **Have a cup of hibiscus tea.** Researchers in Iran studied fifty-three people with type 2 diabetes, dividing them into two groups. One group drank a cup of hibiscus tea twice a day; the other drank two cups a day of black tea. (The hibiscus tea was made from *Hibiscus sabdariffa,* which is also known as red sorrel, Jamaican sorrel, Indian sorrel, roselle, and Florida cranberry.)

  Results: After one month, those drinking hibiscus had:
  - ▶ Higher HDL "good" cholesterol
  - ▶ Lower LDL "bad" cholesterol
  - ▶ Lower total cholesterol
  - ▶ Lower blood pressure

The black tea group didn't have any significant changes in blood fats or blood pressure.

The findings were in the *Journal of Alternative and Complementary Medicine and the Journal of Human Hypertension.*

What to do: Consider drinking a cup or two of hibiscus tea a day, says Hassan Mozaffari-Khosravi, PhD, an assistant professor of nutrition, Shahid Sadoughi University of Medical Sciences, Yazd, Iran, and the study leader.

Seth Baum, MD, medical director of Integrative Heart Care in Boca Raton, Florida, and author of *The Total Guide to a Healthy Heart.* VitalRemedyMD.com.

Kenneth Madden, MD, associate professor of geriatric medicine at the University of British Columbia.

Robb Wolf, owner of NorCal Strength & Conditioning, Chico, California, and author of *The Paleo Solution.*

FOUR MUST-HAVE HEART TESTS

Heart disease is tricky. Like other silent conditions, such as high blood pressure and kidney disease, you may not know that you have it until you're doubled over from a heart attack.

That's because traditional methods of assessing patients for heart disease, such as cholesterol tests and blood pressure measurements, along with questions about smoking and other lifestyle factors, don't always tell a patient's whole story.

Shocking finding: In a recent study, doctors followed nearly six thousand men and women (ages fifty-five to eighty-eight) who had been deemed healthy by standard heart tests for three years and then gave them basic imaging tests.

Result: Sixty percent were found to have atherosclerosis. These study participants were eight times more likely to suffer a heart attack or stroke, compared with subjects without this fatty buildup (plaque) in the arteries.

The Must-Have Tests

Below are four simple tests that can catch arterial damage at the earliest possible stage — when it can still be reversed and before it has a chance to cause a heart attack or stroke.

My advice: Even though doctors don't routinely order these tests, everyone over age fifty should have them at least once — and sometimes more often, depending on the findings. Smokers and people with diabetes, very high cholesterol levels (more than 300 mg/dL), and/or a family history of heart disease should have these tests before age fifty. Having these tests can literally save your life:

- **Coronary calcium computed tomography (CT) scan.** This imaging test checks for calcium deposits in the arteries — a telltale sign of atherosclerosis. People who have little or no calcium in the arteries (a score of zero) have less than a 5 percent risk of having a heart attack over the next three to five years. The risk is twice as high in people with a score of one to ten, and more than nine times higher in those with scores above four hundred.

  While the American College of Cardiology recommends this test for people who haven't been diagnosed with heart disease but have known risk factors, such as high blood pressure and/or a family history of heart disease, I advise everyone to have this test at about age fifty.* The test takes only ten to fifteen minutes and doesn't require the injection of a contrast agent.

* People already diagnosed with heart disease and/or who have had a stent or bypass surgery do not need the coronary calcium CT.

Cost: Ninety-nine dollars and up, which may be covered by insurance.

I use the calcium score as a one-time test. Unless they abandon their healthy habits, people who have a score of zero are unlikely to develop arterial calcification later in life. Those who do have deposits will know what they have to do — exercise, eat a more healthful diet, manage cholesterol and blood pressure, etc.

One drawback, however, is radiation exposure. Even though the dose is low (much less than you'd get during cardiac catheterization, for example), you should always limit your exposure.

My advice: Choose an imaging center with the fastest CT machine. A faster machine (a 256-slice CT, for example) gives less radiation exposure than, say, a 64-slice machine.

- **Carotid intima-media thickness (CIMT).** The intima and media are the innermost linings of blood vessels. Their combined thickness in the carotid arteries in the neck is affected by how much plaque is present. Thickening of these arteries can indicate increased risk for stroke and heart attack.

The beauty of this test is that it's performed with ultrasound. There's no radiation, it's fast (ten minutes), and it's painless. I often recommend it as a follow-up to the coronary calcium test or as an alternative for people who want to avoid the radiation of the coronary calcium CT.

The good news is that you can reduce CIMT with a more healthful diet, more exercise, and the use of statin medications. Pomegranate — the whole fruit, juice, or a supplement — can reduce carotid plaque too. In addition, research has found Kyolic aged garlic (the product brand studied) and vitamin K-2 to also be effective.

Cost: $250 to $350. It may not be covered by insurance.

• **Advanced lipid test.** Traditional cholesterol tests are less helpful than experts once thought, particularly because more than 50 percent of heart attacks occur in patients with normal LDL "bad" cholesterol levels.

Experts have now identified a number of cholesterol subtypes that aren't measured by standard tests. The advanced lipid test (also known as an expanded test) still measures total cholesterol and LDL but also looks at the amounts and sizes of different types of cholesterol.

Suppose that you have a normal LDL reading of 100 mg/dL. You still might have an elevated risk for a heart attack if you happen to have a high number of small, dense LDL particles (found in an advanced LDL particle test), since they can more easily enter the arterial wall.

My advice: Get the advanced lipid test at least once after age fifty. It usually costs thirty-nine dollars and up and may be covered by insurance.

If your readings look good, you can switch to a standard cholesterol test every few years. If the numbers are less than ideal, talk to your doctor about treatment options, which might include statins or niacin, along with lifestyle changes. Helpful supplements include omega-3 fatty acids, vitamin E, and plant sterols.

- **High-sensitivity C-reactive protein (hs-CRP).** This simple blood test has been available for years, but it's not used as often as it should be. Elevated C-reactive protein indicates inflammation in the body, including in the blood vessels. Data from the Physicians' Health Study found that people with elevated CRP were about three times more likely to have a heart attack than those with normal levels.

  If you test low (less than 1 mg/L) or average (1 to 3 mg/L), you can repeat the test every few years. If your CRP is high (above 3 mg/L), I recommend repeating the test at least once a year. It's a good way to measure any progress you may be making from taking medications (such as statins, which reduce inflammation), improving your diet, and getting more exercise.

Cost: About fifty dollars. It's usually covered by insurance.

Joel K. Kahn, MD, a clinical professor of medicine at Wayne State University School of Medicine and director of Cardiac Wellness at Michigan Healthcare Professionals, both in Detroit. He is also a founding member of the International Society of Integrative Metabolic and Functional Cardiovascular Medicine and author of *The Whole Heart Solution.*

ARTERY INFLAMMATION:
SIX SIMPLE, LIFESAVING TESTS

A fire could be smoldering inside your arteries, a type of fire that could erupt at any moment, triggering a heart attack or stroke. In fact, the fire could be building right this minute, and you wouldn't even know it. That's because the usual things doctors look at when gauging cardiovascular risk — cholesterol, blood pressure, blood sugar, weight — can all appear to be fine even when your arteries are dangerously hot.

What does work to detect hot arteries? A set of six simple, inexpensive, and readily available blood and urine tests.

Problem: Few doctors order these tests, and few patients know enough to ask for them. Without the warnings these tests provide, patients often have no way of knowing just how great their risk is for heart attack or stroke and whether or not their preventive treatments are working — until it's too late.

The Body's Army on Attack

Hot arteries are not actually hot (as in very warm). Instead, in this case, "hot" refers to the effects of chronic inflammation. Why call them hot then? Chronic arterial inflammation can put you on the fast track to developing vascular disease by speeding up the aging of your arteries. It's so dangerous to the arterial lining that it's worse than having high

LDL cholesterol. And if your arteries are already clogged with plaque — which acts as kindling for a heart attack or stroke — inflammation is what lights the match.

Inflammation in the body isn't always bad, of course. In fact, it's an important aspect of healing. When something in your body is under attack, the immune system sends in troops of white blood cells to repair and fight off the attacker, and temporary inflammation results. That's why when you cut yourself, for example, you'll see swelling at the site of the injury — it's a sign that your white blood cells are at work for your benefit.

But: When an attack against your body persists (for instance, as occurs when you have an ongoing infection of the gums), your white blood cells continue to drive inflammation. When it turns chronic, inflammation becomes highly damaging to many tissues, including the arteries.

Normally, the endothelium (lining of the arteries) serves as a protective barrier between blood and the deeper layers of the arterial wall. However, when that lining is inflamed, it can't function well, and it gets sticky, almost like flypaper, trapping white blood cells on their way through the body. The inflamed endothelium becomes leaky too, allowing LDL "bad" cholesterol to penetrate into the wall of the artery. The white blood cells then gobble up the cholesterol, forming fatty streaks that ultimately turn into plaque, a condition called atherosclerosis. Then when the plaque itself becomes inflamed, it can rupture, tearing through the endothelium into the channel of the artery where blood flows. This material triggers the formation of a blood clot — a clot that could end up blocking blood flow to the heart or brain.

The Six-Part Fire Panel

Just as firefighters have ways of determining whether a blaze is hiding within the walls of a building, certain tests can reveal whether inflammation is lurking within the walls of your arteries. I use a set of six tests that I call the "fire panel." Each reveals different risk factors, and for several of the tests, too-high scores can have more than one cause — so it's important to get all six tests, not just one or two.

The fire panel can identify people at risk for developing atherosclerosis, reveal whether patients who already have atherosclerosis have dangerously hot arteries that could lead to a heart attack or stroke, and evaluate patients who have survived a heart attack or stroke to see whether their current treatments are working to reduce the inflammation that threatens their lives. Your individual test results will help determine your most appropriate course of treatment.

I recommend that all adults have this panel

of tests done at least every twelve months, or every three to six months for patients at high risk for heart attack or stroke. All of these tests are readily available, are inexpensive and usually covered by insurance, and can be ordered by your regular doctor. Here are the six tests:

- **F2 isoprostanes.** My nickname for this blood test is the "lifestyle lie detector," because it reveals whether or not patients are practicing heart-healthy habits. The test, which measures a biomarker of oxidative stress, helps determine how fast your body's cells are oxidizing or breaking down. According to one study, people who have the highest levels of F2 isoprostanes are nine times more likely to have blockages in their coronary arteries than people with the lowest levels.

  The score you want: A normal score is less than 0.86 ng/L; an optimal score is less than 0.25 ng/L.

- **Fibrinogen.** An abnormally high level of this sticky, fibrous protein in your blood can contribute to the formation of clots. It's also a marker of inflammation. One study divided people into four groups (quartiles) based on their fibrinogen levels and found that stroke risk rose by nearly 50 percent for each quartile. High fibrinogen is particularly dangerous for people who also have high blood pressure, because both conditions damage the blood vessel lining and make it easier for plaque to burrow inside.

Normal range: 440 mg/dL or lower.

- **High-sensitivity C-reactive protein (hs-CRP).** Your liver produces C-reactive protein, and the amount of it in your blood rises when there is inflammation in your body — so an elevated hs-CRP level generally is considered a precursor to cardiovascular disease. The large-scale Harvard Women's Health Study cited this test as being more accurate than cholesterol in predicting risk for cardiovascular disease, while another study of women found that those with high scores were up to four times more likely to have a heart attack or stroke than women with lower scores. A high hs-CRP score is especially worrisome for a person with a large waist. Excess belly fat is often a sign of insulin resistance (in which cells don't readily accept insulin), a condition that further magnifies heart attack and stroke risk.

The score you're aiming for: Under 1.0 mg/L is normal; 0.5 mg/L is optimal.

- **Microalbumin/creatinine urine ratio (MACR).** This test looks for albumin in the urine. Albumin is a large protein molecule that circulates in the blood and shouldn't spill from capillaries in the kidneys into the urine, so its presence suggests dysfunction of the endothelium. Though this test provides valuable information about arterial wall health, doctors rarely use it for this purpose.

Important: New evidence shows that MACR levels that have traditionally been considered normal can signal increased risk for cardiovascular events.

Optimal ratios, according to the latest research: 7.5 or lower for women and 4.0 or lower for men.

- **Lipoprotein-associated phospholipase A2 (Lp-PLA2).** This enzyme in the blood is attached to LDL "bad" cholesterol and rises when artery walls become inflamed. Recent research suggests that it plays a key role in the atherosclerosis disease process, contributing to the formation of plaque as well as to the plaque's vulnerability to rupture. People with periodontal (gum) disease are especially likely to have elevated Lp-PLA2 scores — chronic inflammation can start in unhealthy gums and, from there, spread to the arteries.

  Normal range: Less than 200 ng/ml.

- **Myeloperoxidase (MPO).** This immune system enzyme normally is found at elevated levels only at the site of an infection. When it is elevated in the bloodstream, it must be assumed that it's due to significant inflammation in the artery walls and leaking through the endothelium. This is a very bad sign. MPO produces numerous oxidants that make all cholesterol compounds, including HDL "good" cholesterol, more inflammatory. If your blood levels of MPO are high, HDL goes rogue and joins the gang of inflammatory thugs. It also interacts with another substance in the bloodstream to produce an acid that can eat holes in blood vessel walls. Smokers are particularly prone to high MPO levels.

Normal range: Less than 420 pmol/L.

How to Put Out the Fires

While the fire panel tests above may seem exotic, the solution to the hot artery problem, for most of us, is not. That's because the best way to combat chronic inflammation is simply to maintain a healthful lifestyle. You just have to do it! Key factors include:

- Following a heart-healthy Mediterranean-style diet
- Managing stress
- Getting plenty of exercise
- Guarding against insulin resistance
- Taking good care of your teeth and gums
- Not smoking

In some cases, lifestyle changes alone are enough to quell the flames of chronic inflammation and to put your arteries on the road to recovery. In other cases, patients also need medication such as statins and/or dietary supplements such as niacin and fish oil. Either way, the good news is that once you shut the inflammation off, the body has a chance to heal whatever disease and damage has occurred, so you're no longer on the fast track to a heart attack or stroke.

Bradley Bale, MD, medical director, Grace Clinic Heart Health Program, Lubbock, Texas, and cofounder, Heart Attack & Stroke Prevention Center, Spokane. He is coauthor, with Amy Doneen, ARNP, and Lisa Collier Cool, of *Beat the Heart Attack Gene: The Revolutionary Plan to Prevent Heart Disease, Stroke and Diabetes.*

HOSPITALIZED FOR HEART ATTACK? MAKE SURE THEY CHECK YOU FOR DIABETES

It's well-known among health-conscious people that heart disease and diabetes are linked, so it seems a shame to be hearing news from the American Heart Association that 10 percent of Americans who've had a heart attack probably have undiagnosed diabetes. What's worse, though, is news that doctors are missing opportunities to detect and treat diabetes in people even when they are hospitalized for a heart attack.

Are so many doctors this clueless? Although it might be a great challenge for health-care professionals to identify everyone with diabetes before complications, such as heart attack, occur, a basic precaution can at least help those who do land in the hospital because of heart attack. So if you've had a heart attack or have cardiovascular disease — or you want to be prepared to give yourself the best odds if you ever have a heart attack in the future — here's what you need to insist that your medical-care team does for you, especially if you land in the hospital.

A Simple Overlooked Test

It comes down to getting a simple blood test. Doctors who order a hemoglobin A1C test when a patient is being treated for heart attack are making the right move to ensure that diabetes won't be missed and the heart attack can be treated correctly, says Suzanne V. Arnold, MD, MHA, an assistant professor at the University of Missouri in Kansas City. She led a study on undiagnosed diabetes in heart attack patients that was reported at last year's American Heart Association meeting. The hemoglobin A1C test shows average blood sugar levels for the preceding three months and is widely used to diagnose both type 1 and type 2 diabetes and monitor how well blood sugar is being controlled after diagnosis.

In her study, Dr. Arnold and her team took 2,854 patients who were hospitalized for heart attacks but had never received a diabetes diagnosis and arranged for them to have the hemoglobin A1C test. Both the hospitalized patients and the doctors treating them were kept in the dark ("blinded" in scientific speak) about the test results, and doctors were left to their business-as-usual patient care. Diabetes was considered recognized by the researchers if a patient either received diabetes education while hospitalized and/or diabetes medication when sent home.

The study results were a real eye-opener. Sure, Dr. Arnold's team discovered that 10 percent of these patients had diabetes and didn't know it, but the far bigger issue that patients and their families need to know about was that doctors failed to recognize diabetes in 69 percent of these previously undiagnosed patients.

That's a major fail — especially when all it took for the treating doctors themselves to discover diabetes was to order the same simple, inexpensive A1C test that Dr. Arnold's team had already ordered for their study.

Six months down the road, the researchers checked in on the patients they themselves knew had diabetes. They found that 71 percent of the patients whose diabetes had also been discovered by a doctor during their hospital stays were getting diabetes care. As for the patients whose diabetes had not been discovered by doctors treating them in the hospital, only 7 percent were getting diabetes care, meaning that the likelihood was strong that no one, except Dr. Arnold's team, had yet checked these folks for diabetes. This left them at high risk for more cardiovascular complications, including additional heart attacks.

Knowledge That Can Also Guide Heart Attack Treatment

Knowing that a heart attack patient has type 2 diabetes is important in the moment because it determines treatment decisions, explains Dr. Arnold. For example, patients with multivessel coronary artery disease and diabetes may do better with bypass surgery (rather than stents) and particular blood pressure medications, such as ACE inhibitors.

Dr. Arnold's advice for people who have heart attacks and survive but don't know whether they have diabetes is that they insist on having a hemoglobin A1C test during their hospitalization. She does not advocate routine hemoglobin A1C screening for everyone, though, calling it "impractical," although it's certainly something you can bring up with your doctor if you know you have heart disease. And although you may be in the know about diabetes and heart disease prevention, this seems like a good place to include a refresher for you or a loved one. You can assess your risks and the warning signs of diabetes with these checklists from the American Diabetes Association.

Your chances of diabetes increase if you:

- Have a family history of type 2 diabetes
- Don't get much exercise and are otherwise physically inactive
- Are overweight
- Have high blood pressure
- Have low HDL "good" cholesterol and high triglycerides
- Don't watch your diet and feast on high-calorie, fatty, sugary, and low-fiber foods
- Smoke
- For women, had diabetes during pregnancy

These are warning signs of diabetes:

- Unquenchable thirst
- Excessive urination
- Increased appetite, despite eating
- Unexpected weight loss
- Tingling, pain, and/or numbness in your hands and/or feet
- Blurred vision
- Cuts and bruises that take a long time to heal
- Extreme fatigue

It's not very challenging for health-conscious people to avoid type 2 diabetes and heart disease, but keeping this bit of information on a simple blood test in mind can protect you or a loved one even more.

Suzanne V. Arnold, MD, MHA, assistant professor at Saint Luke's Mid America Heart Institute and the University of Missouri at Kansas City. Her study was presented at the 2014 annual meeting of the American Heart Association.

NEW HEART ATTACK RISK

In a recent finding, low blood sugar levels overnight may trigger prolonged slow heart rates during sleep in people with diabetes. This could lead to abnormal heart rhythms, which increase risk for heart attack.

If you have diabetes (especially if you also have cardiovascular disease): Talk to your doctor about ways to stabilize your blood sugar overnight, such as adjusting the timing, dose, and/or type of medication you take.

Simon Heller, MD, professor of clinical diabetes, University of Sheffield, UK.

SIX SECRETS TO
HOLISTIC HEART CARE

You don't smoke, your cholesterol levels look good, and your blood pressure is under control. This means that you're off the hook when it comes to having a heart attack or developing heart disease, right? Maybe not.

Surprising statistic: About 20 percent of people with heart disease do not have any of the classic risk factors, such as those described above.

The missing link: While most conventional medical doctors prescribe medications and other treatments to help patients control the big risk factors for heart disease, holistic cardiologists also suggest small lifestyle changes that over time make a significant difference in heart disease risk.* My secrets for preventing heart disease:

Secret #1: Stand up! You may not think of standing as a form of exercise. However, it's more effective than most people realize.

Think about what you're doing when you're not standing. Unless you're asleep, you're probably sitting. While sitting, your body's metabolism slows, your insulin becomes less effective, and you're likely to experience a gradual drop in HDL "good" cholesterol.

* To find a holistic cardiologist, go to the website of the American Board of Integrative Holistic Medicine, www.abihm.org, and search the database of certified integrative physicians.

A study that tracked the long-term health of more than 123,000 Americans found that those who sat for six hours or more a day had an overall death rate that was higher — 18 percent higher for men and 37 percent for women — than those who sat for less than three hours.

What's so great about standing? When you're on your feet, you move more. You pace, fidget, move your arms, and walk from room to room. This type of activity improves metabolism and can easily burn hundreds of extra calories a day. Standing also increases your insulin sensitivity to help prevent diabetes. So stand up and move around when talking on the phone, checking e-mail, and watching television.

Secret #2: Count your breaths. Slow, deep breathing is an effective way to help prevent high blood pressure — one of the leading causes of heart disease. For people who already have high blood pressure, doing this technique a few times a day has been shown to lower blood pressure by five to ten points within five minutes. And the pressure may stay lower for up to twenty-four hours.

During a breathing exercise, you want to slow your breathing down from the usual twelve to sixteen breaths a minute that most people take to about three breaths. I use the "4-7-8 sequence" whenever I feel stressed.

What to do: Inhale through your nose for

four seconds, hold the breath in for seven seconds, then exhale through the mouth for eight seconds.

Also helpful: A HeartMath software package, which you can load on your computer or smart phone, includes breathing exercises to help lower your heart rate and levels of stress hormones. Cost: $129 and up, at HeartMath .com. You can also sign up for some free tools on this website.

Secret #3: **Practice "loving kindness."** This is an easy form of meditation that reduces stress, thus allowing you to keep your heart rate and blood pressure at healthy levels.

Research has shown that people who meditate regularly are 48 percent less likely to have a heart attack or stroke than those who don't meditate. Loving kindness meditation is particularly effective at promoting relaxation — it lowers levels of the stress hormones adrenaline and cortisol while raising levels of the healing hormone oxytocin.

What to do: Sit quietly, with your eyes closed. For a few minutes, focus on just your breathing. Then imagine one person in your life whom you find exceptionally easy to love. Imagine this person in front of you. Fill your heart with a warm, loving feeling, think about how you both want to be happy and avoid suffering, and imagine that a feeling of peace travels from your heart to that person's heart in the form of white light. Dwell on the image for a few minutes. This meditation will also help you practice small acts of kindness in your daily life — for example, giving a hand to someone who needs help crossing the street.

Secret #4: **Don't neglect sex.** Men who have sex at least two times a week have a 50 percent lower risk for a heart attack than those who abstain. Similar research hasn't been done on women, but it's likely that they get a comparable benefit.

Why does sex help keep your heart healthy? It probably has more to do with intimacy than the physical activity itself. Couples who continue to have sex tend to be the ones with more intimacy in their marriages. Happy people who bond with others have fewer heart attacks — and recover more quickly if they've had one — than those without close relationships.

Secret #5: **Be happy!** People who are happy and who feel a sense of purpose and connection with others tend to have lower blood pressure and live longer than those who are isolated. Research shows that two keys to happiness are to help others be happy — for example, by being a volunteer — and to reach out to friends and neighbors. Actually, any shared activity, such as going to church or doing group hobbies, can increase survival among heart patients by about 50 percent.

Secret #6: **Try Waon (pronounced waown) therapy.** With this Japanese form of "warmth therapy," you sit in an infrared (dry) sauna for fifteen minutes then retreat to a resting area for half an hour, where you wrap yourself in towels and drink plenty of water. Studies show that vascular function improves after such therapy due to the extra release of nitric oxide, the master molecule in blood vessels that helps them relax.

Some health clubs offer Waon treatments, but the dry saunas at many gyms should offer similar benefits. I do not recommend steam rooms — moist heat places extra demands on the heart and can be dangerous for some people.

Joel K. Kahn, MD, clinical professor of medicine at Wayne State University School of Medicine in Detroit and director of Cardiac Wellness at Michigan Healthcare Professionals. He is a founding member of the International Society of Integrative Metabolic and Functional Cardiovascular Medicine and author of *The Whole Heart Solution.* DrJoelKahn.com.

You Can Cure Heart Disease (and Fight Diabetes) — with Plant-Based Nutrition

In the mid-1980s, seventeen people with severe heart disease had just about given up hope. They had undergone every available treatment, including drugs and surgery — all had failed. The group had experienced forty-nine cardiovascular events, including four heart attacks, three strokes, fifteen cases of increased angina, and seven bypass surgeries. Five of the patients were expected to die within a year.

Twelve years later, every one of the seventeen was alive. They had had no cardiovascular events. The progression of their heart disease had been stopped — and, in many cases, reversed. Their angina went away — for some, within three weeks. In fact, they became virtually heart-attack-proof. And there are hundreds of other patients with heart disease who have achieved the same remarkable results.

How the Damage Is Done

Every year, more than half a million Americans die of coronary artery disease (CAD). Three times that number suffer heart attacks. In total, half of American men and one-third of women will have some form of heart disease during their lifetimes.

Heart disease develops in the endothelium, the lining of the arteries. There, endothelial cells manufacture a compound called nitric oxide that accomplishes four tasks crucial for healthy circulation:

- **Keeps blood smoothly flowing,** rather than becoming sticky and clotted.
- **Allows arteries to widen** when the heart needs more blood, such as when you run up a flight of stairs.
- **Stops muscle cells in arteries from growing into plaque** — the fatty gunk that blocks blood vessels.
- **Decreases inflammation in the plaque** — the process that can trigger a rupture in the cap or surface of a plaque, starting the clot-forming, artery-clogging cascade that causes a heart attack.

The type and amount of fat in the typical Western diet — from animal products, dairy foods, and concentrated oils — assaults endothelial cells, cutting their production of nitric oxide.

Study: A researcher at University of Maryland School of Medicine fed a nine-hundred-calorie fast-food breakfast containing 50 g of fat (mostly from sausages and hash browns) to a group of students and then measured their endothelial function. For six hours, the students had severely compromised endothelial function and decreased nitric oxide production. Another group of students ate a nine-hundred-calorie, no-fat breakfast — and had no significant change in endothelial function.

If a single meal can do that kind of damage, imagine the damage done by three fatty meals a day, seven days a week, fifty-two weeks a year.

Plant-Based Nutrition

You can prevent, stop, or reverse heart disease with a plant-based diet. Here's what you can't eat — and what you can.

What you cannot eat:

- **Meat, poultry, fish, or eggs.** You will get plenty of protein from plant-based sources.
- **Dairy products.** That means no butter, cheese, cream, ice cream, yogurt, or milk — even skim milk, which, though lower in fat, still contains animal protein.
- **Oil of any kind — not a drop.** That includes all oils, even virgin olive oil and canola.

   What you may not know: At least 14 percent of olive oil is saturated fat — every bit as aggressive in promoting heart disease as the saturated fat in roast beef. A diet that includes oils — including monounsaturated oils from olive oil and canola oil — may slow the progression of heart disease, but it will not stop or reverse the disease.

- **Generally, nuts or avocados.** If you are eating a plant-based diet to prevent heart disease, you can have moderate amounts of nuts and avocados as long as your total cholesterol remains below 150 mg/dL. If you have heart disease and want to stop or reverse it, you should not eat these foods.

What you can eat:

- **All vegetables.**
- **Legumes** — beans, peas, lentils.
- **Whole grains and products that are made from them, such as bread and pasta** — as long as they do not contain added fats. Do not eat refined grains, which have been stripped of much of their fiber and nutrients. Avoid white rice and enriched flour products, which are found in many pastas, breads, bagels, and baked goods.
- **Fruits** — but heart patients should limit consumption to three pieces a day and avoid drinking pure fruit juices. Too much

fruit rapidly raises blood sugar, triggering a surge of insulin from the pancreas — which stimulates the liver to manufacture more cholesterol.

- **Certain beverages,** including water, seltzer water, oat milk, hazelnut milk, almond milk, no-fat soy milk, coffee, and tea. Alcohol is fine in moderation (no more than two servings a day for men and one for women).

Supplements

For maximum health, take five supplements daily:

- **Multivitamin/mineral supplement.**
- **Vitamin B-12** — 1,000 mcg.
- **Calcium** — 1,000 mg (1,200 mg if you're over sixty).
- **Vitamin D-3** — 1,000 IU.
- **Flaxseed meal (ground flaxseed)** — one tablespoon for the omega-3 fatty acids it provides. Sprinkle it on cereal.

The Cholesterol Connection

If you eat the typical, high-fat Western diet, even if you also take a cholesterol-lowering statin drug, you will not protect yourself from heart disease — because the fat in the diet will damage the endothelium cells that produce nitric oxide.

In a study in the *New England Journal of Medicine,* patients took huge doses of statin drugs to lower total cholesterol below 150 but didn't change their diets — and 25 percent experienced a new cardiovascular event or died within the next thirty months.

Recommended: Eat a plant-based diet, and ask your doctor if you should also take a cholesterol-lowering medication. Strive to maintain a total cholesterol of less than 150 and LDL "bad" cholesterol below 85.

Moderation Doesn't Work

The most common objection physicians have to this diet is that their patients will not follow it. But many patients with heart disease who find out that they have a choice — between invasive surgery and nutritional changes that will stop and reverse the disease — willingly adopt the diet.

Why not eat a less demanding diet, such as the low-fat diet recommended by the American Heart Association or the Mediterranean diet?

Surprising: Research shows that people who maintain a so-called low-fat diet of 29 percent of calories from fat have the same rate of heart attacks and strokes as people who don't.

Plant-based nutrition is the only diet that can effectively prevent, stop, and reverse heart disease. It also offers protection against stroke, high blood pressure, osteoporosis, diabetes, senile mental impairment, erectile dysfunction, and cancers of the breast, prostate, colon, rectum, uterus, and ovaries.

Caldwell B. Esselstyn, Jr., MD, surgeon, clinician, and researcher at the Cleveland Clinic for more than thirty-five years. He is author of *Prevent and Reverse Heart Disease: The Revolutionary, Scientifically Proven, Nutrition-Based Cure.* DrEsselstyn .com.

DIABETIC EYE DISEASE MAY PREDICT HEART FAILURE

Diabetic eye disease may predict heart failure, says Tien Y. Wong, MD, PhD. According to a recent study, people who have diabetic retinopathy — diabetes-related damage to blood vessels in the retina — have more than double the risk for heart failure than diabetes patients with healthy retinas.

Self-defense: Everyone who has diabetes needs a comprehensive, dilated eye exam at least once a year. People in whom retinopathy is detected should have a complete cardiac exam and regular follow-ups.

Tien Y. Wong, MD, PhD, professor of ophthalmology, National University of Singapore, and director, Singapore National Eye Centre, and senior author of a study of 1,021 adults with type 2 diabetes, published in *Journal of the American College of Cardiology.*

DIABETES DOUBLES YOUR RISK FOR PERIPHERAL ARTERY DISEASE

How serious is peripheral artery disease (PAD)? We all know that plaque in arteries near the heart can lead to heart attack, and plaque in the arteries of the neck and brain can lead to stroke.

With PAD, plaque is typically found in arteries that supply blood to the legs — an indication that blood flow also may be inhibited throughout the body, which increases risk for heart attack and stroke, as well as severe disability or loss of a limb.

Doctors have long been aware of PAD, but the disease has received relatively little attention, because patients either don't have symptoms or have only mild or moderate ones that are wrongly attributed to normal signs of aging.

What's new: The link between PAD and cardiovascular disease is now so strong that virtually all doctors agree that a diagnosis of PAD warrants a checkup and monitoring by a vascular specialist.

Are You at Risk?

PAD is surprisingly common. It affects up to ten million Americans. Because PAD is associated with the same risk factors as heart attack and stroke, the risk for PAD is higher among adults who are over age fifty and/or people who have elevated cholesterol or high blood pressure.

Having diabetes doubles the risk of developing PAD. Prediabetes also increases risk. But the greatest risk comes from smoking. At least 80 percent of people with PAD are current or former smokers. Statistically, the worst combination is smoking and having diabetes — when combined, they increase the risk of developing PAD fivefold.

Symptoms Can Be Tricky

PAD is dangerous because it can creep up on you without causing symptoms. In fact, up to half of people with PAD do not have symptoms.

When symptoms do occur, they start out mild and may be easy to dismiss. Because blood flow is compromised, activities that involve the use of the legs — walking, for example — can become more difficult and feel more tiring.

As plaque blockages become more severe, PAD causes intermittent claudication — legs become painful or achy or cramp up while walking.

At first, a person with PAD may experience symptoms of intermittent claudication only after walking long distances or up a hill or while climbing stairs. The discomfort usually goes away after sitting down and resting for a few minutes. If the condition is left untreated, even a short stroll will trigger the pain.

What most people don't know: In rare cases, PAD can occur in the hands and arms, leading to symptoms such as aching or cramping in the arms.

Getting a Proper Diagnosis

Not all doctors agree on who should be screened for PAD. However, it's wise to be tested if any of the following risk factors developed by the American College of Cardiology and the American Heart Association apply to you.

- *Younger than age fifty:* If you have diabetes and one additional risk factor (such as smoking or high blood pressure).
- *Age fifty to sixty-nine:* If you have a history of smoking or diabetes.
- *Age seventy and older:* Even if you have no known risk factors.

Many experts believe that screening also is warranted — regardless of your age — if you have the following:

- **Leg symptoms,** such as aches and cramping with exertion.
- **Diagnosis of atherosclerosis,** fatty buildup in the walls of the arteries, includ-

553

ing those in the heart and neck.

- **Numbness, tingling, or loss of sensation in the feet** or cold feet or areas of color change (bluish or dark color, for example) on your toes — an indication of compromised blood flow.
- **High blood levels of C-reactive protein (CRP),** an inflammation marker.

The Tests You Need

If you meet one of the criteria described above, ask your doctor to test you for PAD. He/she will perform a measurement called an ankle-brachial index to get a sense of whether blood pumps equally through your arms and your legs. To perform this test, your doctor will measure your blood pressure in your ankle as well as in your arm and compare the two numbers.

Best Treatment Options

There is no medication that will dissolve PAD plaque, so you should work with your doctor to manage your risk factors. If you're a smoker, stopping smoking is the most important step you can take to help control PAD.

Everyone with PAD should do the following:

- **Get the right kind of exercise.** Surprising as it might sound, walking is the most beneficial form of exercise for PAD sufferers. It won't get rid of the plaque, but it can improve your stamina and make walking less painful.

What to do: Walk on flat ground every day, or try a treadmill if you prefer.

- **Use your level of leg pain to determine the amount of time you walk.** For example, walk until the leg pain reaches a moderate level, stop walking until the pain is relieved, then resume walking. This approach trains the muscle to be more efficient in using its blood supply. Try to work your way up to fifty minutes of walking at least five days a week.

  Be sure to consult your doctor before starting a walking program, especially if you have other conditions, such as heart disease, arthritis, or spine disease. Supervised exercise, such as that offered at rehab centers, has been shown to be the most effective for PAD patients — perhaps because people are more likely to stick to a walking program in these settings.

- **Monitor other risk factors.** It is critically important to pay attention to all your other health-related risk factors. For example, if you have diabetes, monitor and keep glucose levels under control. If you have elevated cholesterol or high blood pressure, talk with your doctor about medication.

To reduce the risk for blood clots, which could lead to limb damage, heart attack, or stroke, your doctor may suggest a daily aspirin (81 mg) or a medication that prevents clotting, such as clopidogrel. A statin also may be prescribed. Statins not only lower cholesterol, but also lower levels of the inflammation marker CRP.

When Additional Treatment Is Needed

In about 30 percent of PAD patients, the condition causes severe pain that affects their quality of life, or the amount of blockage significantly restricts blood flow. In these cases, your doctor may recommend a more invasive measure, such as angioplasty or bypass surgery, to improve blood flow in the affected artery.

With angioplasty, a tiny balloon and, possibly, stents are inserted via a catheter into the artery to widen the artery as much as possible. Bypass surgery involves creating a blood-flow "detour" around a blockage, allowing the blood to flow more freely.

Important: Treatment for PAD is highly individualized. If you've been diagnosed with the condition, you should see your doctor at least once or twice each year.

For more information on PAD and vascular

specialists, visit www.vascularcures.org or see the Resources section at the back of the book.

Michael S. Conte, MD, a vascular surgeon and professor and chief of the division of vascular and endovascular surgery and codirector of the Heart and Vascular Center at the University of California, San Francisco. He is a former recipient of the Distinguished Achievement Award from the New York Weill Cornell Medical Center Alumni Council and is on the editorial boards of *Vascular and Endovascular Surgery* and *Vascular Medicine.*

NATURAL TREATMENTS FOR
PERIPHERAL ARTERY DISEASE

You are walking or climbing up a set of stairs, and suddenly, you notice a dull, cramping pain in your leg. Before you write off the pain as simply a sign of overexertion or just a normal part of growing older, consider this: you may have intermittent claudication, the most common symptom of peripheral artery disease (PAD).

PAD, also known as peripheral vascular disease, is a condition in which arteries and veins in your limbs, usually in the legs and feet, are blocked or narrowed by fatty deposits that reduce blood flow.

Intermittent claudication, leg discomfort (typically in the calf) that occurs during exertion or exercise and is relieved by rest, is usually the first symptom of PAD. But other possible symptoms may include leg sores that won't heal (chronic venous ulcers), varicose veins (chronic venous insufficiency), paleness (pallor) or discoloration (a blue tint) of the legs, or cold legs.

Why is "a little leg trouble" so significant? If it's due to PAD, you have got a red flag that other arteries, including those in the heart and brain, may also be blocked. In fact, people with PAD have a two- to sixfold increased risk for heart attack or stroke.

An estimated eight to twelve million Americans — including up to one in five people age sixty or older — are believed to have PAD. While many individuals who have PAD experience the symptoms described earlier, some have no symptoms at all.

Those at greatest risk: Anyone who smokes or has elevated cholesterol, high blood pressure, or diabetes is at increased risk for PAD.

Better Treatment Results

The standard treatment for PAD typically includes lifestyle changes (such as quitting smoking, getting regular exercise, and eating a healthful diet). Medical treatment may include medication, such as one of the two drugs approved by the FDA for PAD — pentoxifylline and cilostazol — and, in severe cases, surgery.

For even better results: Strong scientific evidence now indicates that several natural therapies — used in conjunction with these treatments — may help slow the progression of PAD and improve a variety of symptoms more effectively than standard treatment alone can.

Important: Before trying any of the following therapies, talk to your doctor to determine which might work best for you, what the most effective dose is for you, and what side effects and drug interactions may occur.

Do not take more than one of the following therapies at the same time — this will increase bleeding risk.

Among the most effective natural therapies

for PAD are:

- **Ginkgo biloba.** A standardized extract from the leaf of the ginkgo tree, which is commonly taken to improve memory, is one of the top-selling herbs in the United States. But the strongest scientific evidence for *Ginkgo biloba* may well be in the treatment of PAD.

  Scientific evidence: Numerous studies currently show that *Ginkgo biloba* extract can decrease leg pain that occurs with exercise or at rest. The daily doses used in the studies ranged from 80 to 320 mg.

  Warning: Because it thins the blood and may increase risk for bleeding, *Ginkgo biloba* should be used with caution if you also take a blood thinner, such as warfarin or aspirin. In addition, *Ginkgo biloba* should not be taken within two weeks of undergoing surgery.

- **Grape seed extract.** Grapes, including the fruit, leaves, and seeds, have been used medicinally since the time of the ancient Greeks. Grape seed extract is rich in oligomeric proanthocyanidins, antioxidants that integrative practitioners in Europe use to treat varicose veins, chronic leg ulcers, and other symptoms of PAD.

  Scientific evidence: In several recent studies, grape seed extract was found to reduce the symptoms of poor circulation in leg veins, which can include nighttime cramps, swelling, heaviness, itching, tingling, burning, numbness, and nerve pain.

Caution: Don't use this supplement if you're allergic to grapes. It should be used with caution if you take a blood thinner.

- **Hesperidin.** This flavonoid is found in unripe citrus fruits, such as oranges, grapefruits, lemons, and tangerines.

  Scientific evidence: Research now shows that hesperidin may strengthen veins and tiny blood vessels called capillaries, easing the symptoms of venous insufficiency. Hesperidin has also been shown to reduce leg symptoms such as pain, cramps, heaviness, and neuropathy (burning, tingling, and numbness). Some hesperidin products also contain diosmin, a prescription medication that is used to treat venous disease, vitamin C, or the herb butcher's broom, all of which strengthen the effects of hesperidin.

  Caution: Many drugs can react with hesperidin. If you take a diabetes medication, antihypertensive, blood thinner, muscle relaxant, antacid, or antinausea medication, be sure to use this supplement cautiously, and promptly alert your doctor if you experience any new symptoms after starting to use hesperidin.

- **Horse chestnut seed extract.** The seeds, leaves, bark, and flowers of this tree, which is native to Europe, have been used for centuries in herbal medicine.

Scientific evidence: Several studies now indicate that horse chestnut seed extract may be helpful for venous insufficiency, decreasing leg pain, fatigue, itchiness, and swelling.

Caution: Horse chestnut may lower blood sugar and interfere with diabetes medication.

- **L-carnitine.** Also known as acetyl-L-carnitine, this amino acid may improve circulation and help with PAD symptoms.

   Recent finding: Taking L-carnitine in addition to the PAD medication cilostazol increased walking distance in people with intermittent claudication up to 46 percent more than taking cilostazol alone, reported researchers from the University of Colorado School of Medicine in a recent issue of *Vascular Medicine.*

- **Inositol nicotinate.** This is a form of niacin (vitamin B-3) that is less likely to create the typical flushing (redness and heat) that is produced by high doses of niacin.

   Scientific evidence: Several studies show that it is helpful in treating PAD. It is commonly used in the UK to treat intermittent claudication.

- **Policosanol.** This is a natural cholesterol-lowering compound made primarily from the wax of cane sugar. Comparative studies show that policosanol treats intermittent claudication as effectively as the prescription blood thinner ticlopidine and more effectively than the cholesterol-lowering statin lovastatin.

Other Therapies

You may read or hear that acupuncture, biofeedback, chelation therapy, garlic, omega-3 fatty acids, and vitamin E can help with PAD.

However: The effectiveness of these particular therapies is uncertain at this time. For this reason, it is best to forgo these approaches until more scientific evidence becomes available.

Catherine Ulbricht, PharmD, cofounder of the Somerville, Massachusetts–based Natural Standard Research Collaboration, which collects data on natural therapies, and senior attending pharmacist at Massachusetts General Hospital in Boston. She is also author of *Natural Standard Herbal Pharmacotherapy* and *Natural Standard Medical Conditions Reference* and editor-in-chief of the *Journal of Dietary Supplements.*

TAKE THIS TEST
BEFORE STARTING A STATIN

Before starting a statin, have a coronary artery calcium (CAC) test, advises Khurram Nasir, MD, MPH. The CAC test more accurately predicts cardiovascular risk than factors such as cholesterol, blood pressure, current smoking, and diabetes. In 35 percent of people considered high risk according to those factors, a CAC test showed that risk was relatively low and could be managed by lifestyle modifications instead of medication. The test is widely available, takes about three minutes, and may be covered by insurance.

Khurram Nasir, MD, MPH, a cardiovascular disease specialist and director of Center for Prevention and Wellness at Baptist Health South Florida, Miami Beach. He is senior author of a study published in *European Heart Journal*.

MAKE CHOLESTEROL
A LAUGHING MATTER

Laughter is great medicine — it's not just a platitude. Nor should this come as a surprise, since previous studies regarding laughter have noted its impact on cardiovascular risk, blood pressure, and stress. The latest finding is that it even can lower cholesterol.

In research presented at the 2009 meeting of the American Physiological Society, twenty high-risk diabetic patients who had both hypertension and high cholesterol were divided into two groups. One group received standard pharmaceutical treatments for diabetes (metformin, TZD, and glipizide), hypertension (ACE inhibitors), and high cholesterol (statin drugs), while the second group received the same medication but also were instructed to watch thirty minutes a day of humorous videos. Since different people find different things funny, participants were able to select their own.

Laughing All the Way to Good Health

By the end of the second month, the benefits were already evident. By the end of one year, the laughter group had increased their "good" cholesterol by 26 percent (compared with 3 percent for the control group) while also decreasing C-reactive protein, an inflammatory marker, by 66 percent (versus 26 percent in the control group). In addition, over the course of the yearlong study, only one patient in the laughter group suffered a heart attack — compared with three in the control group.

"The benefits we see with laughter are very similar to what we see with moderate exercise," notes researchers Lee Berk, DrPH, of Loma Linda University and Stanley Tan, MD, PhD, of Oak Crest Research Institute. Dr. Berk has even coined a term — Laughercise — to describe the benefits of therapeutic laughter. This newest finding builds upon previous research by the same team in which laughter was found to boost blood flow to the heart. Dr. Berk says that further studies are planned to determine how long this positive effect will last.

Healing Power of Laughter
Dr. Berk says that "it's clear that the repetitive use of laughter produces physiological changes that lower stress hormones, increase endorphins, and — in our studies — lower risk factors for heart disease, including inflammation and cholesterol."

Lee Berk, MPH, DrPH, associate professor of Allied Health and Pathology, Schools of Allied Health Professions and Medicine, Loma Linda University, Loma Linda, California.

SMALL DROPS IN BLOOD PRESSURE CAN REDUCE RISK OF DYING BY ONE-FIFTH

Type 2 diabetes is now considered a global pandemic, which is alarming, since many people who have this disease will eventually be disabled by or even die from complications of it. That's the bad news. The good news is that you can reduce your risk of heart attack, stroke, and kidney disease — three common complications, often fatal — by bringing your blood pressure down, even by just a little. About 73 percent of adults with diabetes have high blood pressure (defined in this case as greater than or equal to 130/80 mmHg) or use prescription medications for hypertension. Research demonstrates that treatment with blood pressure drugs can reduce the risk of dying by one-fifth, generally with few side effects.

Lower Blood Sugar = Better Outcomes

People with diabetes are extrasensitive to changes in blood pressure, explains Anne Peters, MD, director of the University of Southern California (USC) Westside Center for Diabetes in Beverly Hills. The ADVANCE (Action in Diabetes and Vascular Disease) trial, involving more than eleven thousand people with type 2 diabetes from twenty countries, clearly demonstrated that lowering blood pressure significantly improved certain outcomes. It should be noted that the trial was funded by Servier, the manufacturer of Preterax, and the National Health and Medical Research Council of Australia.

Participants were randomly given the blood pressure drug Preterax — a combination of the ACE inhibitor perindopril and the diuretic indapamide — or a placebo and were followed for more than four years. Researchers found that treatment with Preterax significantly reduced the risk of serious complications of diabetes. Specifically, those who took Preterax:

• Reduced their risk of death from cardiovascular disease by 18 percent
• Cut their risk of kidney-related events by 21 percent
• Lowered their risk of death from any cause by 14 percent

The findings were published online in the September 2, 2007, issue of *The Lancet.*

More Aggressive Treatment Required For People With Diabetes

Commenting on the study, Dr. Peters says that in her view, the improvements were small and actually less than she would have expected. She says that physicians treat blood pressure more aggressively in people with diabetes, typically prescribing medications for those whose pressure is above 130/80. Participants in the ADVANCE trial had a far higher mean starting blood pressure of 145/81 and were only treated to an average of 135/75 — an improvement, to be sure, but one that doesn't go far enough to reach target levels for people with diabetes.

That said, Dr. Peters notes that the study does add to the literature that even small reductions in blood pressure are beneficial. Also, she says, ACE inhibitors and diuretics have long track records for safety and effectiveness in people with diabetes, as well as those who don't have the disease. Generic versions of these blood pressure–lowering drugs are also available.

We asked naturopathic doctor Andrew Rubman, ND, whether these results could be achieved without pharmaceutical drugs. He believes they could and suggests beginning with dietary and lifestyle modifications. "Specifically, calcium and magnesium are important for both hypertension and adult-onset diabetes," he says but notes that managing blood pressure to target levels for a person with diabetes is complicated and requires specialized care. "Just as you'd not take heart medications without oversight from a cardiologist, you can't treat a medical condition with supplements without specialist oversight."

Anne Peters, MD, professor of clinical medicine, Keck School of Medicine of the University of Southern California in Los Angeles, and director of the USC Westside Center for Diabetes. She is author of *Conquering Diabetes — A Cutting Edge, Comprehensive Program for Prevention and Treatment.*

Five Foods That Fight High Blood Pressure (You Might Not Even Need Medication)

Is your blood pressure on the high side? Your doctor might write a prescription when it creeps above 140/90, but you may be able to forgo medication. Lifestyle changes still are considered the best starting treatment for mild hypertension. These include not smoking, regular exercise, and a healthy diet. In addition to eating less salt, you want to include potent pressure-lowering foods, including the following.

Raisins

Raisins are basically dehydrated grapes, but they provide a much more concentrated dose of nutrients and fiber. They are high in potassium, with 220 mg in a small box (1.5 ounces). Potassium helps counteract the blood pressure–raising effects of salt. The more potassium we consume, the more sodium our bodies excrete. Researchers also speculate that the fiber and antioxidants in raisins change the biochemistry of blood vessels, making them more pliable — important for healthy blood pressure. Opt for dark raisins over light-colored ones, because dark raisins have more catechins, a powerful type of antioxidant that can increase blood flow.

Researchers at Louisville Metabolic and

Atherosclerosis Research Center compared people who snacked on raisins with those who ate other packaged snacks. Those in the raisin group had drops in systolic pressure (the top number) ranging from 4.8 points (after four weeks) to 10.2 points (after twelve weeks). Blood pressure barely budged in the no-raisin group. Some people worry about the sugar in raisins, but it is natural sugar (not added sugar) and will not adversely affect your health (though people with diabetes need to be cautious with portion sizes).

My advice: Aim to consume a few ounces of raisins every day. Prunes are an alternative.

Beets

Beets too are high in potassium, with about 519 mg per cup. They're delicious, easy to cook (see the tasty recipe on page 132), and very effective for lowering blood pressure.

A study at the London Medical School found that people who drank about eight ounces of beet juice averaged a ten-point drop in blood pressure during the next twenty-four hours. The blood pressure–lowering effect was most pronounced at three to six hours past drinking but remained lower for the entire twenty-four hours.

Eating whole beets might be even better, because you will get extra fiber.

Along with fiber and potassium, beets are also high in nitrate. The nitrate is converted first to nitrite in the blood, then to nitric oxide. Nitric oxide is a gas that relaxes blood vessel walls and lowers blood pressure.

My advice: Eat beets several times a week. Look for beets that are dark red. They contain more protective phytochemicals than the gold or white beets. Cooked spinach and kale are alternatives.

Dairy

In research involving nearly forty-five thousand people, researchers found that those who consumed low-fat "fluid" dairy foods, such as yogurt and low-fat milk, were 16 percent less likely to develop high blood pressure. Higher-fat forms of dairy, such as cheese and ice cream, had no blood pressure benefits. The study was published in *Journal of Human Hypertension.*

In another study, published in the *New England Journal of Medicine,* researchers found that people who included low-fat or fat-free dairy in a diet high in fruits and vegetables had double the blood pressure–lowering benefits of those who just ate the fruits and veggies.

Low-fat dairy is high in calcium, another blood pressure–lowering mineral that should be included in your diet. When you don't have enough calcium in your diet, a "calcium leak" occurs in your kidneys. This means that the kidneys excrete more calcium in the urine, disturbing the balance of mineral metabolism involved in blood pressure regulation.

My advice: Aim for at least one serving of low-fat or nonfat milk or yogurt every day. If you don't care for cow's milk or can't drink it, switch to fortified soy milk. It has just as much calcium and protein and also contains phytoestrogens, compounds that are good for the heart.

Flaxseed

Flaxseed contains alpha-linolenic acid (ALA), an omega-3 fatty acid that helps prevent heart and vascular disease. Flaxseed also contains magnesium. A shortage of magnesium in our diet throws off the balance of sodium, potassium, and calcium, which causes the blood vessels to constrict.

Flaxseed is also high in flavonoids, the same antioxidants that have boosted the popularity of dark chocolate, kale, and red wine. Flavonoids are bioactive chemicals that reduce inflammation throughout the body, including in the arteries. Arterial inflammation is thought to be the trigger that leads to high blood pressure, blood clots, and heart attacks.

In a large-scale observational study linking dietary magnesium intake with better heart health and longevity, nearly fifty-nine thousand healthy Japanese people were followed for fifteen years. The scientists found that the people with the highest dietary intake of magnesium had a 50 percent reduced risk for death from heart disease (heart attack and stroke). According to the researchers, magnesium's heart-healthy benefit is linked to its ability to improve blood pressure, suppress irregular heartbeats, and inhibit inflammation.

My advice: Add one or two tablespoons of ground flaxseed to breakfast cereals. You also can sprinkle flaxseed on yogurt or whip it into a breakfast smoothie. Or try chia seeds.

Walnuts

Yale researchers found that people who ate two ounces of walnuts a day had improved blood flow and drops in blood pressure (a 3.5-point drop in systolic blood pressure and a 2.8-point drop in diastolic blood pressure). The mechanisms through which walnuts elicit a blood pressure–lowering response are believed to involve their high content of monounsaturated fatty acids, omega-3 ALA, magnesium, and fiber and their low levels of sodium and saturated fatty acids.

Bonus: Despite the reputation of nuts as a "fat snack," the people who ate them didn't gain weight.

The magnesium in walnuts is particularly important. It limits the amount of calcium that enters muscle cells inside artery walls. Ingesting the right amount of calcium (not too much and not too little) on a daily basis is essential for optimal blood pressure regulation. Magnesium regulates calcium's movement across the membranes of the smooth muscle cells, deep within the artery walls.

If your body doesn't have enough magnesium, too much calcium will enter the smooth muscle cells, which causes the arterial muscles to tighten, putting a squeeze on the arteries and raising blood pressure. Magnesium works like the popular calcium channel blockers, drugs that block entry of calcium into arterial walls, lowering blood pressure.

My advice: Eat two ounces of walnuts every day. Or choose other nuts such as almonds and pecans.

Janet Bond Brill, PhD, RDN, FAND, is a registered dietitian/nutritionist, a fellow of the Academy of Nutrition and Dietetics, and a nationally recognized nutrition, health, and fitness expert who specializes in cardiovascular disease prevention. Based in Hellertown, Pennsylvania, Dr. Brill is author of *Blood Pressure Down: The 10-Step Plan to Lower Your Blood Pressure in 4 Weeks — Without Prescription Drugs, Prevent a Second Heart Attack: 8 Foods, 8 Weeks to Reverse Heart Disease,* and *Cholesterol Down: 10 Simple Steps to Lower Your Cholesterol in 4 Weeks — Without Prescription Drugs.* DrJanet.com.

LOWER BLOOD PRESSURE
WITH THIS VITAMIN

Many of us swallow a daily multivitamin and assume that we're getting all the vitamin C that we need.

After all, most multivitamins provide 100 percent of the USDA's recommended Dietary Reference Intake (DRI) per day for vitamin C — 75 to 90 mg.

So we're all set, right?

Well, a recent analysis from Johns Hopkins University in Baltimore shows that getting even more than the DRI each day might go a long way in terms of reducing blood pressure or maintaining healthy blood pressure.

But how much is enough?

"C" Is for Controlling Pressure

Scouring forty-five years of medical literature, lead investigator Stephen Juraschek, MD, and his colleagues looked at twenty-nine clinical trials comparing blood pressure measurements among participants taking vitamin C supplements with those taking placebos. The range of supplementation taken was 60 to 4,000 mg per day — the median amount was 500 mg per day — so most subjects were taking far more than the USDA's recommended amount. Subjects took the supplements for, on average, eight weeks. Some had high blood pressure, and some didn't.

Results: Participants with normal blood

pressure who took vitamin C had 3.8 points lower systolic blood pressure (the top number of the reading), on average, than the placebo group and 1.5 points lower diastolic blood pressure (the bottom number of the reading), on average, and those with high blood pressure who took vitamin C had 4.9 points lower systolic, on average, and 1.7 points lower diastolic, on average.

These reductions may not be as significant as the results you might get from blood pressure medications, but if your blood pressure is only slightly high, the vitamin might help keep your pressure in a healthy range or help you take less or no medication.

Juraschek says that the dips in blood pressure are thought to result from vitamin C's action as a diuretic — it prompts the kidneys to excrete more salt and water from the body, which can relax blood vessels.

May Help, Won't Harm

Again, this research was a meta-analysis of many studies, and each study was conducted slightly differently, so Juraschek can't tell us exactly how much vitamin C is the ideal amount to take.

But since the people in the study were taking more than the USDA's recommended amount of vitamin C and their blood pressure was lowered, then should we all be taking more than 75 to 90 mg per day?

There's mixed advice from experts on the topic.

Juraschek takes a very cautious approach, saying that more research is needed before people increase how much vitamin C they take. He warns that doses larger than the USDA's recommendation could lead to diarrhea or kidney stones in some people, such as those prone to those problems.

But we're talking about vitamin C here! A vitamin that's good for you that is naturally in many healthy foods. Is so much caution necessary, given that vitamin C is, generally speaking, quite benign?

Excess vitamin C is excreted in urine, so how dangerous could it really be for most people? We spoke to naturopathic doctor Andrew Rubman, ND, medical director of the Southbury Clinic for Traditional Medicines in Southbury, Connecticut, to find out the answers.

Dr. Rubman says that people who are prone to diarrhea or kidney stones might have problems consuming extra vitamin C, so those people, in particular, may want to be cautious. "But that's not most of us," he says. "Chances are that most people — especially those who are prehypertensive (blood pressure between 120/80 and 139/89) or hypertensive (blood pressure of 140/90 or higher) — would benefit from taking more than 75 to 90 mg per day."

If you're interested in taking more vitamin C than you already do as a way of controlling blood pressure, discuss it with your doctor, especially if you have diabetes or another chronic condition.

Stephen Juraschek, MD, lead investigator, department of epidemiology, Johns Hopkins University, Baltimore. Juraschek et al., "Effects of Vitamin C Supplementation on Blood Pressure: A Meta-Analysis of Randomized Controlled Trials," *The American Journal of Clinical Nutrition* (April 4, 2012). Andrew Rubman, ND, medical director, Southbury Clinic for Traditional Medicines, Southbury, Connecticut.

STRESS BUSTERS THAT HELP
BEAT HIGH BLOOD PRESSURE

We don't mean to cause undue alarm — especially since the point of this article is to reduce stress, not add to it — but a disturbing set of facts needs to be brought to light. It's the reality that high blood pressure is becoming an increasingly significant problem for women.

A recent study in the journal *Circulation* found this alarming trend — that rates of uncontrolled hypertension are increasing among women even as rates among men are decreasing.

The Centers for Disease Control and Prevention report that more than one-third of women age forty-five to fifty-four now have high blood pressure, while among women age seventy-five and older, 80 percent do!

A more recent report from the National Center for Health Statistics states that, in the past decade, there has been a 62 percent increase in the number of visits to the doctor due to high blood pressure.

How much the lousy economy might be contributing to the problem (though studies have shown that worries about job stability increase a person's risk for high blood pressure) is up for debate. Other research has shown that chronic stress is a significant contributor to hypertension. As C. Tissa Kappagoda, MBBS, PhD, a professor in the preventive cardiology program at the University of California, Davis, explained, "Chronic stress raises blood pressure by increasing levels of adrenaline and cortisol, hormones that promote artery spasm and salt retention. It also increases vascular resistance, the resistance to flow that must be overcome to move blood through the blood vessels, which is a primary cause of hypertension." Stress also can impede basic self-care, such as eating healthfully and exercising — which probably explains why stress is such a "massive multiplier of the effects of conventional risk factors," Dr. Kappagoda added.

Though high blood pressure doesn't cause pain or other obvious symptoms, it does damage arteries — increasing the risk for heart attack, diabetes, stroke, and kidney problems. How high is too high? Hypertension is diagnosed when blood pressure hits 140/90 mmHg or higher, but doctors now realize that prehypertension (blood pressure between 120/80 and 139/89) is also risky.

Of course, it's important to follow your doctor's advice regarding blood pressure-lowering lifestyle changes, such as limiting salt and alcohol and losing excess weight. But stress reduction should be a priority too, Dr. Kappagoda said — and may reduce the need for hypertension medication. That's good, because these drugs can have side effects, such as dizziness, chronic cough, and muscle cramps, and often are taken for the rest of a person's life.

Research shows that the following stress-lowering techniques help reduce blood pressure. If you have hypertension or prehypertension, consider:

- **Breathing control.** When you're relaxed, your breathing naturally slows, and if you slow down your breathing, your body naturally relaxes. This encourages constricted blood vessels to dilate, improving blood flow.

  Target: Practice slow breathing for fifteen minutes twice daily, aiming to take six breaths per minute.

  If you find it difficult (or even stressful!) to count and time your breaths, consider using a biofeedback device instead. One example designed for home use is RESPeR-ATE, which looks like a portable CD player with headphones and uses musical tones to guide you to an optimal breathing pattern. Typically, it's used for fifteen minutes three or four times per week, and results are seen within several weeks. In studies, users experienced significant reductions in systolic pressure (the top number of a blood pressure reading) and diastolic pressure (bottom number). There are many similar and effective devices, said Dr. Kappagoda, so ask your doctor about the options. Biofeedback devices are safe and have no side effects.

- **Meditation.** A recent analysis of nine clinical trials, published in *American Journal of Hypertension,* found that regular practice of transcendental meditation reduced blood pressure, on average, by 4.7 mmHg systolic and 3.2 mmHg diastolic. Though these results are for transcendental meditation specifically, many experts believe that any type of meditation works.

  Goal: Meditate for twenty minutes daily.

- **Exercise.** Regular physical activity reduces blood pressure not only by alleviating stress, but also by promoting weight loss and improving heart and blood vessel health. Research shows that becoming more active can reduce systolic pressure by 5 to 10 mmHg, on average. An excellent all-around exercise is walking, Dr. Kappagoda said, so with your doctor's OK, take a thirty-minute walk at least three times weekly.

  Caution: Weight training can trigger a temporary increase in blood pressure during the exercise, especially when heavy weights are used. To minimize this blood pressure spike, use lighter weights to do more repetitions, and don't hold your breath during the exertion.

The late C. Tissa Kappagoda, MBBS, PhD, professor of medicine in the Preventive Cardiology Program at the University of California, Davis. Dr. Kappagoda published more than two hundred medical journal articles on matters relating to cardiology and cardiovascular health.

REDUCE HIGH BLOOD PRESSURE
BY TAPPING YOUR TOES

There's a killer running rampant among us — and its name is high blood pressure.

Overly dramatic? Not really.

High blood pressure increases your risk not only for heart attack, heart failure, and stroke, but also for grave maladies that you may never have considered, such as kidney failure, dementia, aneurysm, blindness, and osteoporosis.

Yes, medications help reduce blood pressure, but their nasty side effects can include joint pain, headache, weakness, dizziness, heart palpitations, coughing, asthma, constipation, diarrhea, insomnia, depression, and erectile dysfunction!

But there's a promising alternative therapy that's completely risk-free — and costs nothing.

We're talking about tapping, which is based on the principles of Chinese medicine.

Something Old, Something New

The tapping method was described by Ann Marie Chiasson, MD, of the Arizona Center for Integrative Medicine. For her own patients with high blood pressure, Dr. Chiasson has adapted a tapping technique that is part of the ancient Chinese practice called qigong.

Qigong involves simple movements, including tapping on the body's meridians or "highways" of energy movement. These meridians are the same as those used during acupuncture and acupressure treatments. According to a review of nine studies published in the *Journal of Alternative and Complementary Medicine,* qigong reduced systolic blood pressure (the top number) by an average of seventeen points and diastolic blood pressure (the bottom number) by an average of ten points. Those are big reductions! In fact, they are comparable to the reductions achieved with drugs — but the qigong had no unwanted side effects.

Though Dr. Chiasson has not conducted a clinical trial on her tapping protocol, she has observed reductions in blood pressure among her patients who practice tapping. The technique she recommends could also conceivably benefit people who do not have high blood pressure if it reduces stress and thus helps lower the risk of developing high blood pressure.

Tap Away

Some tapping routines are complicated, involving tapping the top of the head, around the eyes, side of the hand, and under the nose, chin, and/or arms. But Dr. Chiasson's technique is a simpler toe-and-torso method that is quite easy to learn. It is safe and can be done in the privacy of your own home, so if it might help you, why not give it a try?

First, you may want to get a blood pressure reading so you can do a comparison later on. If the tapping technique is helpful, you eventually may be able to reduce or even discontinue your high blood pressure drugs (of course, for safety's sake, you should not stop taking any drugs without first talking to your doctor about it).

Dr. Chiasson's plan: Each day, do five minutes of toe tapping (instructions below), five minutes of belly tapping, and five minutes of chest tapping. You may experience tingling or a sensation of warmth in the part of the body being tapped and/or in your hands, which is normal. You can listen to rhythmic music during your tapping if you like. As you tap, try to think as little as possible, Dr. Chiasson says — just focus on your body, tapping, and breath.

Rate: For each tapping location, aim for a rate of about one to two taps per second.

- **Toe tapping.** Lie flat on your back on the bed or floor. Keeping your whole body relaxed, quickly rotate your legs inward and outward from the hips (like windshield wipers), tapping the sides of your big toes together with each inward rotation. Tap as softly or as vigorously as you like.

- **Belly tapping.** Stand with your feet a little wider than shoulder-width apart. Staying relaxed, gently bounce up and down by slightly bending your knees. At the same time, tap softly with gently closed fists on the area below your belly button and above your pubic bone. Try to synchronize your movements to give one tap per knee bend.
- **Chest tapping.** Sit or stand comfortably. Using your fingertips, open hands, or gently closed fists, tap all over your chest area, including the armpits. Tap as softly or as vigorously as you like without pushing past your comfort level.

Cautions: If you are recovering from hip or knee surgery, skip the toe tapping (which might strain your joint) and do only the belly tapping and chest tapping. If you are pregnant, stick with just the chest tapping — lying on your back during toe tapping could reduce blood flow to the fetus, and tapping on your belly may not feel comfortable and could stimulate the acupressure points used to induce labor, Dr. Chiasson says.

Follow-up: Continue your tapping routine for eight weeks, then get another blood pressure reading to see whether your numbers have improved. If they have — or if you simply enjoy the relaxing effects of the tapping — you might want to continue indefinitely.

Ann Marie Chiasson, MD, family practitioner and clinical assistant professor of medicine, Arizona Center for Integrative Medicine, University of Tucson. She is author of *Energy Healing: The Essentials of Self-Care.* Her video *Energy Healing for Beginners: Ten Essential Practices for Self-Care,* which includes a tapping demo, can be downloaded from www.AnnMarieChiasson MD.com/Publications.html.

ALPHA-LIPOIC ACID HELPS REDUCE DIABETES AND HEART DISEASE RISK

Alpha-lipoic acid, which is found in foods such as red meat and liver, works as an antioxidant, so it fights disease all over the body. It also regenerates other antioxidants, such as vitamins A and E, and improves insulin sensitivity, so it reduces your risk for cardiovascular disease and diabetes, and it may help reduce blood sugar levels. Dr. Horowitz typically prescribes 300 to 600 mg per day in pill form, while those patients with diabetes and/or cardiovascular risk factors will often be prescribed up to 1,200 mg per day.

Richard Horowitz, MD, Hudson Valley Healing Arts Center, Hyde Park, New York.

STROKE: YOU CAN DO MUCH MORE TO PROTECT YOURSELF

No one likes to think about having a stroke. But maybe you should. The grim reality: stroke strikes about eight hundred thousand Americans each year and is the leading cause of disability. And having diabetes increases your stroke risk.

Now for the remarkable part: About 80 percent of strokes can be prevented. You may think that you've heard it all when it comes to preventing strokes — it's about controlling your blood pressure, eating a good diet, and getting some exercise, right? Actually, that's only part of what you can be doing to protect yourself. Read the surprising recent findings on stroke — and the latest advice on how to avoid it:

• **Even "low" high blood pressure is a red flag.** High blood pressure — a reading of 140/90 mmHg or higher — is widely known to increase one's odds of having a stroke. But even slight elevations in blood pressure may also be a problem.

  An important recent study that looked at data from more than half a million patients found that those with blood pressure readings that were just slightly higher than a normal reading of 120/80 mmHg were more likely to have a stroke.

  Any increase in blood pressure is worrisome. In fact, the risk for a stroke or heart attack doubles for each twenty-point rise in systolic (the top number) pressure above 115/75 mmHg, and for each ten-point rise in diastolic (the bottom number) pressure.

My advice: Don't wait for your doctor to recommend treatment if your blood pressure is even a few points higher than normal. Tell him/ her that you are concerned. Lifestyle changes — such as getting adequate exercise, avoiding excess alcohol, and maintaining a healthful diet — often reverse slightly elevated blood pressure. Blood pressure consistently above 140/90 mmHg generally requires medication.

- **Sleep can be dangerous.** People who are sleep deprived — generally defined as getting less than six hours of sleep per night — are at increased risk for stroke.

What most people don't realize is that getting too much sleep is also a problem. When researchers at the University of Cambridge tracked the sleep habits of nearly ten thousand people over a ten-year period, they found that those who slept more than eight hours a night were 46 percent more likely to have a stroke than those who slept six to eight hours.

It is possible that people who spend less/ more time sleeping have other, unrecognized conditions that affect both sleep and stroke risk.

Example: Sleep apnea, a breathing disorder that interferes with sleep, causes an increase in blood pressure that can lead to stroke. Meanwhile, sleeping too much can be a symptom of depression — another stroke risk factor.

My advice: See a doctor if you tend to wake up unrefreshed, are a loud snorer, or often snort or thrash while you sleep. You may have sleep apnea. (For more on this condition, see page 321.) If you sleep too much, also talk to your doctor to see if you are suffering from depression or some other condition that may increase your stroke risk.

What's the sweet spot for nightly shut-eye? When it comes to stroke risk, it's six to eight hours per night.

- **What you drink matters too.** A Mediterranean-style diet — plenty of whole grains, legumes, nuts, fish, produce, and olive oil — is perhaps the best diet going when it comes to minimizing stroke risk. A recent study concluded that about 30 percent of strokes could be prevented if people simply switched to this diet.

But there's more you can do. Research has found that people who drank six cups of green or black tea a day were 42 percent less likely to have strokes than people who did not drink tea. With three daily cups, risk dropped by 21 percent. The antioxidant epigallocatechin gallate or the amino acid

L-theanine may be responsible.

- **Emotional stress shouldn't be pooh-poohed.** If you're prone to angry outbursts, don't assume it's no big deal. Emotional stress triggers the release of cortisol, adrenaline, and other so-called stress hormones that can increase blood pressure and heart rate, leading to stroke.

    In one study, about 30 percent of stroke patients had heightened negative emotions (such as anger) in the two hours preceding the stroke.

    My advice: Don't ignore your mental health — especially anger (it's often a sign of depression, a potent stroke risk factor). If you're suffering from negative emotions, exercise regularly, try relaxation strategies (such as meditation), and don't hesitate to get professional help.

- **Be alert for subtle signs of stroke.** The acronym *FAST* helps people identify signs of stroke. *F* stands for facial drooping — does one side of the face droop, or is it numb? Is the person's smile uneven? *A* stands for arm weakness — ask the person to raise both arms. Does one arm drift downward? *S* stands for speech difficulty — is speech slurred? Is the person unable to speak or hard to understand? Can he/she repeat a simple sentence such as, "The sky is blue" correctly? *T* stands for time — if a person shows any of these symptoms (even if they go away), call 911 immediately. Note the time so that you know when symptoms first appeared.

But stroke can also cause one symptom that isn't widely known — a loss of touch sensation. This can occur if a stroke causes injury to the parts of the brain that detect touch. If you suddenly can't feel your fingers or toes — or have trouble with simple tasks such as buttoning a shirt — you could be having a stroke. You might notice that you can't feel temperatures or that you can't feel it when your feet touch the floor.

It's never normal to lose your sense of touch for an unknown reason — or to have unexpected difficulty seeing, hearing, and/or speaking. Get to an emergency room!

Also important: If you think you're having a stroke, don't waste time calling your regular doctor. Call an ambulance, and ask to be taken to the nearest hospital with a primary stroke center. You'll get much better care than you would at a regular hospital emergency room.

A meta-analysis found that there were 21 percent fewer deaths among patients treated at stroke centers, and the surviving patients had faster recoveries and fewer stroke-related complications.

My advice: If you have any stroke risk factors, including high blood pressure, diabetes, or elevated cholesterol, find out now which hospitals in your area have stroke centers. To find one near you, go to heart.org/myhealthcare.

Ralph L. Sacco, MD, chairman of neurology, the Olemberg Family Chair in Neurological Disorders, and the Miller Professor of Neurology, Epidemiology, and Public Health, Human Genetics and Neurosurgery at the Miller School of Medicine at the University of Miami, where he is the executive director of the Evelyn McKnight Brain Institute. He is also the chief of the Neurology Service at Jackson Memorial Hospital and the 2014 recipient of the American Heart Association's Cor Vitae Stroke Award.

9
HEALTHY LIFE HABITS THAT KEEP DIABETES AWAY FOREVER

Now that you have diabetes, how do you stay your healthy, vibrant self?

Anyone, at any age, must become more diligent and aware once they've been diagnosed. However, older readers have many other considerations to contend with, and the balance between everything can seem overwhelming. What can you do to keep yourself on the right track?

Some advice is surprisingly simple, and some will have never been considered: take the stairs, try yoga, get rid of diet soda drinks, etc. These pages contain various tips and secrets that can become part of your daily routine and easily make sure that your diabetes is not going ignored.

GOURMET COOKING SECRETS FOR PEOPLE WITH DIABETES

Can people with diabetes eat healthfully and enjoy their meals at the same time? The answer is a resounding yes, says Chris Smith, author of *The Diabetic Chef's Year-Round Cookbook*. Smith uses fresh, seasonal ingredients to create healthy, interesting meals full of flavor for individuals with diabetes and everyone else at the table, while reducing the salt, sugar, and fat that many have come to rely upon to add taste.

Healthy Eating . . . With Diabetes

Just like the rest of us, people with diabetes should eat nutritious meals that are low in fat (especially saturated and trans fat), moderate in salt, and very sparing in sugar, while emphasizing whole grains, vegetables, and fruit. However, because people with diabetes are at a greater risk for life-threatening complications such as hypertension, heart disease, and stroke, it's particularly important that they keep blood glucose control while maintaining normal levels of blood pressure and blood lipids (cholesterol). It can be challenging to do all that while still preparing flavorful and appealing food. Here, the Diabetic Chef shares his secrets for preparing foods that are appropriate for people with diabetes and delicious enough for everyone.

Herbs and Spices Are Essential

Liven up your meals with garden-fresh herbs, many of which are available year-round. Fresh herbs are densely packed with flavor.

You can use herbs in a variety of ways throughout the seasons.

- **Fine herbs, such as thyme, oregano, dill, basil, and chives, are usually available in the spring and summer.** These should be added as a finish (at the end of the cooking process) to release their delicate flavors and aromatic qualities. "Use fresh basil with summer tomatoes and olive oil for pasta or as a finish to a tomato sauce," says Smith. "Use chives as a delicate finish to soups, salads, and sauces."
- **Hearty herbs (rosemary, sage), available year-round,** can be added earlier on in the cooking process. Use them with stews, soups, and Crock-Pot dishes. They can withstand the heat of cooking without losing flavor and, in fact, the longer they're cooked, the more mellow and flavorful they are, says Smith.
- **Dried herbs must be rehydrated,** so use at the beginning of the cooking process (adding as you sauté onions for a sauce, for example). Your homemade tomato sauce with dried oregano and basil tastes better the next day as the flavor of the dried herbs fully blooms and combines with the other ingredients.

Herb typically describes the leaves of a plant, while spices are derived from any other part — including the root, seeds, bark, or buds. Spices can be used to create a medley of flavors and can be evocative of different types of ethnic cuisines. "Spices bring great diversity to food," Smith says.

Other Tips for Healthful Eating

Overall, Smith points out that healthful eating is a matter of practicing what he calls "Nutritional MVP," which stands for moderation, variety, and portion control.

From his cookbook, another suggestion is to learn how to do template cooking. Template cooking is taking one recipe and adapting it in different ways by using the same cooking method but substituting different ingredients, says Smith. "It gives you the freedom to be creative, which is the essence of good cooking." It also brings much-needed diversity to meals, so you are not forever serving the same old thing. One example of a template recipe is the Herbed Chicken Breast (see page 117). "There are only seven ingredients in this recipe, but you can vary it with fresh, seasonal ingredients," says Smith. "For instance, in springtime, you can exchange the olive oil for sesame oil and use lemongrass rather than garlic to create an Asian flavor. In summer, substitute fresh cilantro for the rosemary."

Try different cooking techniques to bring out the essence of foods.

- **Grill, broil, roast, sauté, or steam food to enhance flavor without added fat or salt.** Slow-roast vegetables with a drizzle of olive oil in a four-hundred-degree oven to bring out their true flavors. Many develop a natural sweetness when roasted. Season with garlic or add herbs to vary the taste. Rather than sautéing garlic or onions with butter or oil before adding them to soups or stews, try roasting in the oven.
- **Marinate foods in a few ingredients.** "The herbs, lemon, and spice in the Simple Chicken Breast recipe create a vibrant flavor, and the extra-virgin olive oil allows the herbs and spices to reach their full bouquet," says Smith.
- **Sear meat (brown on both sides in a pan for a few minutes before placing it in the oven)** to enhance flavor without adding extra fat or salt. "Any kind and cut of meat can be seared," says Smith.
- **Pair dishes with colorful sides.** Instead of a plate full of brown items such as chicken and rice, liven up your plate with deeply colored fruits and vegetables that add variety and important phytonutrients (components of fruits and vegetables that are thought to promote health) to your diet.
- **Keep the pantry stocked with these healthy ingredients.**
  - ▶ *Oils:* extra-virgin olive oil, sesame oil, and grapeseed oil.

▶ *Vinegars:* balsamic, champagne, rice, and aged sherry vinegar.

▶ *Essential spices:* cayenne pepper, chili powder, cinnamon, mustard, nutmeg, paprika, and pepper.

▶ *Essential dried herbs:* bay leaves, dill, basil, oregano, rosemary, thyme, and sage.

▶ *Other essential products:* chicken, vegetable, and beef broth, dried beans, whole gluten-free grains such as quinoa and amaranth.

▶ *Essential fresh ingredients:* lemons, limes, oranges, garlic, onions, shallots, carrots, tomatoes, potatoes, mushrooms, butter (salt free), sour cream (fat free), eggs, hard cheeses (Parmesan and Romano), mustard (grain, Dijon), capers, and olives.

Chris Smith, the Diabetic Chef, is an executive chef working in the healthcare field. Author of two cookbooks, *Cooking with the Diabetic Chef* and *The Diabetic Chef's Year-Round Cookbook,* he lectures widely about cooking for people with diabetes.

EAT LIKE A VIKING
TO MANAGE DIABETES

Have you heard about the "new" Nordic diet? It turns out that Scandinavians who follow their countrymen's traditional way of eating seem to live longer. But, sorry to tell you, the key is not Danish pastries and Swedish meatballs. They eat a lot of wholegrain rye bread — real rye bread, not the mushy "rye" found alongside white bread in supermarkets — and cabbage. But there's more to the Nordic diet than that.

Live Like a Viking

Anja Olsen, PhD, a researcher at the Danish Cancer Society, and a team of researchers collected information about the diets and lifestyles of approximately fifty-seven thousand Danes ages fifty to sixty-four. Over the twelve-year study period, 4,126 died. After accounting for lifestyle differences (such as exercise, weight, smoking, alcohol use, and education), the researchers found a strong correlation between eating traditional Nordic foods and length of life. For instance, men who followed the traditional Nordic diet most closely had a nearly 36 percent lower risk of dying during the twelve years of follow-up. And women who ate the most Nordic staples reduced their risk for death by 25 percent. These results appeared in the *Journal of Nutrition*.

Wholegrain rye bread, which most study participants ate daily (the median amount was two and a half slices) appeared to have the strongest protective effect, especially in men. This is not the prepackaged rye bread with additives and sugars found in most supermarkets.

Adding further to the chance of living longer, both wholegrain rye and cabbage help in the battle against obesity. And cabbage has been related to a decreased risk for both cancer and heart disease.

However, as in other Western countries, many Nordic folk today eat too much processed and/or fatty food, including pasta, french fries, pizza, and sugary desserts, and, as a result, may suffer from high rates of heart disease, diabetes, and cancer.

Danish Modern . . . Not?

To encourage better health, Dr. Olsen recommends that we focus on old-style dietary habits as they've long existed in most traditional cultures, be they Nordic or from other countries. They tend to emphasize natural, whole, and often wild foods — in contrast to our modern approach of eating highly refined foods.

Luckily, you don't have to be a Dane, Swede, or Norwegian to eat like one. Here are some ways you can enjoy the benefits of the healthy Nordic diet:

- **Eat real rye bread.** Whole grains such as rye, barley, and oats abound in dietary fiber, minerals, and antioxidants that protect against heart disease, type 2 diabetes, and cancer. In this study, wholegrain rye had the most positive impact on health — but it's important to realize that this is not the rye bread we grew up with in the United States.

  Instead, in this country, you'll most easily find this European-style rye by looking for German wholegrain rye, such as the Mestemacher brand, usually found in the deli section of grocery stores, and also in health-food stores, health-oriented markets such as Whole Foods, and even online.
- **Cut up some cabbage.** Cabbage is packed with fiber and isothiocyanates (the sulphur-containing compounds found in cruciferous vegetables). Enjoy both red and green cabbage shredded raw in salads and slaws or lightly steamed.
- **Root for root vegetables.** Root vegetables, especially carrots, are rich in phytochemicals such as carotenes, which neutralize free radicals that damage cells in your body and may cause cancer. Parsnips and turnips are also good choices.
- **Enjoy apples, pears, and wild berries.** Wild berries, which are easily available in Scandinavia, are especially rich sources of substances such as omega-3 fatty acids, es-

607

sential to normal growth and development, as well as antioxidants and phytoestrogens such as lignans, which help lower cancer risk. But even though wild berries contain many more of these healthful components, the berries you find in U.S. grocery stores — i.e., cultivated ones — are still a good source of these important nutrients.

Anja Olsen, PhD, researcher, Institute of Cancer Epidemiology, Danish Cancer Society, Copenhagen, Denmark.

SUREFIRE WAY TO STOP OVEREATING: THE FIVE-POINT HUNGER SCALE

It happened again. You sat down to a meal or started to snack and, despite your intention not to overindulge, somehow kept eating until you were stuffed. Curses! Perhaps you've tried that "mindful eating" business in the past — paying attention to the physical and emotional sensations during every moment with food — because you've heard that it helps people avoid overeating. The problem is, that "every moment" aspect is tough to pull off. After all, sometimes you want to converse with your meal companions or look at the newspaper or just gaze out the window while you eat, rather than focusing fully on every single bite.

Well, there's an easier way to achieve the same kind of control that mindful eating provides. It's called the five-point hunger scale. The idea is to simply rate your hunger on the following scale:

1. Starved
2. Hungry
3. Comfortable
4. Full
5. Stuffed

The beautiful simplicity of the five-point scale is that, rather than thinking about it constantly while you eat, you need only give it a moment's focus three times — before, midway through, and after any given meal or snack. Here's what to do.

When you're tempted to eat, before you begin, rate your hunger, asking yourself:

- **Are you feeling ravenous, spacey, or light-headed?** Do you feel like almost any kind of food would satisfy you? You're at point one, starving, and you must eat — in fact, you have waited too long. When you're feeling starved, self-control becomes extremely difficult, and you're likely to end up overeating, after which you'll feel guilty, so you'll starve yourself again. In essence, you bounce back and forth from starving to stuffed all day, without ever feeling truly comfortable and satisfied.

  Best: Don't let your hunger reach point one.

- **Is your stomach growling, letting you know that your body needs fuel?** Has the feeling come on gradually? You're at point two, hungry. Hunger is a slow sensation. It doesn't jump into your brain all of a sudden, and it usually occurs around the same time that you're used to having breakfast, lunch, or supper.

  Remember: Point two is the perfect point at which to eat.

- **Are you physically comfortable but still feel like eating — with a specific type of food in mind?** You're at point three, and you're facing a craving, not true hunger. A craving is a psychological issue rather than a physical one, a spark sensation that comes on suddenly.

What to do: Don't jump right into eating. Instead, consider what emotion is driving your urge to eat. Then try to satisfy that need with a food-free activity to see whether the craving goes away. Feeling lonely? Pick up the phone. Bored? Tackle a crossword puzzle, or clear some clutter out of your garage or closet. Stressed? Soak in the tub, or take a hike. If you still desire that particular food afterward, go ahead and indulge in moderation, eating only as much as you need to satisfy the craving.

Halfway through your meal: After you've been eating for five to ten minutes, put down your fork and rate your hunger again:

• **Have your physical sensations of hunger lessened but still linger?** You're just past point two, on your way to three. Some people stop here, especially when they want to lose weight. But this backfires because it usually triggers a second eating period not much later.

Better: Keep eating!

• **Do you feel pleasantly sated?** You're at point three, comfortable — which is ideal, especially if you're trying to lose weight. If you stop now, you should have enough energy to last until your next scheduled meal. But if you're enjoying your food, you don't have to stop yet. It's OK to keep eating slowly for a few more minutes.

- **Are you on your way to discomfort?** Is your waistband starting to feel snug? You're at point four, full — and you should definitely stop eating now. Remember, it takes fifteen to twenty minutes for your stomach to send the signal to your brain that it is full. If you eat until your stomach feels full, you will be beyond full — in fact, you'll be painfully stuffed, point five — by the time your brain gets that signal.

Twenty minutes after your meal: Rate your hunger level one last time:

- **Is your belly a bit distended but not painful?** Congratulations — you're at point four, full. You stopped eating in time.
- **Do you feel the urge to groan or lie down?** Are you so full that you couldn't put another bite into your mouth? You're at point five, stuffed, and you definitely went too far. Your body would have been satisfied if you had stopped several hundred calories sooner, and you would have avoided the discomfort and weight gain that come with overeating.

Helpful: Don't starve yourself for the rest of the day, but at your next meal, do pay closer attention to your midmeal hunger rating, and stop when you're at point three.

For the first few weeks: While you're learning to recognize how your body feels at each point, keep a written log of your hunger scale scores before, midway through, and after each meal. If you need a reminder, set a timer or program your cell phone to beep. Keep it up, and you'll soon become adept at waiting to reach point two before you start eating (without delaying too long and hitting point one) and at stopping when you reach point three or four (without ever hitting point five). Once that happens, you're on your way to a lifetime of sensible, pleasurable eating and easy weight control — an essential part of living well with diabetes.

Osama Hamdy, MD, PhD, medical director, Obesity Clinical Program, Joslin Diabetes Center, and assistant professor of medicine, Harvard Medical School, both in Boston. He is a coauthor of *The Diabetes Breakthrough: Based on a Scientifically Proven Plan to Lose Weight and Cut Medications.* TheDiabetesBreakthrough.com.

TIMING MATTERS!

When you eat is almost as important as what you eat:

- **Plan on eating four or five daily meals** — breakfast between six a.m. and eight a.m., an optional (and light) late-morning snack, lunch between 11:00 a.m. and 12:30 p.m., a midafternoon snack, and supper between 5:00 p.m. and 7:00 p.m.
- **Plan your meals so that you get more protein at supper.** It will stimulate the release of growth hormone, which burns fat while you sleep.
- **Avoid all food three hours before bedtime.** Eating late in the evening causes increases in blood sugar and insulin that can lead to weight gain — even if you consume a lower-calorie diet (1,200 to 1,500 calories a day).

Ridha Arem, MD, an endocrinologist, director of the Texas Thyroid Institute and clinical professor of medicine at Baylor College of Medicine, both in Houston. He is a former chief of endocrinology and metabolism at Houston's Ben Taub General Hospital and is author of *The Thyroid Solution Diet.* AremWellness.com.

THE RIGHT WAY TO
TAKE YOUR VITAMINS

Many of us take vitamins and other nutritional supplements. In fact, researchers from Harvard analyzed data from nearly 125,000 middle-aged and older people and found that an astounding 88 percent of women and 81 percent of men took supplements.

Unfortunately, a lot of us take nutritional supplements wrong.*

We don't take high enough doses, or we take them at the wrong time of day, or we combine them with other supplements, foods, or drugs that can block absorption.

Good news: I've counseled thousands of patients on the best ways to take vitamins, and I can assure you that taking them correctly can be simple and straightforward.

What you might be doing wrong — and how to quickly fix the problem:

Vitamin mistake #1: **You take a dose that's too low.** There are many nutrient-nutrient interactions that can reduce the absorption of individual nutrients by 5 to 10 percent. Example: iron cuts the absorption of zinc — the more iron in a supplement, the less zinc you're likely to absorb.

My advice: Don't take a multivitamin that

---

* Be sure to check supplement dosage amounts with your doctor, especially if you have diabetes or another chronic condition.

supplies 100 percent of the daily value of nutrients, a level intended only to prevent deficiency diseases. Instead, take a multivitamin that supplies an optimal amount of nutrients — an amount that will easily overcome every absorption issue caused by nutrient-nutrient interactions.

For simplicity, use the B vitamins as your reference point. Look for a product that supplies about 40 mg each of thiamin, riboflavin, niacin, and vitamin B6 (pyridoxine), and 200 mcg of vitamin B12. These levels are safe and therapeutic, improving energy and mental clarity. When a product contains the above levels of these nutrients, it usually will have optimal levels of other nutrients as well.

Vitamin mistake #2: **You take a dose that's too high.** It can be detrimental to your health to take high doses of vitamin A and vitamin E. Reasons: taking more than 3,000 IU of vitamin A (retinol) daily can increase your risk for osteoporosis, the bone-eroding disease. Vitamin E is actually a family of eight compounds called tocopherols and tocotrienols. Alpha-tocopherol — the compound commonly found in multivitamins — can be toxic in doses higher than 100 IU daily.

My advice: Take a multivitamin that contains no more than 3,000 IU of vitamin A total, with approximately one-half from retinol and one-half from beta-carotene (which turns into vitamin A in the body and does not cause osteoporosis).

Choose a multivitamin with no more than 100 IU of vitamin E. If you take the nutrient as a separate supplement for a specific condition, such as for breast tenderness, take it in the form of mixed tocopherols and tocotrienols.

Vitamin mistake #3: **You try to take vitamins two or three times a day.** Taking vitamins in divided doses — two or even three times a day — is ideal because the body sustains higher blood levels of the nutrients. But very few people can stick with this type of regimen.

My advice: Take vitamins first thing in the morning, with breakfast. (The fat in the meal will help you absorb vitamins A, D, and E, which are fat-soluble.) Yes, there's a tiny trade-off of effectiveness for convenience, but it's worth it.

Exception: If you take magnesium as a separate supplement, you might want to take it at bedtime for deeper sleep. Avoid magnesium oxide and magnesium hydroxide, both of which are poorly absorbed. Magnesium glycinate or magnesium malate is preferred.

Vitamin mistake #4: **You take a second-rate formulation.** Vitamins come in a range of forms — tablets, caplets, capsules, chewables, softgels, liquids, powders — and some are better than others.

Vitamin tablets, for example, are a poor choice. They may not dissolve completely — and you can't absorb any nutrients from a pill that doesn't dissolve. Tablets (and some of the other forms listed above) also may contain binders, fillers, and other additives. These supposedly inert compounds may have all kinds of unknown effects on the body.

My advice: I recommend powders, which are highly absorbable. Just add water and stir. My favorite is the Energy Revitalization System, from Enzymatic Therapy, which I formulated. (So that I can't be accused of profiting from my recommendation, I donate 100 percent of my royalties from sales to charity.) I recommend one scoop each morning combined with 5 g of ribose (a naturally occurring sugar) to optimize energy.

Don't like drinks? Try a combination of My Favorite Multiple Take One by Natrol plus two tablets of Jigsaw Sustained Release Magnesium plus two chewable ribose tablets (2 to 3 g each).

Vitamin mistake #5: **You take calcium.** One-third of people who take supplements take calcium — and I think just about every one of those people is making a mistake. The scientific evidence shows that taking a calcium supplement provides little or no protection against bone fractures, and research now links calcium supplements to increased risk for heart attacks and strokes.

My advice: I strongly recommend that you get your calcium from food, eating one or two servings of dairy a day. Almonds, broccoli, and green leafy vegetables such as kale are also good calcium sources. Unlike supplemental calcium, calcium from food is safe. If you decide to take a calcium supplement for stronger bones, take no more than 100 to 200 mg daily, and always combine it with other bone-supporting nutrients, such as vitamin D, magnesium, and vitamin K. Take these at night to help sleep.

Vitamin mistake #6: **You don't realize that your medication can cause a nutrient deficiency.** Some medications block the absorption of specific nutrients. In my clinical experience, the two worst offenders are:

- **The diabetes drug metformin**, which can cause a B12 deficiency.

  What to do: Metformin is an excellent medication, but be sure to take a multivitamin containing at least 200 mcg of B12 daily.

- **Proton pump inhibitors** such as esomeprazole, which block the production of stomach acid and are prescribed for heartburn, ulcers, and other gastrointestinal problems. Long-term use can cause deficiencies of magnesium and B12.

What to do: Take a multivitamin with 200 mcg of B12 and additional magnesium (200 mg daily), and talk to your doctor about getting off the drug. (A gradual decrease in dosage is safest.) Proton pump inhibitors are toxic when used long-term and addictive, causing rebound acid hypersecretion when stopped. The solution? Improve digestion using plant-based digestive enzymes, deglycyrrhizinated licorice (DGL), marshmallow root, and other stomach-healing supplements. Follow directions on the labels.

Jacob Teitelbaum, MD, board-certified internist, holistic physician, and nationally known expert in the fields of chronic fatigue syndrome, fibromyalgia, sleep, and pain. Based in Hawaii, he is author of numerous books, including *The Fatigue and Fibromyalgia Solution, Pain-Free 1–2-3,* and *Real Cause, Real Cure,* as well as the popular free iPhone and Android application "Cures A–Z." Vitality101.com.

TEN HYDROPHILIC FOODS THAT SATISFY HUNGER AND HELP YOU LOSE WEIGHT

What if you could swallow a pill right before dining that would make your stomach swell like a balloon so you would feel artificially full? Well, such a pill is in the works, but there's a much better solution for you — hydrophilic foods. They attract and absorb water, which makes them swell in size — in a natural process — so you naturally feel satisfied and automatically consume fewer calories. Plus, unlike a weird new diet pill or other diet gimmicks, they are full of nutrients that your body needs. And besides helping you lose or maintain weight, hydrophilic foods — because they contain digestible soluble fiber — also help control blood sugar and cholesterol.

And it's all real food. What more could you want?

The Top Ten Hydrophilic Foods

- **Chia seeds.** Chia seeds are the perfect example of a hydrophilic food. They start out as tiny, crunchy, nutty-tasting seeds (just a little bigger than poppy seeds), but each seed can absorb up to twelve times its weight in water, so they form a gel that's filling and extremely nutrient-rich — each seed is supercharged with omega-3s and packed with antioxidants, fiber, iron, magnesium, calcium, and potassium! So sprinkle a tablespoon into your smoothie for breakfast, add some to soups and porridges, or use them in place of breadcrumbs to bind meatballs. You can even make a simple and nutritious pudding by combining two tablespoons of chia seeds per cup of almond milk or other liquid, sweetening to taste, and refrigerating overnight — no cooking needed.

- **Okra.** OK, okra might be a turnoff for some people because it gets sappy — or downright slimy — when cooked, but that texture speaks volumes about its soluble fiber, which, along with a host of vitamins and minerals, turns okra into a dietary powerhouse. Add sliced okra to soups and stews, where the consistency doesn't stand out so much and, in fact, the okra acts as a natural thickener. Also consider cooking okra at high heat (in a wok, for example), or slicing it lengthwise and grilling it — both cooking styles will reduce the vegetable's slipperiness. To use it raw, slice and toss into salads, or dress with oil and vinegar all on its own. It's tasty, with a good crunch, and its slight sappiness enhances the texture of the dressing.

- **Oatmeal.** Oatmeal is a hydrophilic food you might already be filling up on since it's well-known for its cholesterol-controlling abilities. Just picture the way raw oats absorb water while they cook, and you'll understand why they make my top-ten list of hydrophilic foods. Don't like oatmeal? Maybe it's because the only kind you know is rolled oats — the kind that look flattened and may have even been partially cooked before you buy them. Rolled oats can cook up mushy and without much natural flavor. Try steel-cut oats. They cook up into a hearty, pleasantly toothsome, and nutty-tasting dish.

• **Pears.** Pears are naturally full of pectin, a type of soluble fiber found in the walls of plant cells. If you've ever made jam, you've probably added pectin powder to thicken it. In addition to helping you feel full, pectin acts as a detoxifier, a gastrointestinal tract regulator, and an immune system stimulant. Grab a pear for a juicy snack, or try these delicious ways to use them — add thin slices to sandwiches, toss into salads, or cut them in half, core them, and either grill or roast them. To grill, simply place them, cut side down, on a lightly oiled stovetop grill until they are seared. To roast, place them, cut side down, in a baking pan, warm up a half cup of apple juice and a tablespoon or two of honey, pour the apple juice over the pears, and bake at 400°F for thirty minutes.

• **Barley.** Like oats, barley absorbs a substantial amount of water as it cooks — and like oats, it also expands further in your stomach, providing heart-healthy nutrition and natural fullness. Americans aren't very familiar with barley and don't use it very much in their kitchens, which is ironic, since it was one of the original foods grown by the Pilgrims and may have been eaten at the first Thanksgiving. Beyond the standard beef-barley stew (which, by the way, can be a very healthful meal), it's actually very easy to use and enjoy barley. Just follow cooking instructions on the package, and then use barley as the base in your favorite wholegrain salad recipe (instead of wheat berries, for example) or instead of small pastas in soups (it lends an earthier tone than pasta), or sauté it with some butter and sliced mushrooms, salt, and pepper. You can even cook barley like risotto — barley's soluble fiber creates the right kind of creaminess for risotto-like dishes.

- **Brussels sprouts.** Serving for serving, Brussels sprouts are among the vegetables highest in soluble fiber. For a taste revelation, try tossing fresh Brussels sprouts with olive oil and salt, then roasting in the oven at 400°F for thirty to forty minutes or until they are softened and caramelized, or shred them raw and use in slaw. You can also make an easy, delicious boiled Brussels sprouts dish. Cut the sprouts in half, then boil them with a variety of herbs such as garlic, basil, thyme, and rosemary in one-part wine vinegar and one-part water until they are tender. Drain, then dress with balsamic vinegar and olive oil, salt, pepper, and more herbs to taste. Let cool and serve at room temperature.

- **Kidney beans.** Like all beans, kidney beans soak up water as they cook and keep doing it after you eat them. I especially favor kidney beans because their red color indicates a high level of disease-fighting antioxidants — the darker red, the better. Of course, they are a great addition to chilies, salads, and soups such as minestrone. You might also like to partly mash a cup and a half of cooked kidney beans and mix them with olive oil, a dash of balsamic vinegar, salt, garlic, and other spices to taste for a delicious bean spread served with crostini or Italian bread.

- **Chickpeas.** Also called garbanzo beans, these might be the single easiest and most versatile food on this top-ten list. You know you can toss them onto any salad, but you don't even need the salad. You can simply open a can of chickpeas, drain, add any salad dressing, and start eating — and if you like this idea, don't miss trying them in Caesar dressing with Parmesan cheese sprinkled on top. If you have a little more time, purée chickpeas with garlic, cumin, tahini, olive oil, and lemon juice for a healthy, homemade hummus. For a portable snack, toss chickpeas with a bit of olive oil and your favorite spice blend, then roast until irresistibly crunchy. Or make pasta e fagiole — the Italian version of rice and beans — by adding cooked chickpeas and small pasta to a saucy sauté of diced onions, carrots, celery or fennel, zucchini, and stewed tomatoes and their juice.

- **Oranges.** That an orange easily fits in a purse or jacket pocket makes it one of my favorite snacks. Besides the famous vitamin C content, oranges are packed with soluble fiber. To get the most nutritional (and weight-loss) benefit, don't peel off all the pith — the white substance beneath the peel. It's got loads of pectin and almost as much vitamin C as the juicy fruit it covers.

- **Agar.** Unless you are really into baking or fancy cooking, agar (also called agar-agar) is the hydrophilic food you're least likely to have in your pantry, but you might want to consider stocking it. It's a gelling agent made from seaweed that has a whopping 80 percent soluble fiber with no fat and virtually no calories, carbs, or sugar. If you want a homemade sweet, agar is the perfect ingredient for making custards, puddings, and fruit gels. And it couldn't be easier to use — just substitute it for gelatin in recipes. Bon appétit to your health and waistline!

Keren Gilbert, MS, RD, nutritionist and the founder and president of Decision Nutrition, a nutrition consulting firm in Great Neck, New York, and author of *The HD Diet: Achieve Lifelong Weight Loss with Chia Seeds and Other Water-Absorbent Foods.*

The phrase "addictive white powder" probably makes you think of illegal drugs. Add sugar to that addictive group. Americans consume vast quantities — and suffer withdrawal symptoms when they don't get it. In fact, animal studies indicate that sugar is more addictive than cocaine.

Excess sugar has been linked to obesity, cancer, diabetes, and dementia.

Sugar, Sugar, Everywhere

In the United States, the average person consumes about 142 pounds of sugar each year, the equivalent of forty-eight teaspoons a day. Of that amount, seventy-four pounds are added sugar — about twenty-three teaspoons every day. Added sugars are defined as those sugars added to foods and beverages during processing or home preparation as opposed to sugars that occur naturally.

People who want to cut back on sweeteners usually start with the sugar bowl. They spoon less sugar on their breakfast cereal, for example, or use a sugar substitute in their coffee.

This doesn't help very much. The vast majority of added sugar in the diet comes from packaged foods, including foods that we think are healthful.

For example, eight ounces of one brand of sweetened apple yogurt contains 44 g of sugar, according to the nutrition facts label. Four grams equals one teaspoon, so that's eleven teaspoons of sugar. (You cannot tell from the label how much sugar is from the yogurt, how much is from the apples, and how much is added sugar.)

Most of the added sugar that we consume comes from regular soft drinks (there are about ten teaspoons of sugar in twelve ounces of nondiet soda), candy, pies, cookies, cakes, fruit drinks, and milk-based desserts and products (ice cream, sweetened yogurt).

If you look carefully at ingredients labels, which list ingredients in order of quantity, you will see that the first two or three ingredients are often forms of sugar, but many have innocuous-sounding names, such as barley malt, galactose, and agave nectar. Other forms of sugar include honey, maple syrup, corn syrup, corn sweetener, dextrine, rice syrup, glucose, sucrose, and dextrose.

Dangerous Imbalance

The difference between sickness and health lies in the body's ability to maintain homeostasis, the proper balance and performance of all of the internal functions. Excess sugar disturbs this balance by impairing immunity, disrupting the production and release of hormones, and creating an acidic internal environment.

It's not healthy to maintain a highly acidic

state. The body tries to offset this by making itself more alkaline. It does this, in part, by removing calcium and other minerals from the bones.

Result: People who eat too much sugar experience disruptions in insulin and other hormones. They have an elevated risk for osteoporosis due to calcium depletion. They also tend to have elevated levels of cholesterol and triglycerides (blood fats), which increase the risk for heart disease.

Break the Cycle

Sugar, like drugs and alcohol, is addictive because it briefly elevates levels of serotonin, a neurotransmitter that produces positive feelings. When a sugar addict doesn't eat sugar, serotonin declines to low levels. This makes the person feel worse than before. He/she then eats more sugar to try to feel better, and the vicious cycle goes on.

For the best chance of breaking a sugar addiction, you need to ease out of it. This is usually more effective than going cold turkey. Once you've given up sugar entirely and the addiction is past, you'll be able to enjoy small amounts of sugar if you choose, although some people find that they lose their taste for it. Here's how to break the habit:

• **Divide sugar from all sources in half.** Do this for one week.

Examples: If you've been drinking two soft drinks a day, cut back to one. Eat half as much dessert. Eat a breakfast cereal that has only half as much sugar as your usual brand, or mix a low-sugar brand in with your higher-sugar brand.

- **Limit yourself to one sweet bite.** The second week, allow yourself to have only one taste of only one very sweet food daily. This might be ice cream, sweetened cereal, or a breakfast muffin. That small hit of sugar will prevent serotonin from dropping too low, too fast.

  After about two weeks with little or no sugar, your internal chemistry, including levels of serotonin and other neurotransmitters, will stabilize at a healthier level.

- **Eat fresh fruits and vegetables.** These foods help restore the body's natural acid-alkaline balance. This will help reduce sugar cravings and promote better digestion. Be sure to substitute fresh fruits for juices. Whole fruit is better, because the fiber slows the absorption of sugars into the bloodstream. The fiber is also filling, which is why few people will sit down and eat four oranges, the number you would need to squeeze to get one eight-ounce glass of juice.

  Helpful: All fruits are healthful, but melons and berries have less sugar than other fruits.

Nancy Appleton, PhD, a clinical nutritionist in San Diego. She is author, with G. N. Jacobs, of *Suicide by Sugar: A Startling Look at Our #1 National Addiction.*

KICK THE SUGAR HABIT: FOUR-WEEK PLAN

The average American consumes forty-eight teaspoons of added sugar per day. That's right — forty-eight teaspoons a day.

We all know that sugar can lead to weight gain, but that's just the beginning. People who eat a lot of sugar have nearly double the risk for heart disease as those who eat less, according to data from the Harvard Nurses' Health Study. They're more likely to develop insulin resistance and diabetes. They also tend to look older, because sugar triggers the production of advanced glycation end products (AGEs), chemical compounds that accelerate skin aging.

If you want to avoid these problems, it's not enough to merely cut back on sugar. In my experience, patients need to eliminate it from their diets — at least at the beginning — just like addicts have to eliminate drugs from their lives. In fact, a study showed that sugar cravings are actually more intense than the cravings for cocaine.

You don't have to give up sugar indefinitely. Once the cravings are gone, you can enjoy sweet foods again — although you probably will be happy consuming far less than before. After a sugar-free "washing out" period, you'll be more sensitive to sweet tastes. You won't want as much.

Bonus: Some people who have completed

the four-week diet and stayed on the maintenance program for four or five months lost thirty-five pounds or more.

First Step: Three-Day Sugar Fix

For sugar lovers, three days without sweet stuff can seem like forever. But it's an essential part of the sugar detox diet, because when you go three days without any sugar, your palate readjusts. When you eat an apple after the three-day period, you'll think it's the sweetest thing you've ever tasted. You'll even notice the natural sweetness in a glass of whole or 2 percent milk (which contains about three teaspoons of naturally occurring sugar).

You may experience withdrawal symptoms during the first three days. These can include fatigue, headache, fogginess, and irritability, but soon, you'll feel better than you have in years.

Caution: If you have any type of blood sugar problem, including hypoglycemia, insulin resistance, or diabetes, you must consult your physician before starting any type of diet, including the sugar detox diet. In addition, if you are on insulin or an oral medication to control blood sugar, it is likely that your dosage will need to be adjusted if you lower your daily sugar intake.

During the three days, follow these guidelines:

- **No foods or drinks with added sugar.** No candy, cookies, cake, doughnuts, etc. — not even a teaspoon of sugar in your morning coffee.
- **No artificial sweeteners of any kind, including diet soft drinks.** Artificial sweeteners contribute to the sweetness overload that diminishes our ability to taste sugar.
- **No starches.** This includes pasta, cereal, crackers, bread, potatoes, and rice.
- **No fruit, except a little lemon or lime for cooking or to flavor a glass of water or tea.** I hesitate to discourage people from eating fruit, because it's such a healthy food, but it provides too much sugar when you're detoxing.
- **No dairy.** No milk, cream, yogurt, or cheese. You can have a little (one to two teaspoons) butter for cooking.
- **Plenty of protein,** including lean red meat, chicken, fish, tofu, and eggs.
- **Most vegetables,** such as asparagus, broccoli, cauliflower, celery, peppers, kale, lettuce, and more — but no corn, potatoes, sweet potatoes, winter squash, beets, or other starchy vegetables.
- **Nuts** — two one-ounce servings a day. Almonds, walnuts, cashews, and other nuts are high in protein and fat, both of which will help you feel full. Nuts also will keep your hands (and mouth) busy when you're

craving a sugary snack.

- **Lots of water, but no alcohol.** It's a carbohydrate that contains more sugar than you might think. You can drink alcohol later (see below).

Next Step: A Four-Week Plan

This is the fun part. During the three-day sugar fix, you focused on not eating certain foods. Now you'll spend a month adding tasty but nutritious foods back into your diet. You'll continue to avoid overly sweet foods — and you'll use no added sugar — but you can begin eating whole grains, dairy, and fresh fruits.

Week 1: **Wine and cheese.** You'll continue to eat healthy foods, but you now can add one apple a day and one daily serving of dairy, in addition to having a splash of milk or cream in your coffee or tea if you like. A serving of dairy could consist of one ounce of cheese, five ounces of plain yogurt, or one-half cup of cottage cheese. You also can have one serving a day of high-fiber crackers, such as Finn Crisp Hi-Fibre or Triscuit Whole Grain crackers.

You also can start drinking red wine if you wish — up to three four-ounce servings during the first week. Other alcoholic beverages such as white wine, beer, and liquor should be avoided. Red wine is allowed because it is high in resveratrol and other antioxidants.

Week 2: **More dairy, plus fruit.** This is when you really start adding natural sugar back into your diet. You can have two servings of dairy daily if you wish and one serving of fruit in addition to an apple a day. You can have one-half cup of blackberries, blueberries, cantaloupe, raspberries, or strawberries each day. Or you can have a grapefruit half. You'll be surprised how sweet fruit really is. You also are allowed one small sweet potato or yam (one-half cup cubed) daily.

Weeks 3 and 4: **Whole grains and more.** The third and fourth weeks are very satisfying, because you can start eating grains again. But make sure it's whole grain. Carbohydrates such as white bread, white pasta, and white rice are stripped of their fiber during processing, so they are easily broken down into sugar. Whole grains are high in fiber and nutrients and won't give the sugar kick that you would get from processed grains.

Examples: A daily serving of barley, buckwheat, oatmeal (not instant), quinoa, wholegrain pasta, whole-wheat bread, or brown rice.

You might find yourself craving something that's deliciously sweet. Indulge yourself with a small daily serving (one ounce) of dark chocolate.

DEADLY DIET DRINKS

Drinking two or more diet sodas or diet fruit drinks a day resulted in a 30 percent greater risk for heart attack or stroke than rarely or never consuming these diet drinks, an eight-year observational study of nearly sixty thousand women (average age sixty-two) has found.

Theory: Diet sodas and diet fruit drinks (as well as the nondiet versions) have been linked to weight gain and metabolic syndrome, which raise risk for heart disease.

Ankur Vyas, MD, cardiovascular diseases fellow, University of Iowa Health Care, Iowa City.

Patricia Farris, MD, FAAD, clinical associate professor at Tulane University, New Orleans, and member of the media-expert team for the American Academy of Dermatology. She is coauthor, with Brooke Alpert, MS, RD, CDN, of *The Sugar Detox: Lose the Sugar, Lose the Weight, Look and Feel Great.*

GET RID OF STUBBORN BELLY FAT THAT INCREASES DIABETES RISK

Don't count on the latest diet to shrink an expanding waistline. Belly fat is stubborn. Unlike fat in the thighs, buttocks, and hips, which visibly diminishes when you cut calories, belly fat tends to stick around. Even strenuous exercise might not make a dent.

The persistence of a belly bulge isn't merely cosmetic. Beneath the subcutaneous fat that you can pinch with your fingers, fat deep in the abdomen is metabolically different from normal fat. Known as visceral fat, it secretes inflammatory substances that increase the risk for type 2 diabetes, as well as risk for heart attack and some cancers. Even if you're not overweight, a larger-than-average waistline increases health risks.

Surprisingly, even thin people can have a high percentage of visceral fat. It might not be visible, but the risks are the same.

Weight-loss diets can certainly help you drop pounds, and some of that weight will come from the deep abdominal area. But unless you take a broader approach than the standard diet and exercise advice, it's very difficult to maintain visceral fat reductions over the long haul. Here are better approaches to shrink your belly:

- **Don't stress over losing weight.** Everyone knows about stress eating. After a fight with your spouse or a hard day at work, food can be a welcome distraction. What people don't realize is that the struggle to lose weight may itself be highly stressful and that it can cause your belly fat to stick around.

How this happens: Cortisol, one of the main stress-related hormones, increases appetite and makes you less mindful of what you eat. It causes the body to store more fat, particularly visceral fat. People who worry a lot about their weight actually may find themselves eating more.

Take action to reduce stress by practicing yoga (see page 319), meditation, or tai chi (see page 183) for even just a few minutes a day. One study found that there was little or no obesity among more than two hundred women over age forty-five who had practiced yoga for many years. The key is regular practice — it's better to do ten minutes of yoga a day than a ninety-minute class once a week.

Also helpful: Belly breathing. Sit up straight in a chair or lie down on your back, close your eyes, and tune into your breathing. Breathe in and out through your nose slowly and deeply but without straining. You'll feel your belly gently moving out as you inhale and then in as you exhale.

This type of breathing is an effective form of stress control. Try it for one to five minutes once or twice a day or anytime you're feeling stressed.

- **Cultivate mindfulness in your everyday life.** According to yoga and Ayurvedic medicine (a system of healing that originated in India), an overly busy mind can play as big a role in weight gain as diet or exercise. We all need to step back from the chaos of life and give our nervous system a chance to unwind. Take it one step at a time. Do less multitasking. Try to move a little more slowly and deliberately. Spend less time on the internet and watching television — especially when you're eating. Although these activities may seem relaxing, they can stimulate the mind and the nervous system and lead to overeating.

  Bonus: When you eat mindfully, you'll enjoy your food more and need less to feel satisfied.

- **Exercise, but don't go crazy.** Exercise, particularly aerobic exercise, can obviously be good for weight loss. But for many people, the intensity at which they exercise becomes yet another source of stress.

  Example: One of my medical colleagues described a "type A" patient who was an exercise fanatic. Despite her strenuous fitness program, she had a stubborn ten pounds that she couldn't get rid of. He suggested that she might have more luck if she'd simply relax a bit. She ignored his advice — until she broke a leg and had to take a break. The ten pounds melted away.

My advice: Get plenty of exercise, but enjoy it. Don't let it be stressful — make it a soothing part of your day. Go for a bike ride, swim in a lake, or take a hike in nature. Exercise that is relaxing may burn just as many calories as a do-or-die gym workout but without the stress-related rise in cortisol.

Tip: If you've practiced belly breathing (see above), try to bring that kind of breath focus to your exercise. It's even possible to slowly train yourself to breathe through your nose while you exercise, potentially lowering cortisol levels and the rebound hunger that is so common after a workout.

• **Eat more fresh, unprocessed food.** What really matters for health and healthy weight is the quality of your food. Many diets that have been shown to be effective — such as the low-fat vegetarian Ornish program, the Mediterranean diet, and some high-protein plans — disagree with one another, but they all emphasize old-fashioned unprocessed food.

My advice: Worry less about micronutrients such as specific vitamins, minerals, and types of fat or your protein/carbohydrate balance, and instead focus on eating more fresh vegetables, legumes, whole grains, fruit, nuts, and seeds. If you eat animal foods, choose free-range and pasture-raised meat and dairy products, organic if possible.

• **Cut back on refined sugar.** If you follow the advice above and avoid processed foods, you'll naturally consume less sugar, refined grains (such as white bread), and other simple carbohydrates. This will help prevent insulin surges that can lead to more visceral fat.

As always, balance is important. I don't advise anyone to give up all sources of sugar or all carbohydrates. After all, a plum is loaded with the sugar fructose — and fruits are good for you! It's the added sugar in junk and fast food that's the problem. Just be aware that any processed food — including many snacks that are marketed as healthier alternatives — will make it harder to control your weight.

Timothy McCall, MD, an internist and medical editor of *Yoga Journal.* He is author of *Yoga As Medicine: The Yogic Prescription for Health and Healing,* in which he reports on the connection between stress and weight gain. DrMcCall.com.

FIVE TRICKS TO MAKE YOURSELF EXERCISE

Seven out of ten Americans can't make exercise a habit, despite their best intentions and obvious health risks — especially diabetes. But you can learn to motivate yourself to make exercise a regular part of your life. Elite athletes as well as everyday people who have made a successful commitment to lifelong fitness use these insider tips. Here are their secrets:

• **Make your first experience positive.** The more fun and satisfaction you have while exercising, the more you'll want to pursue it and work even harder to develop your skills. Even if your first experience was negative, it's never too late to start fresh. Choose a sport you enjoy, and work to improve your skill level.

The key is finding a strong beginner-level coach who enjoys working with novices. For instance, the YMCA offers beginner swim lessons, and instructors are armed with strategies for teaching in a fun, nonintimidating way.

If your friends have a favorite dance class, play racquetball, or practice karate, ask them for a referral to an approachable teacher. City recreation departments also often host beginner-level classes for a variety of indoor and outdoor activities. You might also try a private lesson. The confidence you gain will motivate you to try it out in a group setting next.

- **Focus on fun, not fitness.** Forcing yourself to hit the gym four times a week sounds like a chore, and you'll likely stop going before you have the chance to begin building your fitness level. But lawn bowling, dancing, Frisbee throwing, hiking, even table tennis — those all sound fun, and you'll still be getting physical activity that helps promote weight control; reduced risk for heart disease, diabetes, and cancer; stronger bones; and improved mood. As you start to have more fun, you'll want to become more involved, and your fitness level will improve over time.

  No strategy is more crucial than this: Get hooked on the fun, and you'll get hooked on the activity for life.

- **Find your competitive streak.** We all have one, and you can tap into it, no matter what activity you choose. Jogging outside? Make it a game by spotting landmarks in the near distance, like trees or homes, and push yourself to pass them in a certain number of seconds. Swimming laps? Try to match the pace of the slightly faster swimmer in the next lane. Or keep track of the time it takes to swim ten laps, and try to beat your time. Even riding the recumbent bicycle at the gym can be turned into a competition by moving your workout to the spin studio, where you can privately compete against other class members for pace or intensity.

- **Practice the art of the con.** If you've ever overheard a pair of weight lifters in the gym, you'll recognize this tip. The spotter encourages the lifter, "One more, just one more!" and then after the lifter completes one more lift, the spotter again urges, "Now one more!" Make this tip work for you by learning how to self-con. Let's say you're too tired to work out. Tell yourself, *I'll just drive to the gym and park. If I'm still tired, I can leave.* This is often enough to kick-start your workout. And while swimming laps, tell yourself you'll just do five, then two more, then just three more.

- **Cultivate a mind-set of continuous improvement.** Tennis great Jimmy Connors once shared what keeps athletes motivated — "Getting better." Lifelong exercisers have a yearning to improve that acts as both a motivator and a goal.

- **Help yourself get better by educating yourself about your sport.** To do this, read books by or about professional athletes, read articles about them in magazines, newspapers, and online, and even book a private lesson to have your running gait/ golf swing/ basketball shot analyzed.

Also, offer yourself rewards for hitting

certain benchmarks. Treat yourself to a massage after your first three months of walking your dog nightly for thirty minutes, or book a trip to a luxury ski lodge to celebrate your first year of skiing. You earned it!

Robert Hopper, PhD, a Santa Barbara–based exercise physiologist and author of *Stick with Exercise for a Lifetime: How to Enjoy Every Minute of It!*

Test (and Fix!) Your Fitness for a Long, Healthy Life

We all know that exercise is good for us, but some ways of exercising are particularly effective, and they don't require time-consuming maneuvers or expensive equipment.

Are you out of breath after walking up a flight of stairs? Do you feel discomfort or pain when looking over your shoulder as you back up a car? Is it becoming difficult to reach the top shelves of closets? Or after having sat through a movie, do you feel pain or stiffness when you stand up? Any yes answer means that exercise would be especially beneficial for you.

To Increase Flexibility

Test: Put one arm over your shoulder, and reach behind your back. Then bring your other arm up behind your back, and try to touch the fingers of the hand that went over your shoulder.

Goal: To increase the flexibility of your arms, especially your shoulders.

Exercise: The test is also an exercise. Perform it several times a day, holding the stretch for thirty seconds, then reversing your arms. Soon, your fingers will easily touch. At that point, it's OK to reduce the frequency until you reach a level where you can consistently touch fingers.

648

Exercise for lower back and hamstring muscles: Sit toward the front of a chair with one leg stretched out straight with toes pulled toward you and the other leg bent to a right angle at the hip and knee. With one hand on top of the other, reach your hands toward the toes of the straight leg.

Important: If you have osteoporosis or have had an upper-back fracture, do not do this exercise.

For Better Posture

Test: Stand with your back as flush as possible against a wall and both heels touching it. When you're in that position, does your head easily touch the wall? If it doesn't, you could use some work on posture, which can be vital to overall physical health.

Goal: To improve posture as quickly as possible.

Exercise: Once or twice daily, sit in a supportive chair, chin tucked in toward your chest. Breathe in as you bend your elbows at your sides and close your fingers in a relaxed fist. Gently press your elbows back into the chair. Stay in that position for ten seconds as you continue to breathe deeply. Do not move. Breathe in again as you release the position slowly. Begin with three repetitions, and build to ten or twenty.

Once your head effortlessly touches a wall when you stand against it, you'll know that your posture has improved. At that point, reduce the number of times you perform the exercise.

By experimenting with the frequency of the exercise, you can determine how many times you need to do it in order to maintain good posture. Keep in mind, however, that as you age, the number of times required will nearly always increase slightly from year to year.

For More Strength

Test: In thirty seconds, how many times can you stand up from and sit down in a chair with your arms crossed on your chest?

Goal: Women between the ages of sixty and sixty-four should be able to stand and sit twelve to seventeen times in thirty seconds. Men of that age should be able to perform the task fifteen to twenty times. The benchmark drops slightly as your age increases.

Exercise: Perform the test two or three times a day until you can easily stand and sit within the benchmark range. Then do the exercise once every other day to keep in shape.

Also helpful: Unless you have problems with your hips and knees, walk up and down a flight of stairs two or three more times a day than you normally would.

To strengthen the arms, weighted dumbbells may be used. You should seek the guidance of a physical therapist before you start any weight training so that you perform the motions correctly and also use the correct amount of weight. An alternative to using weights is using elastic bands that can be cut into appropriate lengths for both arm and leg exercises. (See my book *Age-Defying Fitness* for many exercises with weights and elastic bands.)

Advantages of elastic bands: Unlike weights, there's no danger in dropping an elastic band when you exercise. Also, you can easily take an elastic strip with you when you travel. TheraBand strips, about six inches wide, are available from many retailers that sell exercise equipment and from distributors.

How to do it: Run the elastic band under the seat of an armless chair from side to side. Sit in the chair, and hold one end of the band in each hand. Then raise your arms high over your head, stretching the band as you do so and also breathing out. Cut the TheraBand strip to a length that lets you perform a set of eight to twelve stretches before tiring. Perform one or two sets of these exercises three times a week.

For Better Balance

Test: Cross your arms on your chest, then see how long you can stand on one leg. Then test the other leg.

Goal: To remain standing for at least thirty

seconds. If you can't, your balance needs improving.

Exercise: Hold on to the counter with one hand and stand on your toes. Then bend one knee back so that you're standing on your toes with one leg. After doing it only a few times, you may not need to hold on to the counter with your hand. Also try to rise up and down on your toes five to ten times while standing on one leg.

To Increase Endurance

Test: Assuming that you do not have any heart or lung problems, try to march in place for two minutes, bringing your knees about halfway up to the level of your hips. Count only the number of times you bring your right knee up.

Goal: In two minutes, women ages sixty to sixty-four should be able to bring up the right knee between 75 and 107 times. For men of that age, the benchmark is between 87 and 115 times.

Exercise: March in place several times a week, slowly increasing the number of steps you take in each two-minute period. Traditional exercises, such as walking, running, and bicycling, are also effective in building up endurance. Or use a treadmill or stationary bike. Whatever your choice of endurance exercise, you should gradually build up to thirty to forty-five minutes each session anywhere from three to seven days a week.

Getting Started

Note: If you're new to exercise, consult a physical therapist who will guide you through an appropriate exercise program. If you have heart, blood pressure, or lung problems, also consult your physician before starting the program. To find a physical therapist, contact the American Physical Therapy Association or your state's physical therapy association.

Marilyn Moffat, PhD, PT, a professor of physical therapy at New York University in New York City and a former president of the American Physical Therapy Association. She is coauthor of *Age-Defying Fitness*.

IF YOU'RE STARTING TO EXERCISE, EXPECT TO BE MISERABLE

We all know that exercise is perhaps the single most beneficial action we can take to protect our health. So why are two of every three American adults still sedentary — meaning they get little or no exercise?

Live Three Years Longer!

Most people who want to start exercising do so because it's good for them. But to stay motivated, you should know exactly why you want to start exercising.

For example, compared with people who exercise regularly, sedentary people are three times more likely to develop metabolic syndrome — a constellation of risk factors including high blood pressure (hypertension), elevated LDL "bad" cholesterol, high blood sugar, and obesity. Regular physical activity also has been found to reduce risk for cognitive decline.

And if that doesn't keep you motivated, consider this: People who regularly exercise briskly live an average of three years longer than those who are sedentary. "Briskly" means exercising at an intensity that makes you perspire and breathe a little heavily while still being able to carry on a conversation. This is known as the talk test.

How Much Exercise?

It's a common misconception that you must exercise daily to achieve significant health benefits.

In a study of ten thousand men and three thousand women conducted at the Cooper Aerobics Center's clinic, we found that walking just two miles in less than thirty minutes three days a week is all that's needed to achieve a moderate level of fitness, which lowers risk for all causes of death and disease.

For a less demanding workout that confers the same benefits, you could walk two miles in thirty-five minutes four days a week, or walk two miles in forty minutes five days a week. If you prefer other forms of exercise, such as biking or swimming, use these frequency guidelines, plus the talk test (described above) to achieve a moderate fitness level. By increasing the frequency and/or intensity, you'll achieve even greater health benefits.

Hit the Six-Week Mark

If you have not exercised regularly in the last six months and/or are overweight (for women, having a waist size of thirty-five inches or more; for men, forty inches or more), the basic exercise requirement described above may be too much. You may want to start by walking only to the end of the block for a few days, then gradually increase the distance.

Aim for an increase of up to 10 percent weekly — for example, from ten minutes per week to eleven minutes the next week and so on.

Helpful: Expect the first few weeks to be miserable — you'll feel some muscle soreness for a while. Accept it — but make the commitment to keep going.

Important: If your muscle pain doesn't go away within several weeks, see your doctor to rule out an underlying condition, such as arthritis.

We've found at the Cooper Aerobics Center that few people quit after they've performed a program of physical activity for six weeks. Once people reach the four to six-month mark, adherence to an exercise program approaches 100 percent for the long term.

Determine Your Baseline

If you've been sedentary, be sure to get a comprehensive medical checkup before starting an exercise program. This is particularly important for men age forty and older and women age fifty and older — cardiovascular disease risk rises at these ages.

People of any age with underlying health problems or a family history of diabetes, hypertension, high cholesterol, or heart disease also should get a checkup before starting to exercise.

Ask your doctor — or a fitness trainer — to

give you baseline measurements for strength, flexibility, and aerobic capacity, which will enable you to track future changes.

Checking these measurements (along with such markers as blood pressure, cholesterol, and blood sugar) again in about three months will give you tangible evidence of your progress and can motivate you to keep exercising.

Tyler C. Cooper, MD, MPH, a preventive medicine specialist at the Dallas-based Cooper Aerobics Center (CooperAerobics.com) and founder of Cooper Ventures, which helps people incorporate healthy living into every aspect of their lives. He is coauthor, with his father, Kenneth H. Cooper, MD, MPH, founder and chairman of Cooper Aerobics Center, of *Start Strong, Finish Strong*.

You Can Exercise Less and Be Just as Healthy

Do you struggle to fit the recommended amount of exercise into your busy schedule? Well, what if we told you that the amount of exercise needed to reap health benefits might be less than you think? Maybe you could free up some of your workout time for other activities that are important to you and beneficial to your health — like playing with your kids or grandkids, volunteering for a favorite charity, or cooking healthful meals.

The Latest in Exercise Research

A recent study published in the *Journal of the American College of Cardiology* found that people lived longest when they ran, on average, for thirty minutes or more, five days a week. Surprisingly, that research also showed that people who jogged at an easy pace for as little as five to ten minutes a day had virtually the same survival benefits as those who pushed themselves harder or longer.

Also surprising: A study recently done at Oregon State University found that one and two-minute bouts of activity that add up to thirty minutes or more per day, such as pacing while talking on the telephone, doing housework, or doing sit-ups during TV commercials, may reduce blood pressure and cholesterol and improve health as effectively as a structured exercise program.

How to Exercise Smarter, Not Harder

Here are four strategies to help you exercise more efficiently:

- **Recognize that some exercise is always better than none.** Even though exercise guidelines from the Centers for Disease Control and Prevention (CDC) call for at least 150 minutes of moderate exercise each week, you'll do well even at lower levels.

  A study in *The Lancet* found that people who walked for just fifteen minutes a day had a 14 percent reduction in death over an average of eight years. Good daily exercises include not only walking but working in the yard, swimming, riding a bike, etc.

  If you're among the multitudes of Americans who have been sedentary in recent years, you'll actually gain the most. Simply making the transition from horrible fitness to below average can reduce your overall risk for premature death by 20 to 40 percent.

- **Go for a run instead of a walk.** The intensity, or associated energy cost, of running is greater than walking. Therefore, running (or walking up a grade or incline) is better for the heart than walking — and it's easier to work into a busy day, because you can get equal benefits in less time.

  For cardiovascular health, a 5-minute run

(5.5 mph to 8 mph) is equal to a 15-minute walk (2 mph to 3.5 mph), and a 25-minute run equals a 105-minute walk.

A 2014 study of runners found that their risk of dying from heart disease was 45 percent lower than nonrunners over a fifteen-year follow-up. In fact, running can add, on average, three extra years to your life.

Caution: If you take running seriously, you should still limit your daily workouts to sixty minutes or less, no more than five days a week. (See below for the dangers of overdoing it.) People with heart symptoms or severely compromised heart function should avoid running. If you have joint problems, check with your doctor.

- **Ease into running.** Don't launch into a running program until you're used to exercise. Make it progressive. Start by walking slowly, say, at about 2 mph. Gradually increase it to 3 mph, then to 3.5 mph, etc. After two or three months, if you are symptom-free during fast walking, you can start to run (slowly at first).

- **Aim for the "upper-middle."** I do not recommend high-intensity workouts for most adults. Strive to exercise at a level you would rate between "fairly light" and "somewhat hard."

How to tell: Check your breathing. It will be slightly labored when you're at a good level of exertion. Nevertheless, you should still be able to carry on a conversation.

Important: Get your doctor's OK before starting vigorous exercise, and don't ignore potential warning symptoms. It's normal to be somewhat winded or to have a little leg discomfort. However, you should never feel dizzy, experience chest pain, or have extreme shortness of breath. If you have any of these symptoms, stop exercise immediately, and see your doctor before resuming activity.

Too Much of a Good Thing?

Most people who run for more than an hour a day, five days a week, are in very good shape. Would they be healthier if they doubled the distance or pushed themselves even harder? Not necessarily. Risks linked to distance running include:

- **Acute right-heart overload.** Researchers at William Beaumont Hospital who looked at distance runners before and immediately after marathon running found that they often had transient decreases in the pumping ability of the right ventricle and elevations of the same enzymes (such as troponin) that increase during a heart attack.
- **Atrial fibrillation.** People who exercise intensely for more than five hours a week may be more likely to develop atrial fibrilla-

tion, a heart-rhythm disturbance that can trigger a stroke.

- **Coronary plaque.** Despite their favorable coronary risk factor profiles, distance runners can have increased amounts of coronary artery calcium and plaque as compared with their less active counterparts.

Watch out: Many hardcore runners love marathons, triathlons, and other competitive events. Be careful. The emotional rush from competition increases levels of epinephrine and other stress hormones. These hormones, combined with hard exertion, can transiently increase heart risks.

Of course, all this doesn't mean that you shouldn't enjoy a daily run or a few long ones — just don't overdo it!

Barry A. Franklin, PhD, director of cardiac rehabilitation at William Beaumont Hospital in Royal Oak, Michigan. He is also coauthor, with Joseph C. Piscatella, of *109 Things You Can Do to Prevent, Halt & Reverse Heart Disease.*

STRENGTH TRAINING FOR BEGINNERS — NO GYM NEEDED

Strength training not only builds muscles, it also improves bone density, speeds up metabolism, promotes balance, and even boosts brain power. You'll also gain mobility, says Cedric X. Bryant, PhD, chief science officer at the American Council on Exercise, who designed the workout below. Translation: this routine will help make everyday movements — such as getting in and out of a car, reaching overhead, bending, and climbing stairs — much easier for you.

And not to worry — you won't be straining under heavy barbells. All the exercises below use just your own body weight or a simple elastic tube for resistance.

Recommended: Opt for a light-resistance tube with handles, available at sporting goods stores and online.

What to do: Get your doctor's OK first, as you should before beginning any new exercise routine. Perform eight to fifteen reps of each of the following moves two to three times per week on nonconsecutive days — muscles need a day between workouts to repair and strengthen, Dr. Bryant notes. Always move in a slow, controlled fashion, without jerking or using momentum. When you can easily do fifteen reps of a particular exercise, advance to the "To progress" variation.

No-Equipment-Needed Exercises

• **Wall squat** — for legs and buttocks.

Start: Stand with head and back against a wall, arms at sides, legs straight, feet hip-width apart and about eighteen inches from wall.

Move: Keeping head and torso upright and your back firmly pressed against the wall, bend knees and slide down the wall about four to eight inches. Knees should be aligned above ankles — do not allow knees to extend past toes. Hold for several seconds. Then, using thigh and buttock muscles, straighten legs and slide back up wall to the start position. Repeat.

To progress: Bend knees more, ideally to a 90° angle so thighs are parallel to floor, as if sitting in a chair.

• **Wall push-up** — for chest, shoulders, and triceps.

Start: Stand facing a wall, feet hip-width apart and about eighteen inches from wall. Place hands on wall at shoulder height, slightly wider than shoulder-width apart.

Move: Tighten abdominal muscles to brace your midsection, keeping spine and legs straight throughout. Slowly bend elbows, bringing face as close to wall as you can. Hold for one second, then straighten arms and return to the start position. Repeat.

To progress: Start with feet farther from wall, and bring face closer to wall during push-up.

- **Supine reverse march** — for abdominals, lower back, and hips.

    Start: Lie face up, knees bent, feet flat on floor, arms out to sides in a T position, palms up, abs contracted.

    Move: Slowly lift left foot off floor, keeping leg bent. Bring knee up and somewhat closer to torso. When left thigh is vertical to floor, stop moving and hold for five to ten seconds. Then slowly lower leg and return foot to floor. Repeat. Switch legs.

    To progress: As knee moves upward, raise both arms toward ceiling. Lower arms as leg lowers.

Moves With Tubes

- **Seated row** — for back, abs, and biceps.

    Start: Sit on floor, torso upright, legs out in front of you, knees slightly bent, feet together. Place center of elastic resistance tube across soles of feet and hold tube handles in hands, arms extended in front of you, elbows straight.

    Move: Bending elbows, slowly pull handles of tube toward chest (do not lean backward, arch back, shrug shoulders, or bend wrists). Hold for several seconds, then slowly straighten arms and return to the start position. Repeat.

To progress: To increase resistance, rather than placing center of tube across soles of feet, anchor it firmly around an immovable object one to three feet in front of you.

- **Lateral raise** — for shoulders.

Start: Stand with feet hip-width apart, anchoring center of elastic resistance tube under both feet. Hold tube handles in hands, arms down at sides.

Move: Keeping elbows very slightly bent and wrists straight, slowly lift arms out to sides so palms face floor and hands reach shoulder height (or as high as you can get them). Lower arms to the start position. Repeat.

To progress: To increase resistance, widen your stance on the tubing.

Cedric X. Bryant, PhD, the chief science officer for the American Council on Exercise. He has written more than 250 articles and columns in fitness magazines and exercise science journals and is author or coauthor of more than thirty books, including *Strength Training for Women.* AceFitness.org, twitter.com/DrCedricBryant.

TAKE THE STAIRS!

Until recently, fitness gurus have advised people to take the stairs mainly as a substitute for do-nothing elevator rides.

Now: Stair-climbing is becoming increasingly popular as a workout that's readily accessible (stairs are everywhere), often climate-controlled (indoor stairs), and free.

It burns more calories than walking, strengthens every muscle in the legs, and is good for your bones as well as your cardiovascular system. It may even extend your life span.

Compelling research: A study found that participants who averaged eight flights of stairs a day had a death rate over a sixteen-year period that was about one-third lower than those who didn't exercise and more than 20 percent lower than that of people who merely walked.

A Concentrated Climb

Walking is mainly a horizontal movement, with an assist from forward momentum. Stair-climbing is a vertical exercise. Your body weight is lifted straight up, against gravity. Climbing stairs also involves more muscles — in the calves, buttocks, and the fronts and backs of the thighs — than walking. Even the arms get a workout. Canadian researchers found that it required double the exertion of walking on level ground and 50 percent more than walking up an incline.

As a weight-loss tool, stair-climbing is hard to beat. An hour of climbing (for a 160-pound person) will burn about 650 calories. That compares with 400 calories an hour for a fifteen-minute-mile power walk and 204 calories for a leisurely stroll.

It's Easy to Start

Inconvenience is one of the biggest barriers to exercise. It sometimes feels like a hassle to change into workout clothes and drive to a health club or even exercise at home. But you can always find a set of stairs — in your neighborhood, at work, at the mall, or at home.

You don't need fancy workout gear to climb stairs (uncarpeted stairs are preferred). Because it doesn't involve side to side movements, you don't necessarily need to invest in specialized shoes. You can do it in any pair of athletic shoes or even work shoes, as long as they don't have high heels.

How to Climb

When getting started, begin with a single flight of stairs. When that feels easy, take additional flights or increase the intensity by going a little faster. Work up to five minutes, then slowly increase that to ten, fifteen and twenty minutes, if possible, three times a week. Here are some other tips:

668

- **Keep your upper body straight.** There's a natural tendency to lean forward when you climb stairs, particularly because a forward-leaning position feels easier. Remind yourself to stand straight when you're climbing and descending. It will give your legs a better workout, strengthen your abdominal and other core muscles, and help improve your balance.
- **Swing your arms.** You don't need an exaggerated swing, but keep your arms moving — it helps with balance and provides exercise for your arms and shoulders. You'll often see stair-climbers with their hands or arms on the rails. It's OK to use the rails if you need the support, but it reduces the intensity of the exercise. It also causes the stooped posture that you want to avoid.
- **One step at a time.** Unless you're a competitive stair-climber, you'll probably do best by taking just one step at a time. Ascending stairs is a concentric exercise that increases muscle power; it's also the part of the workout that gives most of the cardiovascular benefit. Coming down the stairs is an eccentric (also called negative) movement that puts more stress on the muscles and increases strength.

  Important: Descend the stairs slowly, and keep jolts to a minimum. It sounds counterintuitive, but the descents cause more muscle soreness than the climbs.

You can take two steps at a time on the ascent if your balance is good and you're bored with single-step plodding. The faster pace will increase the intensity of your workout, particularly when you give your arms a more exaggerated swing. To minimize jolt and maximize safety, however, stick to single steps on the descent.

To End Your Workout

The "Figure 4 Stretch" is a great way to conclude a stair-climbing workout. It stretches the calves, hamstrings, gluteals, low back, and upper back.

What to do: While sitting on the floor with your right leg straight, bend your left leg so that your left foot touches your right thigh, making a *4.* Slowly reach your right hand toward your right foot. Then grasp your foot, ankle, or lower leg, and hold for twenty seconds. Repeat on the other side.

Caution: Stair-climbing should be avoided if you have serious arthritis or other joint problems. It's less jarring than jogging, but it's still a weight-bearing exercise that can stress the joints. People with joint issues might do better with supported exercises, such as cycling, rowing, or swimming.

Before taking up stair-climbing as a form of exercise, check with your doctor if you're middle-aged or older, have arthritis or a history of heart or lung disease, or if you've been mainly sedentary and aren't confident of your muscle strength — or your sense of balance.

Stair-Stepping Without a Staircase

If you want to climb stairs without using a staircase, consider buying a commercial stepper, such as those from StairMaster. Some have components that work the arms as well as the legs. Stair-steppers, however, don't provide the benefit of actual stair-climbing, which uses more muscles because of the descent. These machines can be costly (at least $2,500 for a new one but much less for a used one on Craigslist or eBay). They typically hold up for years of hard use.

Caution: I don't recommend mini-steppers that sell for as little as fifty dollars. They have hydraulics, bands, or other systems that cause the steps to go up and down, but the equipment usually breaks quickly.

Wayne L. Westcott, PhD, a professor of exercise science at Quincy College in Quincy, Massachusetts, and a strength-training consultant for the American Council on Exercise and the American Senior Fitness Association. He is also coauthor of several books, including *Strength Training Past 50.*

SEVEN MISTAKES THAT CAN SABOTAGE YOUR WALKING WORKOUT

We all know that walking is very good for us. Studies have shown that walking promotes heart health, strengthens bones, spurs weight loss, boosts mood, and even cuts risk for diabetes, cancer, and Alzheimer's.

But what most people don't realize is that they could significantly improve the health benefits of their walks by tweaking their walking techniques and using the right equipment.

Here are common walking mistakes — and what you should be doing instead.

Mistake #1: **Tilting forward.** Some walkers tilt their upper bodies forward, as though they're walking into the wind. They think that this position increases speed. It does not — and it greatly increases pressure on the lower back while straining the shins.

Better: Walk with your head high and still, shoulders relaxed, and chest slightly out. In this position, you can rotate your eyes downward to survey the path and look ahead to view the scenery around you.

Mistake #2: **Swinging the arms inefficiently.** Many walkers waste energy by swinging their arms side to side or pumping their arms up and down. These exaggerated movements add little to cardiovascular fitness and make walking less efficient, because arm

672

energy is directed upward or sideways rather than straight ahead.

Better: For maximum efficiency, pump your arms straight ahead on a horizontal plane, like you're reeling in a string through your midsection. This motion improves balance, posture, and walking speed.

Mistake #3: **Using hand and/or ankle weights.** While some people like to walk with weights to boost the intensity of a walking workout, the risk for injury far outweighs the benefits of using weights. The repetitive stress of swinging weights can cause microtears in the soft tissues of the arms and legs.

Better: To increase exertion, walk uphill or on an inclined treadmill.

Another good option: Try Nordic walking for a total-body workout. With this type of walking, you use specially designed walking poles (one in each hand) to help propel your body forward.

Compared with regular walking, Nordic walking can increase your energy expenditure by 20 percent, according to a study from the Cooper Institute. It works the abdominal, arm, and back muscles and reduces stress on the feet, ankles, knees, and hips while improving endurance.

Mistake #4: **Not doing a warm-up.** You're inviting muscle soreness and potential injury if you hit your top speed at the start.

Better: Be sure to warm up. Start slowly, accelerating over the first five to ten minutes, and end slowly, decelerating over the last five minutes. A slow start allows your muscles to warm up and become flexible, while enabling your cardiorespiratory system to get used to higher workloads. A proper cooldown helps eliminate the buildup of lactic acid, which can lead to muscle soreness.

Mistake #5: **Doing the same walk every day.** It's best to alter your routine for maximum health benefits and to maintain motivation.

Better: Do shorter, faster-paced walks some days (cardiovascular conditioning) and longer, moderate-paced walks on other days (calorie burning). Also try walks on steeper terrains and walks that alternate faster intervals with slower intervals.

Mistake #6: **Not keeping a walking log or journal.** Every day, indicate how far and fast you walked and any other observations you wish to record in a notebook or on your computer. Keeping a journal helps foster a sense of accomplishment and self-esteem and is the single most effective method for ensuring that you'll stick to a walking program.

Mistake #7: **Choosing cushy shoes.** A study in the *American Journal of Sports Medicine* found that, on average, expensive, high-tech footwear caused twice the injuries as shoes costing half as much.

Some high-priced, cushiony shoes can make you feel as if you're walking on a foam mattress, but they have an inherent wobble that can cause your foot to move side to side, leading to potential foot, ankle, knee, and hip injuries.

What to do: In addition to walking regularly, start a core-muscle strengthening regimen and a stretching program to tone your hip and leg muscles.

Robert Sweetgall, president of Creative Walking, a McCall, Idaho, company that designs walking and fitness programs for schools, corporations, and other clients. He is the only person to have walked through all fifty states in 365 days, and he has walked/run across the United States seven times. Sweetgall is coauthor, with Barry Franklin, PhD, of *One Heart, Two Feet: Enhancing Heart Health One Step at a Time.* CreativeWalking.com.

WIN THE INNER GAME OF STRESS

Stress creates unproductive panic, inhibits creative thought, contributes to chronic illness, and is just plain exhausting. But no matter what's going on in our lives, we can tap into our inner resources to keep stress from doing its damage.

Different strategies work for different people. Below are some of the most effective ones.

The Inner Game

We all are playing an inner game whether we recognize it or not. That means that while we are all involved in outer games (overcoming obstacles in the outside world to reach our goals), we are at the same time faced with inner obstacles, such as fear, self-doubt, frustration, pain, and distractions. These inner obstacles prevent us from expressing our full range of capabilities and enjoying our time to the utmost.

The secret lies in knowing that you have choices about how you look at external events, how you define them, how you attribute meaning to them, and how you react to them mentally and emotionally. The key is to recognize that every person has the internal wisdom to bypass the frustrations and fears that pull them into the negative cycle of stress.

Become Your Own CEO

Feeling powerless and victimized is among the most common sources of stress. You're likely to feel more in control if you consider yourself the CEO of your life. To do so:

- **Write a mission statement.** What is the primary mission of your life?

   Examples: To create prosperity for myself and my family, to pay attention to my inner life as well as my achievements, to help others in my work or personal life.

- **Identify your main product or service.** What do you provide to others? These could be specific to a particular business or profession.

   Example: As a doctor, my services would include being up-to-date in my knowledge, knowing the best specialists to refer a patient to, seeing patients quickly.

- **List your company's resources.** Include both internal resources — positive personal traits, such as your compassion, intelligence, and humor — and external resources — your financial assets, friends, and possessions. Ask yourself whether you are getting as much from each of these resources as you could.

Lost Control?

Consider whether you have given up too much control of your corporation. What would it cost to buy back some of your shares?

Example: Did you sell too many shares of yourself for your big home? If massive mortgage payments fill you with stress — or force you to remain in a job that fills you with stress — perhaps you should move into a smaller home and take back those shares.

This CEO thought process serves as a reminder that we are not helpless. Your life is yours, and you get to decide everything. It is always your choice, even if you decide to comply with the wishes of someone else. Once you become aware of the limits that you place on your choices, your freedom will evolve, and your stress will ease.

Regaining Control

Trying to control things that are outside our control is enormously stressful — yet many of us unwittingly do this. When you feel stressed, consider:

What don't I control here?

What am I trying to control here?

What could I control here that I'm not currently controlling?

Confronting these questions can help us focus on things that we can accomplish and reduce our stress over things that we cannot.

Example: When a man who is stressed over his wife's poor health asks himself these questions, he realizes that her health is not something that he can control, so he should stop trying to. What he can control is his attitude toward life. By remaining upbeat, he can help his wife remain upbeat.

The Magic Pen

Select a stress-causing situation in your life, then write down your usual inner dialog on this subject. Once you have written everything that comes to mind, take out a new piece of paper, and imagine that your pen has been magically endowed with one of your positive inner resources. This resource might be your clarity, compassion, candor, serenity, or patience — any trait that you consider a personal strength. Try to empty your mind of all thought, then let your magic pen write a message to you about this stressful subject. Don't censor the pen — let it write everything.

Example: A man feels guilty about his grown son, who can't find direction in life. If he endowed his pen with his compassion, the pen might write that he did his best to raise his son and that his son is doing his best to live his life.

John Horton, MD, a physician specializing in preventive medicine and stress, Westlake Village, California. He is coauthor, with sports psychologist W. Timothy Gallwey and stress expert Edd Hanzelik, MD, of *The Inner Game of Stress: Outsmart Life's Challenges and Fulfill Your Potential.*

YOGA CAN CHANGE YOUR LIFE!

Not that long ago, yoga was viewed primarily as an activity for "youngish" health nuts who wanted to round out their exercise regimens.

Now: Older adults — meaning people in their sixties, seventies, eighties, and beyond — are among the most enthusiastic practitioners of this ancient healing system of exercise and controlled breathing.

Yoga Goes Mainstream

Virtually everyone can benefit from yoga. Unfortunately, many people are reluctant to try it because they assume that it's too unconventional and requires extreme flexibility. Neither belief is true.

What's more, its varied health benefits are largely what's making the practice so popular now with older adults. More than one thousand scientific studies have shown that yoga can improve conditions ranging from arthritis, asthma, insomnia, and depression to heart disease, diabetes, and cancer.

You look better too: Yoga is quite useful in helping to prevent rounding (or hunching) of the back, which occurs so often in older adults. This condition can lead to back pain and breathing problems as the rib cage presses against the lungs.

My experience: After teaching yoga to thousands of students, I'm continually amazed at how many tell me that it has literally changed their lives by helping them feel so much better physically and mentally.

Getting Started

If you want to see whether you could benefit from yoga, ask your doctor about trying the following poses, which address common physical complaints. These poses are a good first step before taking a yoga class.* Yoga is best performed in loose, comfortable clothing and in your bare feet, so your feet won't slip. Try these poses:

- **Knees to chest pose.** For low back pain and painful, tight hips.

  What to do: Lie on your back (on carpet or a yoga mat, available at sports-equipment stores for about twenty-five dollars). With your arms, hug both knees in to your chest. Keep your knees together and your elbows pointing out to each side of your body. Slowly rock from elbow to elbow to massage your back and shoulders. Take deep, abdominal breaths while holding your thighs close to your chest, and hold for six complete inhales and exhales.

- **Mecca pose.** This pose also relieves back pain.

* To find a yoga class near you, check your local community center and/or consult the International Association of Yoga Therapists (www.iayt.org).

682

What to do: Begin by kneeling on the floor with your knees together. For added comfort, place a small towel behind your knees. Sit back on your feet, and lean forward from your waist so that your chest and stomach rest atop your thighs. Reach your arms out in front of you, resting your forehead to the floor while stretching your tailbone to your heels. Hold for six complete inhales and exhales.

• **Leg rotation.** For sciatica, a cause of back, pelvic, and leg pain.

What to do: Lie on your back with both legs extended. Slowly bring your right knee to your chest and inhale. Rest your right ankle on the front of your left thigh, and exhale as you slowly slide it down along your left knee, shin, and ankle to toes. This helps "screw" the top of your right thighbone into the hip socket, easing lower back and leg pain. Repeat on other side. Do three times on each side.

To conclude your session: While in a sitting position, press your palms together. Bring your thumbs into your breastbone. Tuck your elbows in and down, and press your breastbone to your thumbs, lifting and opening your chest. Hold for six breaths.

Important: Even when you're not doing yoga, don't forget your breath. Slow, thoughtful, deep breathing is most effective, but don't perform it too quickly. I find the technique to be most effective when you hold the inhalation and exhalation for a certain number of counts.

What to do: Lie on your back, resting your hands on your belly so that your middle fingers touch across your navel. Inhale through your nose for a count of six, pushing your navel out so that your finger-tips separate. Pause, then exhale for a count of nine, pulling your navel back in. Perform these steps two more times (more may make you dizzy). Do this in the morning and at night (deep breathing improves mental focus and can be energizing in the morning and calming at night).

Mary Louise Stefanic, a certified yoga and qigong instructor with a focus on therapeutic yoga. Ms. Stefanic is a staff member at the Loyola Center for Fitness and Loyola University Health System, both in Maywood, Illinois. She has been teaching yoga since 1969.

DANGERS OF SLEEP APNEA

Doctors have long known that obstructive sleep apnea (repeated interruptions in breathing during sleep) can harm the overall health of men and women who suffer from the condition.

Now: Recent research shows that sleep apnea is even more dangerous than experts had previously realized, increasing the sufferer's risk for heart attack, stroke, diabetes, and fatal car crashes.

No Room to Breathe

Sleep apnea occurs about twice as often in men as in women, but it is overlooked more often in women. An estimated 70 percent of people with sleep apnea are overweight. Fat deposited around the neck (men with sleep apnea often wear a size seventeen or larger collar, while women with the disorder often have a neck circumference of sixteen inches or more) compresses the upper airway, reducing air flow and causing the passage to narrow or close. Your brain senses this inability to breathe and briefly awakens you so that you can reopen the airway.

The exact cause of obstructive sleep apnea in people of normal weight is unknown, but it may involve various anatomical characteristics, such as having a narrow throat and upper airway.

Red flag #1: About half of all people who snore loudly have sleep apnea. One telling sign is a gasping, choking kind of snore, during which the sleeper seems to stop breathing. (If you live alone and don't know whether you snore, ask your doctor about recording yourself while you are sleeping to check for snoring and other signs of sleep apnea.)

Red flag #2: Daytime sleepiness is the other most common symptom. Less common symptoms include headache, sore throat and/or dry mouth in the morning, sexual dysfunction, and memory problems.

Dangers of Sleep Apnea

New scientific evidence shows that sleep apnea increases risk for the following:

• **Cardiovascular disease.** Sleep apnea's repeated episodes of interrupted breathing — and the accompanying drop in oxygen levels — takes a toll on the heart and arteries.

   Recent finding: Heart attack risk in sleep apnea sufferers is 30 percent higher than normal over a four- to five-year period, and stroke risk is twice as high in people with sleep apnea.

- **Diabetes.** Sleep apnea (regardless of the sufferer's weight) is linked to increased insulin resistance — a potentially dangerous condition in which the body is resistant to the effects of insulin.

    Recent finding: A Yale study of 593 patients found that over a six-year period, people diagnosed with sleep apnea were more than two and a half times more likely to develop diabetes than those without the sleep disorder.

- **Accidents.** Sleep apnea dramatically increases the risk for a deadly mishap due to sleepiness and impaired alertness.

    Recent finding: A study of sixteen hundred people, presented at an American Thoracic Society meeting, found that the eight hundred sleep apnea sufferers were twice as likely to have a car crash over a three-year period. Surprisingly, those who were unaware of being sleepy were just as likely to crash as those who were aware of being sleepy.

Do You Have Sleep Apnea?

If you think you may have sleep apnea, see a specialist at an accredited sleep center, where a thorough medical history will be taken and you may be asked to undergo a sleep study. This involves spending the night in a sleep laboratory where your breathing, oxygen level, movements, and brain wave activity are measured while you sleep.

Best Treatment Options

The treatment typically prescribed first for sleep apnea is continuous positive airway pressure (CPAP). A stream of air is pumped onto the back of the throat during sleep to keep the airway open. The air is supplied through a mask, most often worn over the nose, which is connected by tubing to a small box that contains a fan.

In recent years, a larger variety of masks have become available, and fan units have become smaller and nearly silent. A number of adjustments may be needed, which may require trying several different devices and more than one visit to a sleep lab.

Other treatments for sleep apnea are usually prescribed to make CPAP more effective, or for people with milder degrees of the disorder who have tried CPAP but were unable or unwilling to use it.

These treatments include:

- **Mouthpieces.** Generally fitted by a dentist and worn at night, these oral appliances adjust the lower jaw and tongue to help keep the airway open.
- **Surgery.** This may be recommended for people who have an anatomical abnormal-

ity that narrows the airway and for whom CPAP doesn't work. The most common operation for sleep apnea is uvulo-palatopharyngoplasty (UPPP), in which excess tissue is removed from the back of the throat. It works about 50 percent of the time.

Helping Yourself

Several measures can make sleep apnea treatment more effective and, in some cases, eliminate the condition altogether. Try these suggestions:

- **Lose weight, if you are overweight.** For every 10 percent of body weight lost, the number of apnea episodes drops by 25 percent.
- **Change your sleep position.** Sleeping on your side — rather than on your back — typically means fewer apnea episodes. Sleeping on your stomach is even better. Some obese people who have sleep apnea do best if they sleep while sitting up.
- **Avoid alcohol.** It relaxes the muscles around the airway, aggravating sleep apnea.
- **Use medication carefully.** Sleep medications can worsen sleep apnea by making it harder for your body to rouse itself when breathing stops. If you have sleep apnea,

make sure a doctor oversees your use of sleep medications (including over-the-counter drugs).

Ralph Downey III, PhD, D, ABSM, adjunct associate clinical professor of medicine and past chief, sleep medicine, Loma Linda University Medical Center, Loma Linda University Children's Hospital.

SLEEP SOUNDLY: SAFE, NATURAL INSOMNIA SOLUTIONS

A good night's sleep. There's nothing more restorative — or elusive — for the 64 percent of Americans who report regularly having trouble sleeping. Poor-quality sleep may even be secretly sabotaging your blood sugar. A disconcertingly high percentage of the sleepless (nearly 20 percent) solve the problem by taking sleeping pills. But sleeping pills can be dangerously addictive, physically and/or emotionally — and swallowing a pill when you want to go to sleep doesn't address the root cause of the problem. What, exactly, is keeping you up at night?

Slow Down

According to Rubin Naiman, PhD, a psychologist and clinical assistant professor of medicine at the University of Arizona's Center for Integrative Medicine, most of our sleep problems have to do not with our bodies, per se, but with our habits. The modern American lifestyle — replete with highly refined foods and caffeine-laden beverages, excessive exposure to artificial light in the evening, and "adrenaline-producing" nighttime activities, such as working until bedtime, watching TV, or surfing the Web — leaves us overstimulated in the evening just when our bodies are designed to slow down and, importantly, to literally cool down as well.

Studies show that a cooler core body temperature — and warmer hands and feet — make you sleepy. "Cooling the body allows the mind and the heart to get quiet," says Dr. Naiman. He believes that this cooling process contributes to the release of melatonin, the hormone that helps to regulate the body's circadian rhythm of sleeping and waking.

Deep Green Sleep

Dr. Naiman has developed an integrative approach to sleep that defines healthy sleep as an interaction between a person and his/her sleep environment. He calls this approach Deep Green Sleep. "My goal was to explore all of the subtleties in a person's life that may be disrupting sleep. This takes into account your physiology, emotions, personal experiences, sleeping and waking patterns, and your attitudes about sleep and the sleeping environment." This approach is unique because it values "the subjective and personal experience of sleep," he says — in contrast with conventional sleep treatment, which tends to rely on "computer printouts of sleep studies — otherwise known as 'treating the chart.' "

It's important to realize that lifestyle habits and attitudes are hard to change, so Dr. Naiman cautions that it often can take weeks, even months, to achieve his Deep Green

Sleep. The good news is that the results are lasting and may even enhance your waking life.

Here are his suggestions on how you can ease into the night:

- **Live a healthful waking life.** "The secret of a good night's sleep is a good day's waking," says Dr. Naiman. This includes getting regular exercise (but not within three hours of bedtime) and eating a balanced, nutritious diet.
- **Cool down in the evening.** It's important to help your mind and body cool down, starting several hours before bedtime, by doing the following:
  - ▶ **Avoid foods and drinks that sharply spike energy,** such as highly refined carbohydrates and anything with caffeine, at least eight hours before bedtime.
  - ▶ **Limit alcohol in the evening** — it interferes with sleep by suppressing melatonin. It also interferes with dreaming and disrupts circadian rhythms.
  - ▶ **Avoid nighttime screen-based activities within an hour of bedtime.** You may think that watching TV or surfing the Web are relaxing things to do, but in reality, these activities are highly stimulating. They engage your brain and expose you to relatively bright light with a strong blue wavelength that "mimics daylight

and suppresses melatonin," says Dr. Naiman.

- **Create a sound sleeping environment.** It is also important that where you sleep be stimulation-free and conducive to rest.

In Your Bedroom

- **Be sure that you have a comfortable mattress, pillow, and bedding.** It's amazing how many people fail to address this basic need — often because their mattress has become worn out slowly, over time, and they haven't noticed.
- **Remove anything unessential from your bedside table** that may tempt you to stay awake, such as the TV remote control or stimulating books.
- **When you are ready to call it a night, turn everything off** — radio, TV, and, of course, the light.
- **Keep the room cool** — 68°F or lower.
- **Let go of waking.** Each day, allow your mind and body to surrender to sleep by engaging in quieting and relaxing activities starting about an hour before bedtime, such as:
  - ▶ Gentle yoga
  - ▶ Meditation
  - ▶ Rhythmic breathing
  - ▶ Reading poetry or other nonstimulating material

▶ Journaling
▶ Taking a hot bath

- **Sex seems to help most people relax and can facilitate sleep,** in part because climaxing triggers a powerful relaxation response, Dr. Naiman says.
- **Consider supplementing with melatonin.** If sleep is still elusive after trying these Deep Green Sleep tips, Dr. Naiman often suggests a melatonin supplement. Dr. Naiman believes that this is better than sleeping pills since melatonin is "the body's own natural chemical messenger of night." "Melatonin does not directly cause sleep but triggers a cascade of events that result in natural sleep and dreams," he says, adding that it is nonaddictive, inexpensive, and generally safe. Not all doctors agree, however, so it is important to check with your doctor first.

Rubin Naiman, PhD, psychologist specializing in sleep and dream medicine and clinical assistant professor of medicine at the University of Arizona's Center for Integrative Medicine. He is author of the book *Healing Night* and coauthor with Dr. Andrew Weil of the audiobook *Healthy Sleep.*

GOOD ORAL HEALTH LOWERS RISK FOR DIABETES AND MORE

Until recently, most people who took good care of their teeth and gums did so to ensure appealing smiles and to perhaps avoid dentures. Now, a significant body of research shows that oral health may play a key role in preventing a wide range of serious health conditions, including heart disease, diabetes, some types of cancer, and perhaps even dementia.

Healthy teeth and gums may also improve longevity. Swedish scientists recently tracked 3,273 adults for sixteen years and found that those with chronic gum infections were significantly more likely to die before age fifty, on average, than were people without gum disease.

What's the connection? Periodontal disease (called gingivitis in mild stages and periodontitis when it becomes more severe) is caused mainly by bacteria that accumulate on the teeth and gums. As the body attempts to battle the bacteria, inflammatory molecules are released (as demonstrated by redness and swelling of the gums). Over time, this complex biological response affects the entire body, causing systemic inflammation that promotes the development of many serious diseases. Scientific evidence links poor oral health to the following conditions:

- **Diabetes.** State University of New York at Buffalo studies and other research show that people with diabetes have an associated risk for periodontitis that is two to three times greater than that of people without diabetes. Conversely, diabetics with periodontal disease generally have poorer control of their blood sugar than diabetics without periodontal disease — a factor that contributes to their having twice the risk of dying of a heart attack and three times the risk of dying of kidney failure.
- **Heart disease.** At least twenty scientific studies have shown links between chronic periodontal disease and an increased risk for heart disease. Most recently, Boston University researchers found that periodontal disease in men younger than age sixty was associated with a twofold increase in angina (chest pain), or nonfatal or fatal heart attack, when compared with men whose teeth and gums are healthy.
- **Cancer.** Chronic gum disease may raise your risk for tongue cancer. State University of New York at Buffalo researchers recently compared men with and without tongue cancer and found that those with cancer had a 65 percent greater loss of alveolar bone (which supports the teeth) — a common measure of periodontitis. Meanwhile,

a Harvard School of Public Health study shows that periodontal disease is associated with a 63 percent higher risk for pancreatic cancer.

- **Rheumatoid arthritis.** In people with rheumatoid arthritis, the condition is linked to an 82 percent increased risk for periodontal disease, compared with people who do not have rheumatoid arthritis.

  Good news: Treating the periodontitis appears to ease rheumatoid arthritis symptoms. In a recent study, nearly 59 percent of patients with rheumatoid arthritis and chronic periodontal disease who had their gums treated experienced less severe arthritis symptoms — possibly because eliminating the periodontitis reduced their systemic inflammation.

- **Dementia.** When Swedish researchers recently reviewed dental and cognitive records for 638 women, they found that tooth loss (a sign of severe gum disease) was linked to a 30 to 40 percent increased risk for dementia over a thirty-two-year period, with the highest dementia rates suffered by women who had the fewest teeth at middle age. More research is needed to confirm and explain this link.

Steps to Improve Your Oral Health

Even though the rate of gum disease significantly increases with age, it's not inevitable. To promote oral health, brush (twice daily with a soft-bristled brush, using gentle, short strokes starting at a forty-five-degree angle to the gums) and floss (once daily, using gentle rubbing motions — do not snap against the gums). In addition:

- **See your dentist at least twice yearly.** Ask at every exam, "Do I have gum disease?" This will serve as a gentle reminder to dentists that you want to be carefully screened for the condition. Most mild to moderate infections can be treated with a nonsurgical procedure that removes plaque and tartar from tooth pockets and smooths the root surfaces. For more severe periodontal disease, your dentist may refer you to a periodontist (a dentist who specializes in the treatment of gum disease).

  Note: Patients with gum disease often need to see a dentist three to four times a year to prevent recurrence of gum disease after the initial treatment.

  Good news: Modern techniques to regenerate bone and soft tissue can reverse much of the damage and halt progression of periodontitis, particularly in patients who have lost no more than 30 percent of the bone to which the teeth are attached.

- **Boost your calcium intake.** Research conducted at the State University of New York at Buffalo has shown that postmenopausal women with osteoporosis typically have more alveolar bone loss and weaker attachments between their teeth and bone, putting them at substantially higher risk for periodontal disease. Other studies have linked low dietary calcium with heightened periodontal risk in both men and women.

  Self-defense: Postmenopausal women and men over age sixty-five should consume 1,000 to 1,200 mg of calcium daily to preserve teeth and bones. Aim for two to three daily servings of dairy products (providing a total of 600 mg of calcium), plus a 600mg calcium supplement with added vitamin D for maximum absorption.

  Helpful: Yogurt may offer an edge over other calcium sources. In a recent Japanese study involving 942 adults, ages forty to seventy-nine, those who ate at least 55 g (about two ounces) of yogurt daily were 40 percent less likely to suffer from severe periodontal disease — perhaps because the "friendly" bacteria and calcium in yogurt make a powerful combination against the infection-causing bacteria of dental disease.

- **Control your weight.** Obesity is also associated with periodontitis, probably because fat cells release chemicals that may contribute to inflammatory conditions anywhere in the body, including the gums.
- **Don't ignore dry mouth.** Aging and many medications, including some antidepressants, antihistamines, high blood pressure drugs, and steroids, can decrease saliva flow, allowing plaque to build up on teeth and gums. If you're taking a drug that leaves your mouth dry, talk to your doctor about possible alternatives. Prescription artificial saliva products — for example, Caphosol or Numoisyn — also can provide some temporary moistening, as can chewing sugarless gum.
- **Relax.** Recent studies reveal a strong link between periodontal disease and stress, depression, anxiety, and loneliness. Researchers are focusing on the stress hormone cortisol as a possible culprit — high levels of cortisol may exacerbate the gum and jawbone destruction caused by oral infections.
- **Sleep.** Japanese researchers recently studied 219 factory workers for four years and found that those who slept seven to eight hours nightly suffered significantly less periodontal disease progression than those

who slept six hours or less. The scientists speculated that lack of sleep lowers the body's ability to fend off infections. However, more research is needed to confirm the results of this small study.

Robert J. Genco, DDS, PhD, distinguished professor in the department of oral biology, School of Dental Medicine, and in the department of microbiology, School of Medicine and Biomedical Sciences at the State University of New York at Buffalo.

DON'T MAKE THESE COMMON MISTAKES WHEN BRUSHING AND FLOSSING

If you're like most Americans, you brush your teeth every day — and may even use floss. But as surprising as it may seem, most people don't do either of these daily rituals correctly and fail to take other small, but highly effective, steps to protect their oral health.

Doing everything you can to care for your teeth and gums is important because, as you probably know, poor oral health has been linked to heart disease and other chronic diseases, such as diabetes and respiratory infections.

Here are some common mistakes to avoid.

Mistake #1: **Assuming that electric toothbrushes are better than manual ones.** It's true that electric and ultrasonic toothbrushes produce more strokes per minute than manual toothbrushes. However, the shape and size of the handle of the typical electric or ultrasonic toothbrush can make it more difficult to access all the teeth, particularly the backs of the last teeth.

My advice: Use both types of toothbrushes. Each time you brush, begin with an electric brush to maximize the strokes per minute, and finish up with a manual one for thirty seconds or so to access teeth you may not have fully reached. Be sure to use a soft-bristle manual brush.

***Mistake #2:* Not brushing long enough.** Most dentists recommend brushing for two minutes in the morning and again in the evening. However, if you have tiny spaces between your teeth or an advanced gum condition, such as periodontitis, you may need to brush for four or even six minutes to adequately clean your teeth.

And don't forget to brush your gums. Regular, gentle brushing can help toughen the gums and keeps the gum tissue more tightly attached to the tooth.

My advice: Brush a minute or so longer than usual (most people don't brush long enough). Then ask your dental hygienist during your next visit if you need to adjust the amount of time you brush.

***Mistake #3:* Not flossing correctly.** Most dentists recommend flossing once daily. But people who have areas in their mouths in which food routinely gets trapped should floss after each meal, as well as after they brush. Flossing after brushing allows you to remove food particles that may have been pushed into any spaces between your teeth with your toothbrush.

My advice: For convenience, keep containers of floss everywhere — in your coat pocket, glove compartment, bag, desk, and near your seat when you watch TV.

Also important: Opt for white floss (waxed or unwaxed is fine). Colored floss makes it hard to see bleeding from the gums, a sign of gum disease.

Mistake #4: **Not considering a dental irrigator.** Dental irrigators, such as those by Waterpik, Oral-B, and Philips, rinse away leftover food particles that brushing and flossing leave behind. Not everyone needs a dental irrigator, but those who have pockets (spaces between the gum and the teeth) of more than 4 mm (as measured by your hygienist) should use one.

My advice: Make irrigating the third step of your daily oral-care routine. As with brushing and flossing, it's important to be gentle. Start with a low setting on the machine, and gradually work up to harder pulsations over a period of days. Ask your hygienist how long you should irrigate each day.

Mistake #5: **Thinking mouthwash can replace flossing.** Mouthwash is easier to use than floss but does not heal gum disease — it should be used only as a supplement to brushing, flossing, and irrigating.

Mouthwash is generally thought of as a breath freshener and bacteria fighter, but some brands that contain added minerals claim to also build enamel. Enamel is composed of minerals, but the mouthwash's "remineralization" occurs only at the surface level.

My advice: If you don't have gum disease, mouthwash is optional. If you do, use mouthwash (either with alcohol or alcohol-free) with an irrigator after each brushing.

Mistake #6: **Forgetting to scrape your tongue.** Bacteria become trapped and breed on the tongue's rough surface, which can lead to bad breath and cavities.

My advice: Scrape your tongue whenever you see a grayish or whitish coating. A healthy tongue is pinkish. Many commercial tongue-scraping tools are available, but you can use a dry toothbrush or even the edge of a spoon.

Important: Each person's specific oral care needs are different, but most people can complete these steps in about three to five minutes each time they brush. If you feel you don't have that much time, ask your hygienist for advice on what areas of your mouth need the most attention and which tools he/she recommends you use most often.

Tom McGuire, DDS, a holistic dentist consultant in Sebastopol, California. He is author of several books, including *Healthy Teeth–Healthy Body: How to Improve Your Oral and Overall Health*. DentalWellness4U.com.

RESOURCES

American Association of Diabetes Educators
800-338-3633
www.diabeteseducator.org

American Board of Integrative Holistic Medicine
www.abihm.org

American Diabetes Association
www.diabetes.org

American Medical ID
800-363-5985
www.americanmedical-id.com

American Physical Therapy Association
800-999-2782
www.apta.org

American Podiatric Medical Association
www.apma.org

Arm Chair Fitness (DVD)
202-882-0974
www.armchairfitness.com

Bright Life Direct
www.brightlifedirect.com

Center for Disease Control and Prevention
https://www.cdc.gov

Diabetic Chef
www.thediabeticchef.com

Dr. Naiman's Deep Green Sleep
www.drnaiman.com

Glaucoma Research Foundation
www.glaucoma.org

ICE
918-592-3722
https://icedot.org

*International Association of Yoga
 Therapists*
www.iayt.org

Medic Alert
888-633-4298
www.medicalert.org

Medical History Bracelet
210-681-3840
http://medicalhistorybracelet.com

One Stop Paleo Shop
www.onestoppaleoshop.com

Open Culture
www.openculture.com/freeonlinecourses

PAD Coalition
www.vascularcures.org

Road ID
800-345-6336
www.roadid.com

USDA Farmer's Market Database
www.usdalocalfooddirectories.com

USDA Food Database
www.nal.usda.gov/fnic/foodcomp/search

University of Michigan
www.med.umich.edu/1libr/mend/
   diabetes-outpatientprocedure.pdf

Vascular Cures
650-368-6022
www.vascularcures.org

INDEX

A

Blood glucose levels. *See also* Diabetes
    drugs; Hypoglycemia; Tests for diabetes
  measuring, premeal, 393
  self-monitoring, 26–27, 348, 352–53, 366,
    390, 393
  during sleep, 537
Blood pressure, high (hypertension),
    177–78, 391. *See also* Heart health
  fibrinogen levels and, 527–28
  foods counteracting, 191, 571–76
  health risks related to, 479–82, 510, 549
  magnesium for, 514
  medication, timing of, 358, 391
  natural treatments for, 319, 334, 514,
    538–42, 559–63, 569, 578–81
  side effects of drugs for, 65, 444, 700
  small drops in, benefits of, 567–70
  stroke risk and, 593–98
  vitamin C for, 578–81
Blood sugar, low. *See* Hypoglycemia
Blood tests, 181–87. *See also* Tests for
    diabetes
Blue-green algae, 253–58
BMI (body mass index), 147, 150–51
Body weight. *See* Weight management
Bone infections, 412–17
BPA (bisphenol A), 108–13
Brain health, 356–62
  Alzheimer's disease, 450–55
  blood sugar control and, 452, 456–58
  decaffeinated coffee for, 459–62
  drug side effects and, 176–77

blood pressure-lowering, 66, 358, 391, 444, 568

cognitive problems linked to, 177

diabetes risk factors and, 62–68, 93–96

dry mouth and, 701

hearing loss caused by, 443–45

statins, 57, 93–95, 463, 547–48, 556, 564

timing of, 358, 361, 391–92

Dry mouth, 701

E

Edema, 319, 464–69

Enoki mushrooms, 233

Exercise

belly fat, getting rid of, 639

for brain health, 454–55, 457

in chilly temperatures, 35–36

choosing the right type of, 85–86, 346–48, 360–61, 364–65

for controlling chronic inflammation, 50

for diabetes prevention, 34–35, 131–32, 151

getting started, 653

for heart health, 90, 512–13, 538–39, 554, 654–57

high-intensity interval training, 323–26

for lowering blood pressure, 585–86

massage after, 139–41

motivating yourself, tips for, 644–47, 654

qigong, 396–98, 587–91

running/jogging, 323–26, 655

simple workout routines, 648–53, 663–66

Ginseng, red, 309–12
Glaucoma, 491–95
Glucose meters, 348, 352–54, 390
Glucose tests. *See* Tests for diabetes
Glutamine, 45–46
Glycemic index (GI), 159–60, 189–90, 219,
    242–43, 452
Goji berries, 234
Goya (bitter melon), 34, 231–32
Grape seed extract, 560–61
Green tea, 247–49, 595–96
Gum disease
  chronic inflammation and, 49–50, 530,
    696
  elevated blood sugar and, 352
  health risks linked to, 530, 696
  tips for improving oral health, 696–702
Gut microbiome, 60, 78–79, 196
Gymnema, 302–4, 327–28

H
Hands, swollen, 464–69
Hands, tingling or numbness in, 43, 179.
    See also Neuropathy
Happiness, 541
Hearing loss, 178, 440–42
Heart health. *See also* Blood pressure, high;
    Cholesterol
  APOE genes and, 54–59
  diabetes, linked to, 88–92, 510–13,
    532–36, 550–57, 567–70

Homocysteine, 184
Horse chestnut seed extract, 561–62
Hunger scale, 609–13
Hydrophilic foods, 621–27
Hypertension. *See* Blood pressure, high
Hypoglycemia, 41–46, 223–24, 387–88, 537
Hypokalemia, 181–82

I

ID bracelets, 380–83
Infections, bone, 412–17
Infections, fungal, 165–66, 414–15, 429–35
Inflammation, chronic, 119
 brain health and, 179
 diabetes link to, 47–48
 methods of reducing, 48–52, 209, 247–49
 oral health and, 49–50, 530, 696
 tests for, 52, 179, 524–31
Inositol nicotinate, 562
Insomnia, 691–95
Insulin injections, 354–55, 361, 366,
 370–71, 377

J

Jerusalem artichokes, 194–99
Jewelry, medical ID, 380–83
Jicama, 232–33
Joint-replacement surgery, complications of,
 412–17
Juicing, 241–43

K

Kidney beans, 625
Kidney disease, 568
  soy foods and, 305–7
  symptoms of, 172–74
  tests for, 349, 376
  walking for, 479–83

L

Latent autoimmune diabetes in adults
     (LADA), 163
Laughter, 565–66
L-carnitine, 420, 426, 562
Leaky gut syndrome, 129–30
Leg pain or cramps, 43, 552–57. *See also*
     Neuropathy
Legs, edema in, 319, 464–69
Legumes. *See* Beans and legumes
Lipoprotein-associated phospholipase A2
     (Lp-PLA2), 529
Low blood sugar (hypoglycemia), 41–46,
     223–24, 387–88, 537
L-Taurine, 453

M

Maca, 337–42
MACR (microalbumin/creatinine urine
     ratio), 528–29
Magnesium, 153
  deficiencies, 70–71, 73–74, 182, 619–20
  for diabetes prevention, 69–74
  foods high in, 72–73, 240, 574–75

for heart health, 71, 516
supplements, 73–74, 182, 619–20
Makeup, 104–7
Managing diabetes, 344. *See also* Exercise;
    Food and diet; Stress; Weight
    management
  chamomile tea, 329, 394–95
  common mistakes, 351–55
  daily schedule for, 356–61, 370
  fasting safely for medical tests, 374–79
  glucose meters, 348, 352–54, 390
  healthy eating habits, 345–46, 599–604
  individualized treatment plans, 369–71,
    388
  insulin injections, 354–55, 361, 366, 370,
    377
  measuring premeal sugar levels, 393
  medical ID jewelry, 380–83
  overtreatment, 384–89
  protein, importance of, 227–29, 363–64
  self-monitoring blood sugar levels, 26–27,
    348, 352–53, 366, 390, 393
  timing of medications, 391–92
Massage, 139–41
Meals, schedule for, 45, 356–61, 370, 392,
    614
Medical ID jewelry, 380–83
Medications. *See* Diabetes drugs; Drugs
Meditation, 540–41, 585
Mediterranean diet, 595
Melon, bitter, 34, 231–32
Memory problems. *See* Brain health

Oral health
  chronic inflammation and, 49–50, 530,
    696
  elevated blood sugar and, 352
  gum disease, health risks linked to, 530,
    696
  tips for improving, 696–702
Oranges, 626
Oregano oil, 433–34
Osteomyelitis, 412–17
Overtreatment of diabetes, 384–89
Oxidation, 202
Oxidative stress analysis, 28

P
Pain, 98–99. *See also* Neuropathy
"Paleolithic" diet, 514–17
Pears, 623
"Pencil Test," 167–68
Peppermint oil, 489
Perfumes, 104–7
Periodontal disease. *See* Gum disease
Peripheral artery disease (PAD), 551–63
Peripheral neuropathy. *See* Neuropathy
Phthalates, 104–7, 115
Pine bark (pycnogenol), 152, 318–21,
    496–97
Plant-based diet, 543–49
Plastics, 108–17
Policosanol, 562–63
Pollution, air, 49
Potassium, 181–82, 191–92, 571

Soft drinks, 84–85, 118–22, 161–62, 638
Soy foods, 305–7
Spices, cooking with, 238, 600–2
Spinach, 229
Spirulina, 253–58
Stair-climbing, 667–71
Standing up and moving, 133, 538–39
Statins, 57, 93–95, 463, 547–48, 556, 564
Stockings, compression, 466
Stomach acid, 125–26
Strength training, 345, 85–86, 347, 360,
    585–86, 650–51, 663–66
Stress, 352
  belly fat and, 639–40
  blood tests and, 182, 184, 185
  negative health effects of, 97–102, 701
  remedies for, 97–102, 539–40, 582–86,
    676–80
  stroke risk and, 596
Stretching, 347, 670
Stroke prevention, 593–98
Sugar, 245, 643. *See also* Artificial
    sweeteners
  controlling cravings for, 121–22, 137, 328,
    628–32
  diabetes connection, 29–31
  fructose, 29–30, 134–38
  health risks of, 134–36, 629–30
  limiting, in diet, 136–38, 628–32
  other names for, 137–38
  soda and fruit drinks, 84–85, 118–22,
    161–62, 638

rural Asian diet, 32–34
sunchokes, 194–99
Vegetarian diet, 58, 184, 543–49
Viagra, 443–44
Vinegar, 125, 211–13, 304–5
Visceral fat, 82–84, 158, 639–43
Vision. *See* Eye health
Vitamin B-6, 45, 184
Vitamin B-12, 179, 358, 420, 423–26, 547,
    619
Vitamin B-complex, 121, 184, 426
Vitamin C, 121, 354, 578–81
Vitamin D, 123, 179, 547
Vitamins, 153, 420, 562, 615–20. *See also*
    Supplements

W
Waist circumference, 84, 157
Walking, 34, 50, 85–86, 345, 466, 479–83,
    554–55, 655, 672–75
Walnuts, 204–7, 575–77
Waon therapy, 542
Water, 161, 345
Weather, changes in, 354, 403
Weight management. *See also* Exercise
  belly fat, 82–84, 158, 639–43
  diabetes prevention and, 37–40, 131–32,
    150–51
  gum disease and, 697
  hydrophilic foods for, 621–27
  insulin-induced weight gain, 365–66
  sleep apnea and, 685, 689

stress and, 100, 639–40
thin and normal-weight people with
    diabetes, 81–86, 639
triglycerides and, 90
weight loss, methods of, 131–32, 151–52,
    159–62, 211, 219, 225–26, 639–43
Weight training. *See* Strength training
Wheat, 160–61
Whey protein, 214–17
Wine, 56, 360, 636–37
Women, health risks for, 440–42, 477–78,
    582
Working out. *See* Exercise

Y
Yoga, 681–84

ABOUT BOTTOM LINE INC.

For more than forty years, **Bottom Line Inc.** (formerly Boardroom Inc.) has provided consumer health and financial insights to more than twenty million readers worldwide. Its vast array of expert-sourced content is published in both subscription-based newsletters and books.

Our mission is to provide the help people need to take on the challenges they face in their lives — how to stay healthy and how to heal when sick, how to make more money, and how to spend it wisely. Simply, how to be happier with their lives.

To empower your life with expert advice, please visit us at BottomLineInc.com.